Advances in Applied Neurological Sciences 2

Editors
R. J. Joynt, Rochester, USA
A. Weindl, Munich, FRG

Senile Dementia of the Alzheimer Type

Early Diagnosis, Neuropathology and Animal Models

Edited by
J. Traber and W. H. Gispen

With 118 Figures

Springer-Verlag
Berlin Heidelberg New York Tokyo

Dr. Jörg Traber
Neurobiology Department
Troponwerke GmbH & Co. KG
Neurather Ring 1
D-5000 Köln 80, FRG

Professor Dr. Willem Hendrik Gispen
Division of Molecular Neurobiology
Rudolf Magnus Institute for Pharmacology
and Institute of Molecular Biology
State University of Utrecht
Padualaan 8
NL-3508 TB Utrecht, The Netherlands

ISBN-13:978-3-642-70646-2 e-ISBN-13:978-3-642-70644-8
DOI: 10.1007/978-3-642-70644-8

Library of Congress Cataloging-in-Publication Data. Main entry under title: Senile dementia of the Alzheimer type. (Advances in applied neurological sciences; 2) Contains the proceedings of the Second International Tropon-Bayer Symposium on Aging of the Brain, held in Cologne in Nov. 1984. Includes index. 1. Alzheimer's disease – Congresses. 2. Brain – Aging – Congresses. 3. Brain – Diseases – Age factors – Congresses. 4. Brain – Diseases – Animal models – Congresses. I. Traber, Jörg. II. Gispen, Willem Hendrik. III. International Tropon-Bayer Symposium on Aging of the Brain (2nd: 1984: Cologne, Germany) IV. Series. [DNLM: 1. Aging – congresses. 2. Alzheimer's Disease – congresses. 3. Brain – congresses. 4. Disease Models, Animal – congresses. W1 AD436AH v.2/WM 220 S477 1984] RC523.S46 1985 618.97'83 85-17229
ISBN-13:978-3-642-70646-2 (U.S.)

2125/3130-543210

Foreword

Society is showing increasing concern for disorders related to aging that lead to a loss of brain function. In view of the enormous proportion of elderly people in our society today, brain aging is more than ever subject to challenge to us all, not only politicians and health authorities, but every individual who is confronted with the difficult situation of watching the mental powers of apparently healthy elderly friends, neighbours, or relatives fail, often with alarming rapidity. This challenge is directed especially toward us scientists. As one of our colleagues succinctly put it 2 years ago at the close of our First International Symposium on Brain Aging: "Do something. We are not dealing here with just another disease; we are concerned with human dignity."

More than any statistics, these words convinced me that Tropon's decision to leave the field of classic CNS pharmacology and move into the field of gerontopsychopharmacology was the right one, even though we knew that success would be uncertain and that, even if it finally comes it will be many years hence.

At this point, let me add a personal comment: each one of us is judged by his or her own success. We live in a competitive society where success counts. This applies not only to the businessman, but also to the scientist, in particular, to those in industry. Considering this pressure, can we expect a young generation of scientists to devote themselves to long-term projects such as the investigation of brain aging? My answer is "yes." In spite of the fact that we can expect to obtain meaningful results only after years of investigation or, perhaps, not at all, it is my belief that the rewards of such a large-scale investment will be proportional to the input.

The International Tropon-Bayer Symposia on Aging of the Brain are meant to encourage and support neuroscientists in their efforts to understand the physiologic and pathologic aspects of brain aging. They are not intended as exclusive gatherings, but are open to all who can in any way contribute to the subject. They are a vehicle for the significant, informal exchange of ideas between clinicians and nonclinicians and between investigators at universities and research institutes and those in industry.

Various people have asked me why we organized a second workshop after only 2 years, considering the long-term scale of research I mentioned above. In response, I would like to point out that, in the meantime, we have worked hard to check the validity of various models. We have tested, rejected, and started again, and in the process, tried completely new approaches. Certainly in the last 2 years, the vast complexity of the pathology underlying abnormal brain aging as well as applications of drug research to gerontological health problems have become increasingly apparent. Hence, it was decided to arrange a meeting on three important, well-defined topics, including the early diagnosis of senile dementia of the Alzheimer type, new insights into the pathology of the aged brain, and animal models in the study of normal and abnormal brain aging.

It is my hope that the discussion of these topics will be instrumental in advancing our knowledge of the brain in normal aging and the malfunctions characterizing the diseased elderly brain.

September, 1985 HARALD HORSTMANN, Cologne

Preface

This volume contains the proceedings of the Second International Tropon-Bayer Symposium on Aging of the Brain, held in Cologne in November 1984.

The program focuses on three topics, the first of which concerns the early diagnosis of senile dementia, especially of the Alzheimer type (SDAT). We would like to thank Dr. Jellemer Jolles for aiding us in organizing this part of the program. Contributions to this subject include the description of clinical phases of senile dementia, the relevance of neuropsychological tests for early diagnosis, and the application of PET and NMR scanning in the diagnosis of diseases related to abnormal brain aging.

The second topic deals with recent developments in the neuropathology of the aged and diseased human brain. The presentations in this area are concerned with both the quantitation of cellular changes occurring in the brain during normal aging and the role of specific neurotransmitters, amino acids, and brain structures in the pathogenesis of SDAT.

The last topic covers the selection and assessment of animal models of "normal" and "abnormal" aging of the human nervous system. These studies describe novel approaches to the study of brain acetylcholine in relation to brain function and assess the usefulness of senescent monkeys and rats in studies of behavioral aspects of brain aging.

A special interest lecture presented by Prof. Stanley Appel of the University of Houston highlights the relevance of trophic factors and neural plasticity to the process of brain aging.

The quality of the presentations was superb and provoked lively discussions on such issues as the cortical as opposed to the subcortical origin of abnormalities in Alzheimer's disease, patient classification, and cultural aspects affecting diagnosis.

We are grateful both to the participants of the symposium and to Dr. Thiekötter of Springer-Verlag for timely publication of the proceedings of this exciting meeting.

We would like to take this opportunity to give special thanks to Mrs. A. Bartz for her skillful and efficient help in organizing this meeting. Furthermore, we are grateful to Mr. H. Demmer and Mr. W. Dreher for their technical assistance during the symposium. Last but not least, we acknowledge Prof. F. Hoffmeister (Bayer) and Dr. H. Horstmann (Tropon) for their valuable comments concerning the program and format of the meeting and Dr. M. Hebler (Tropon) for making it possible to organize this symposium.

We hope that the proceedings will inform the reader about important issues of current research on brain aging and serve as a basis for the design of new experimental or theoretical approaches to understanding the pathogenesis of senile dementia.

September, 1985

Jörg Traber
Willem Hendrik Gispen

Contents

List of Contributors

You will find the addresses at the beginning of the respective contribution

Early Diagnosis of Senile Dementia of the Alzheimer Type
I. Behavioral and Clinical Aspects

Cognitive Function in Normal Aging and Early Dementia

C. FLICKER[1], S. H. FERRIS[1], T. CROOK[2], R. T. BARTUS[3], and B. REISBERG[1]

Both normal aging and senile dementia are associated with a broad array of changes in cognitive function. The objective of this review is to identify and illustrate the most salient features of these changing psychological profiles. Table 1 is a summary of the effects of normal aging and mild to moderate senile dementia upon a variety of psychometric tests, with the test measures assigned to different theoretical categories of cognitive function. The utility of this approach is limited by a number of factors. First, the diffuse nature of the cognitive decline associated with aging and dementia makes it difficult to identify discrete cognitive abilities which are selectively impaired or intact. This problem is greatly magnified in the more advanced stages of senile dementia, where the global nature of the cognitive deterioration makes discrimination between affected and unaffected cognitive processes almost impossible. Virtually any cognitive test will elicit a significant performance decrement in severely demented as opposed to mildly demented subjects. The former subject group is not, therefore, included in Table 1 and this review will be restricted to studies of patients in only the early stages of senile dementia. A second problem with this approach is the relative lack of specificity of the psychometric tests. Since individual test results are normally dependent upon multiple cognitive abilities, it is difficult to attribute a lowered test score solely to a deficit in a particular cognitive function. Finally, the validity of the separate categories of cognitive function as theoretical psychological constructs has also not been adequately established.

Nonetheless, this organization of an extensive body of experimental data reveals consistent patterns of change due to aging or dementia in distinct groups of psychometric tests. To the extent that this perspective accurately reflects our current level of resolution in the delineation of the cognitive profiles of the normal elderly and the mildly demented, the conclusions reached will be of heuristic value.

Normal Aging

Psychomotor Performance

A critical change in cognitive function distinguishing the elderly from the young is a general decay in psychomotor integrity. Deficits are apparent at multiple sen-

1 Department of Psychiatry, New York University Medical Center, 550 First Avenue, New York, NY 10016, USA
2 Center for Study of Mental Health of the Aging, National Institute of Mental Health, 5600 Fishers Lane, Rockville, MD 20857, USA
3 Department of CNS Research, Medical Research Division of American Cyanamid Company, Lederle Laboratories, Pearl River, NY 10965, USA

Senile Dementia of the Alzheimer Type
Ed. by J. Traber and W. H. Gispen

Table 1. Cognitive function in normal aging and early dementia

Function	Normal aging	Early dementia	Measures	References
Sensory acuity	–	– –	Aging: all modalities Dementia: audition, 2-point tactile discrimination No deficit: vision	Corso (1977), Engen (1977), Fozard et al. (1977), Kenshalo (1977), O'Neil and Calhoun (1975)
Peripheral nerve conduction speed	–	–	Ulnar nerve: motor impulse, 10% decrease No deficit: sensory conduction	Levy et al. (1970), Norris et al. (1953), Thomas et al. (1982), Wagman and Lesse (1952)
Sensory-evoked potentials				Goodin et al. (1978), Levy et al. (1971), Michalewski et al. (1980)
latency	+	+ +	All modalities tested: usually late components	
amplitude	–	– –	Increased amplitude: early components, visual stimulus	
Event-related potentials			P 300	Goodin et al. (1978), Pfefferbaum et al. (1982)
latency	+	+ +		
amplitude	–	– –		
Motor speed	–	– –	Finger tapping, ballistic movement	Vrtunski et al. (1983), Welford (1977)
Reaction time				
simple	+	+ +	Including saccadic latency	Ferris et al. (1976), Pirozzolo and Hansch (1981), Spooner et al. (1980), Welford (1977)
choice	+ +	+ + +		Ferris et al. (1976), Vrtunski et al. (1983), Welford (1977)
Attention				
divided attention	–	– –	Dichotic listening	Caird and Englis (1961), Craik (1977), Inglis and Caird (1963), Inglis and Sanderson (1961)
vigilance	0	0	Continuous performance task; aging deficit with fast pace	Thompson et al. (1963)
concentration	0	0	Digit span; aging and dementia deficits: subtracting serial 7s	Caird and Inglis (1961), Craik (1977); Ferris et al. (1985), Fozard (1985), Reed and Reitan (1963), Smith (1967), Wechsler (1981)

Table 1 (continued)

Function	Normal aging	Early dementia	Measures	References
Response inhibition	–	– –	Stroop color-word, Buschke prior-list intrusions, facial recognition: false alarms, reaction time: false alarms	Bettner et al. (1971), Comalli et al. (1962), Ferris et al. (1980), Flicker et al. (1984), Fuld et al. (1982)
Visuospatial praxis	–	– –	Untimed block design, object assembly, Bender-Gestalt, immediate visual reproduction, Minnesota Percepto-Diagnostic Test, Raven Colored Progressive Matrices, mosaic comparisons tests, space test; susceptibility to Muller-Lyer illusion; no aging deficit: perception of verticality, susceptibility to Titchner Circles illusion; no dementia deficit: standardized road map test	Beauvois and Lhermitte (1975), Brilliant and Gynther (1963), Brouwers et al. (1984), Comalli et al. (1959), Crookes (1983), Crookes and Coleman (1973), Horenstein (1971), Muramoto et al. (1984), Rosen (1983), Storandt (1977), Strother et al. (1957), Wapner et al. (1960)
Concept formation/abstract problem solving	–	– –	Poisoned food problems, category test, untimed picture arrangement, picture completion	Arenberg (1982), Rabbitt (1977), Reed and Reitan (1963), Storandt (1977)
Learning	–	– –	Serial, paired associates, mazes	Arenberg and Robertson-Tchabo (1977), Botwinick and Storandt (1974), Brouwers et al. (1984), Caird and Inglis (1961), Miller (1977)
Language	0	–	Confrontation naming, word fluency, symbol referents test; no dementia deficit: comprehension, speech fluency, syntax, vocabulary	Appell et al. (1982), Barker and Lawson (1968), Ferris et al. (1985), Kaplan et al. (1983), Kirshner et al. (1984), Martin and Fedio (1983), Miller and Hague (1975), Reed and Reitan (1963), Rosen (1981, 1983), Schwartz et al. (1979), Strother et al. (1957), Wechsler (1981)
Memory				
sensory	–	– –	Sperling paradigm	Cerella et al. (1982), Miller (1977)
primary	0	0	Digit span, visuospatial recall	Caird and Inglis (1961), Craik (1977), Ferris et al. (1985), Flicker et al. (1984), Fozard (1985), Reed and Reitan (1963), Wechsler (1981)

secondary	–	– –	Paragraph recall, paired associates, shopping list, memory-for-designs, name-face associates, facial recognition, visuospatial recall	Brilliant and Gynther (1963), Craik (1977), Crook et al. (1979), Ferris et al. (1980, 1985), Flicker et al. (1984), Fozard (1985), McCarthy et al. (1981), Miller (1977), Wilson et al. (1982)
tertiary	0	–	Information, new items, famous faces	Fozard (1980), Moscovitch (1982), Reed and Reitan (1963), Squire (1974), Warrington and Sanders (1971), Wechsler (1981), Wilson et al. (1981)

– Indicates a decrease in measures of a given function for aged normals as compared with young normals or for demented subjects as compared with aged normals
– – Indicates a relatively greater decrease in those measures
\+ Indicates an increase in measures of a given function
\+ + Indicates a relatively greater increase in those measures
\+ + + Indicates an increase relative to choice reaction time in aged normals or relative to simple reaction time in demented subjects

sorimotor processing levels. There is a loss of sensory acuity in all modalities including visual (Fozard et al. 1977), auditory (Corso 1977), somatosensory (Kenshalo 1977), gustatory and olfactory (Engen 1977). There is a 10% decrease in peripheral nerve conduction speed for the motor impulse (Norris et al. 1953; Wagman and Lesse 1952), but not for incoming sensory impulses. The latencies of sensory evoked potentials are increased in the elderly (Goodin et al. 1978; Michalewski et al. 1980). It is the late components of these evoked potentials which are prolonged, again suggestive of normal propagation of the sensory impulse in the small-fibered sensory pathways, followed by delays in central synaptic transmission or other aspects of the complex processing of the sensory input. Event-related components of the evoked potential dependent upon higher-level processing of the sensory stimulus, such as the P300, also exhibit prolonged latencies and decreased amplitudes in the elderly (Goodin et al. 1978; Pfefferbaum et al. 1982). These changes are reflected at the behavioral level in their performance of even the simplest psychomotor tasks, as in decreased finger tapping speeds, decreased rates of ballistic movement, and increased reaction times (Ferris et al. 1976; Welford 1977); see Fig. 1.

This diminution of sensorimotor processing speed and efficiency in the elderly can account, at least in part, for many of the decrements observed on tests of cognitive function. For example, it has been established that raw scores on the Wechsler Adult Intelligence Scale (WAIS) performance subtests tend to decline with increasing age whereas raw scores on the verbal subtests are maintained (Botwinick 1977; Wechsler 1981). Thus the digit symbol substitution task is clearly sensitive to age effects whereas the vocabulary subtest is not (see Table 2). Since all of the performance subtests are timed tasks dependent upon motor (or visuomotor) output, a fundamental psychomotor deficit would be expected to affect scores on all of them. Thus further interpretation of impairments on any timed motor task is questionable. For example, the age-related decline in scores

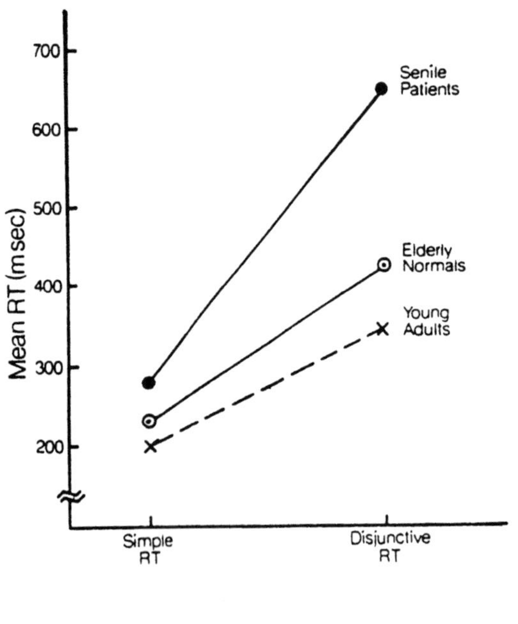

Fig. 1. Simple and choice reaction time in young normal, aged normal, and demented subjects. Choice reaction time is more sensitive than simple reaction time to aging and especially dementia. Reprinted by permission from Ferris et al. (1976)

Table 2. Mean scores of three subject groups on standardized psychometric tests. Reprinted by permission from Ferris et al. (1980)

Measure	Elderly Impaired (N=60)	Elderly Normal (N=44)	Young Normal (N=63)
WAIS			
Vocabulary[a]	13.7 (3.3)	15.4 (2.9)	14.7 (2.9)
Digit Symbol[a]	6.3 (2.7)	8.6 (2.0)	13.3 (2.5)
Digit Span			
Forward	6.8 (1.4)	7.2 (1.3)	7.3 (1.3)
Backward	4.5 (1.1)	5.5 (1.5)	5.7 (1.3)
Guild Memory Test			
Paragraphs:			
Immediate	5.3 (2.9)	9.7 (2.3)	11.1 (3.1)
Delayed	5.0 (3.5)	12.3 (3.0)	14.6 (3.8)
Paired Associates:			
Immediate	1.4 (1.3)	4.6 (1.8)	6.7 (1.9)
Delayed	1.4 (1.4)	5.4 (1.9)	8.1 (2.1)
Memory for Designs	2.4 (1.8)	6.3 (2.5)	8.1 (1.6)

Note: SD's are in parentheses
[a] Standard scaled scores

on the block design subtest cannot be contrued as a valid demonstration of an impairment of visuospatial praxis in the elderly.

Visuospatial Praxis

This is not to suggest that age-specific deficits in psychological processes more complex than sensorimotor function have not been established. With regard to visuospatial praxis, old subjects perform more poorly than young subjects even on an untimed version of the block design subtest (Storandt 1977). Similarly, performance on tests which require immediate untimed visual reproduction of line drawings, such as the Bender-Gestalt Visual Motor Test (Brilliant and Gynther 1963) and the Minnesota Percepto-Diagnostic Test (Crookes and Coleman 1973), also decline with age, indicative of an age-related deficit in constructional abilities. Other indications of an impairment in the perception of spatial relations are apparent in the deficits of aged normals on the space test of the Primary Mental Abilities Test (Strother et al. 1957) and in their susceptibility to the Muller-Lyer illusion (Wapner et al. 1960). In contrast, the elderly are reported to be more accurate in their perception of verticality than the young (Comalli et al. 1959) and to be less susceptible to the Titchner circles illusion (Wapner et al. 1960).

Concept Formation

Other subject-paced tasks reveal age-related deficits in other complex cognitive skills. However, in addition to psychomotor speed, a frequent confounding factor in many tests of higher-level cognitive functions is the memory requirement of the task. For example, a number of concept formation tests, such as poisoned food problems (Arenberg 1982), the untimed picture arrangement subtest of the WAIS (Storandt 1977), and the category test of the Halstead-Reitan battery (Reed and Reitan 1963), elicit age-dependent performance decrements indicative of deficient abstract problem-solving skills in the elderly. But, as pointed out by Rabbitt (1977), all of these tests have a major undifferentiated memory component.

Learning and Attention

Two other areas in which cognitive assessment reveals reliable age-related deficits are learning and attention. In the case of attentional mechanisms, the presence or absence of age-related deficits is dependent upon the operational definition of attention adopted in the test paradigm. Divided attention tasks typically yield marked impairments in the elderly (Craik 1977; Inglis and Caird 1963). Tests of concentration or vigilance, such as the continuous performance task, typically do not, unless the stimulus presentation rate is high (Thompson et al. 1963). It has been cogently argued that the impaired performance of elderly subjects on dichotic listening and other divided attention tasks is secondary to memory dysfunction (Craik 1977). There is an extensive literature documenting age effects upon the performance of a wide variety of learning tasks (Arenberg and Robertson-Tchabo 1977, Botwinick and Storandt 1974). However, since learning deficits in the elderly are also contingent upon age-related memory loss, we will focus on studies which have contributed to the understanding of this underlying dysfunction.

Immediate and Remote Memory

Memory difficulty is the most commonly reported complaint of cognitive decline in the elderly. In the attempt to define more precisely the qualitative nature of the memory loss accompanying normal aging, both subjective and empirical evidence support the conceptual utility of distinguishing between primary (immediate), secondary (recent), and tertiary (remote) memory. One important characteristic of the cognitive profile of the normal elderly is the integrity of their primary memory processes. A classic illustration of this spared function is the relative insensitivity to age of the digit span subtest of the WAIS (see Table 2). A contention which is somewhat more controversial, partly because of the difficulty of designing a properly controlled study of age effects upon remote memory, is that tertiary memory processes are also subject to only modest decline in the elderly (Fozard 1980). As already mentioned, language skills in the elderly are essentially intact, and the remote verbal memory requirements of tests of vocabulary (see Table 2), confrontation naming (see Fig. 3), and verbal fluency (Strother et al. 1957) fail to elicit substantial performance decrements in the aged. However, there is some evidence for a decline in the recall of news items and famous faces from the distant past after age 70 (Squire 1974; Warrington and Sanders 1971).

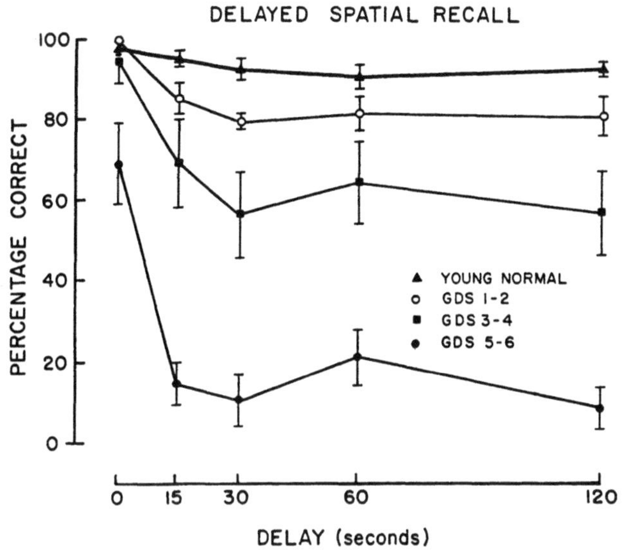

Fig. 2. Effects of delays of between 0 and 120 s on visuospatial recall of young normal, elderly normal, and elderly demented subjects. Subjects were asked to remember which room of a 25-room house, presented on a video monitor, had a lighted window. During the delay inteval, they performed a reaction time task. Ordinate is percentage of correct responses. At the 0-s delay, only the performance of the moderately-to-severely impaired subjects (*GDS 5–6*) differed significantly from that of the mildly-to-moderately impaired subjects (*GDS 3–4*), elderly normal subjects (*GDS 1–2*) or young normal subjects. At 30 s after stimulus, performance level was significantly different among all four groups. Reprinted by permission from Flicker et al. (1984)

Recent Memory

Unlike immediate or remote memory, recent memory is clearly impaired in the normal elderly (Fozard 1980). We have found that this deficit is readily apparent on tests of paragraph recall (see Table 2), paired associates (see Table 2), shopping list recall (McCarthy et al. 1981), memory-for-designs (see Table 2), name-face associates (Ferris et al., to be published), visuospatial recall (see Fig. 2), and facial recognition (Ferris et al. 1980).

Early Senile Dementia

At the present time there is no established set of behavioral indices which can be used to differentiate between the cognitive profiles of the normal and demented elderly. The lack of a straightforward solution to this problem is attributable to the global nature, the probable heterogeneity of etiology, and the ontogenetic characteristics of the cognitive decline associated with senile dementia. First, at least in the advanced stages of dementia, because of the global nature of the cognitive deterioration, virtually any cognitive test will elicit reliable deficits. Second, even in a population of patients who will all receive definitive diagnoses of Alzheimer's disease, there is likely to be considerable variability in the behavioral expression, the sequence of occurrence, and even the presence or absence of underlying neuropathological processes. The third obstacle is discernible in the DSM III definition of primary degenerative dementia, which lists an "insidious onset" as a diagnostic criterion, and thus implies that the early stages of senile dementia consist of a gradual exacerbation of cognitive deficiencies from a paranormal to a pathological level of function. The remainder of this review will concentrate on the initial stages of this decline, since during this period it may be possible to identify aspects of cognitive function which are differentially susceptible to the dementing disorder.

Recent Memory

The available psychometric data, however, seem to suggest that the differences in cognitive function between normal and mildly demented elderly subjects are quantitative rather than qualitative. The primary symptom of senile dementia is a further impairment of the memory for recent events. Results from our studies of recent memory in young normal, elderly normal, and mildly-to-moderately impaired elderly subjects consistently reveal a pattern of significant, progressive decline in performance due to aging and dementia. We have observed this pattern on numerous tests of verbal memory, including recall of paragraphs (see Table 2), shopping lists (McCarthy et al. 1981), and paired associates (see Table 2). Demented subjects are especially prone to perseverative errors of intrusion on list learning tasks (Fuld et al. 1982). Significant differences between young, old, and demented subjects are also apparent on tests of recent visual memory, such as the memory-for-designs test (see Table 2), name-face associates (Ferris et al., to be published) and different tests of visuospatial recall (see Fig. 2). We have previously reported an age effect but no effect of mild cognitive impairment on memory for faces as measured in a continuous recognition paradigm (Ferris et al. 1980). However, in agreement with Wilson et al. (1982) a more recent investigation which included shorter delay intervals between the first and second presentation of the stimulus face revealed significant differences between normal and mildly impaired elderly subjects as well.

Immediate Memory

In the early stages of senile dementia, as in normal aging, tests of primary memory reveal little functional loss. In contrast with the marked deficits on secondary memory tests, digit span is reduced by only about half a character (see Table 2). Immediate recall of the location of a visuospatial stimulus is unimpaired, even though 30 seconds later recall accuracy will be clearly subnormal (see Fig. 2).

Remote Memory

There is at least one study suggesting that there is an impairment of remote memory in the early stages of senile dementia. Wilson et al. (1981) found a deficit in their patients' recall of news items and the names of famous faces two years after onset of the dementing disorder. The conclusion that tertiary memory is impaired in early senile dementia is somewhat controversial. Moscovitch (1982) failed to find a dementia effect using the same famous faces test. In addition, an uncontrolled factor in these studies is the subjects' opportunities for rehearsal subsequent to the onset of the memory impairment. Furthermore, other tests dependent upon remote verbal memory, such as the WAIS vocabulary subtest, are relatively insensitive to early senile dementia (see Table 2). Naming of colors, letters, numbers, and body parts is likewise unimpaired (Rosen 1983).

Language

Elderly subjects with mild to moderate cognitive impairment do, however, exhibit deficient recall from remote verbal memory when tested for visual confrontation naming of objects (see Fig. 3). This word-finding difficulty is also detectable with tests of verbal fluency (Martin and Fedio 1983; Miller and Hague 1975; Rosen 1981) and appears to constitute one of the only established qualitative distinctions between cognitive dysfunction in normal aging and early senile dementia. It has been reported that in some cases this anomia can precede any other sign of memory disturbance (Wechsler 1977). Dysphasia with nominal aphasia has also been reported to be one of the three most common clinical symptoms associated with histopathologically confirmed Alzheimer's disease (Sim and Sussman 1962). Some attempt has been made to specify further the qualitative nature of the language dysfunction associated with senile dementia. However, the naming deficit is still present in demented subjects with otherwise normal scores on the Boston Diagnostic Aphasia Examination (Kirshner et al. 1984). Furthermore, subjects with mild to moderate senile dementia are relatively unimpaired when asked to point out named objects or to point out objects which might be used for a particular task (see Fig. 3). Clearly there is no general disruption of semantic processing. At the present time, the most parsimonious classification of this impairment would characterize it as simply a deficit in retrieval from remote verbal memory.

Visuospatial Praxis

After memory disturbance, the second most common clinical symptom of histopathologically confirmed Alzheimer's disease, according to Sim and Sussman (1962), is temporal and spatial disorientation. Spatial disorientation in the elderly and demented has not yet received adequate quantitative study. As mentioned above, visuospatial memory tests elicit pronounced deficits from subjects with mild to moderate cognitive impairment (see Fig. 2). Tests of visuospatial praxis,

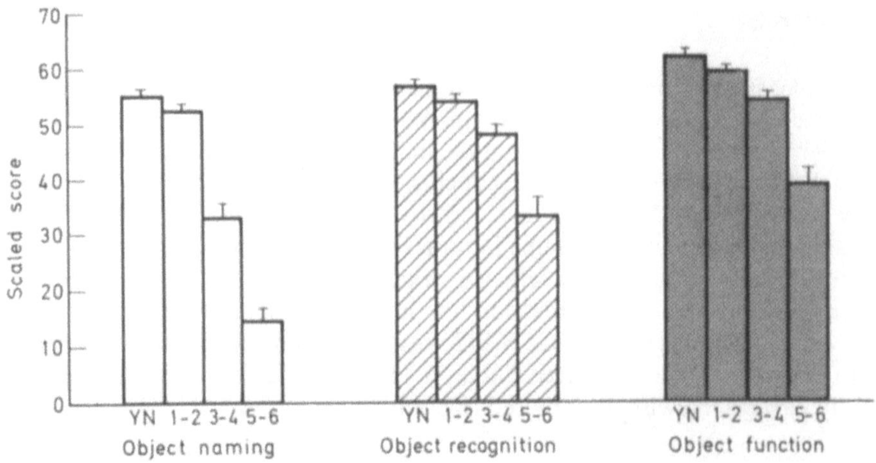

Fig. 3. Effects of aging and dementia on remote memory and language, as measured by tests of object naming, object recognition, and object function recognition. In each task, subjects were presented with line drawings of objects on a video monitor screen. In the naming task, objects were presented individually, and subjects were instructed to supply the name of the object. In the other two tasks, 25 objects were presented simultaneously. In the recognition task, subjects were instructed to point to the object the name of which appeared on the screen. For the function recognition task, subjects were instructed to point to the eight objects which might be used in a particular chore (e.g., dressing). Aged normal subjects (*1–2*) exhibited a slight performance decrement relative to young normal subjects (*YN*) on all three tasks. Moderately-to-severely demented subjects (*5–6*) were markedly impaired on all three tasks. Subjects with mild to moderate senile dementia (*3–4*) were markedly impaired on the naming task only. Numerical designations of the three aged subject groups refer to the Global Deterioration Scale of Reisberg et al. (1982). (Reprinted from C. Flicker, S.H. Ferris, T. Crook, R.T. Bartus, Confrontation naming and other language and remote memory functions in senile dementia of the Alzheimer's type, in preparation)

such as the Minnesota Percepto-Diagnostic Test (Crookes 1983) or other tests requiring the visual reproduction of line drawings (Horenstein 1971; Muramoto et al. 1984; Rosen 1983), of the Rey-Osterrieth Complex Figure (Brouwers et al. 1984), or of gestures or token board designs (Beauvois and Lhermitte 1975) all reveal a deficit in elderly subjects in the early stages of dementia. Horenstein (1971) has concludeded that performance on the Bender-Gestalt of subjects with senile dementia of the Alzheimer type or multi-infarct dementia is qualitatively distinguishable from that of aged normals or brain-damaged subjects. Other tests of the perception of spatial relations, such as the (timed) mosaic comparisons test (Brouwers et al. 1984), are also sensitive to early senile dementia. In contrast, Brouwers et al. (1984) found no dementia effect upon the Standardized Road Map Test, which they interpreted as a demonstration of intact orientation in egocentric as opposed to extrapersonal space. This hypothesis requires further investigation. The effects of dementia upon other tests relevant to spatial orientation, such as map-reading, perceived body position, mental rotation in space, and maze completion, remain to be fully evaluated.

Concept Formation

Concept formation and abstract problem-solving in senile dementia have also received insufficient attention. The Stroop Color Word Test, which requires abstraction and set shifting, yields performance decrements in elderly cognitively impaired subjects (Bettner et al. 1971). Interpretation of this finding is confounded, however, by the use of a time-to-completion measure as the dependent variable derived from this task.

Psychomotor Performance

Both sensorimotor function and cognitive processing speed undergo further deterioration in elderly individuals in the early stages of senile dementia. We have found that both simple and choice reaction time are slower in elderly demented subjects than elderly normals (see Fig. 1). Disjunctive reaction time exhibits significantly more dementia-dependent slowing than simple reaction time, suggesting that decreased higher-level cognitive processing speed might be primarily responsible for the increased latencies, as opposed to slowing of the sensory and motor components of the response (Ferris et al. 1976).

Nonetheless, there is unmistakable evidence of sensorimotor dysfunction independent of more complex cognitive processes in even the earliest stages of senile dementia. There is no change in the speed of peripheral nerve conduction (Levy et al. 1970; Thomas et al. 1982). However, electroencephalographic studies reveal increased latencies and decreased amplitudes of sensory evoked potentials (Levy et al. 1971; Michalewski et al. 1980) and of the P300 wave which occurs in response to a target stimulus (Goodin et al. 1978). At the behavioral level, we have found that relatively pure measures of motor integrity such as finger tapping speed or the isolated "travel time" component of a simple reaction time response are sensitive to even mild cognitive impairment in the elderly (unpublished observations). Vrtunski et al. (1983), based on a fine-grained analysis of the reaction time responses of demented subjects, concluded that senile dementia produces a fundamental disruption of the psychomotor organization of motor outputs. Findings such as these limit the interpretability of deficits on timed complex psychomotor performance tasks such as the digit symbol substitution test (see Table 2).

Summary

In summary, the most prominent alteration in cognitive function produced by advanced age is a decrease in psychomotor speed. This deficit is accompanied by impairments of a number of more complex cognitive abilities, such as visuospatial praxis and concept formation. Aged normal subjects perform worse than young normals on many tasks with a significant memory component. Memory loss in the elderly appears to be restricted to memory for recent events, leaving immediate and remote memory essentially intact.

Cognitive deterioration in the early stages of senile dementia mainly consists of an exacerbation of the cognitive decline associated with normal aging. The primary symptom of dementia is a further impairment of recent memory. There are also significant augmentations of the age-related decrements in cognitive processing speed and psychomotor integrity. Immediate memory seems to remain fairly stable. There is, however, a partial deficit in retrieval from remote memory, which has been most reliably demonstrated on tests of object naming. Other tests of high-level cognitive processes in subjects with incipient senile dementia reveal impaired visuoconstructional abilities and a tendency to make errors of intrusion.

Future Directions

A more accurate description of the cognitive dysfunction associated with the early stages of senile dementia will require a fuller characterization of: (1) the nature of the naming deficit, whether in terms of linguistic or mnestic processes; (2) the differential sensitivity to dementia of the various sub-components of visuospatial praxis and recent memory; (3) the deficits elicited by non-memory tests of concept formation and abstract problem-solving, and (4) the underlying basis of the perseverative tendencies of subjects with early senile dementia.

References

Appell J, Kertesz A, Fisman M (1982) A study of language functioning in Alzheimer patients. Brain Lang 17:73–91

Arenberg D (1982) Changes with age in problem solving. In: Craik FIM, Trehub S (eds) Aging and cognitive processes. Plenum, New York

Arenberg D, Robertson-Tchabo EA (1977) Learning and aging. In: Birren JE, Schaie KW (eds) Handbook of the psychology of aging. Van Nostrand, New York

Barker MG, Lawson JS (1968) Nominal aphasia in dementia. Br J Psychiatry 114:1351–1356

Beauvois MF, Lhermitte F (1975) Selective mnesic deficiency and restricted cortical lesions. Rev Neurol (Paris) 131:3–22

Bettner LG, Jarvik LF, Blum JE (1971) Stroop color-word test, non-psychotic organic brain syndrome and chromosome loss in aged twins. J Gerontol 26:458–469

Botwinick J (1977) Intellectual abilities. In: Birren JE, Schaie KW (eds) Handbook of the psychology of aging. Van Nostrand, New York

Botwinick J, Storandt M (1974) Memory, related functions and age. Thomas, Springfield

Brilliant PJ, Gynther MD (1963) Relationships between performance on three tests for organicity and selected patient variables. J Consult Psychol 27:474–479

Brouwers P, Cox C, Martin A, Chase T, Fedio P (1984) Differential perceptual-spatial impairment in Huntington's and Alzheimer's dementias. Arch Neurol 41:1073–1076

Caird WK, Inglis J (1961) The short-term storage of auditory and visual two-channel digits by elderly patients with memory disorder. J Ment Sci 107:1062–1069

Cerella J, Poon LW, Fozard JL (1982) Age and iconic read-out. J Gerontol 37:197–202

Comalli PE Jr, Wapner S, Werner H (1959) Perception of verticality in middle and old age. J Psychol 47:259–266

Comalli PE Jr, Wapner S, Werner H (1962) Interference effects of Stroop color-word test in childhood, adulthood and aging. J Genet Psychol 100:47–53

Corso JF (1977) Auditory perception and communication. In: Birren JE, Schaie KW (eds) Handbook of the psychology of aging. Van Nostrand, New York
Craik FIM (1977) Age differences in human memory. In: Birren JE, Schaie KW (eds) Handbook of the psychology of aging. Van Nostrand, New York
Crook T, Ferris SH, McCarthy M (1979) The misplaced-objects task: A brief test for memory dysfunction in the aged. J Am Geriatr Soc 27:284–287
Crookes TG (1983) The Minnesota percepto-diagnostic test and presenile dementia. Clin Neurophsychol 5:187–190
Crookes TG, Coleman JA (1973) The Minnesota percepto-diagnostic test (MPD) in adult psychiatric practice. J Clin Psychol 29:204–206
Engen T (1977) Taste and smell. In: Birren JE, Schaie KW (eds) Handbook of the psychology of aging. Van Nostrand, New York
Ferris SH, Crook T, Sathananthan G, Gershon S (1976) Reaction time as a diagnostic measure of cognitive impairment in senility. J Am Geriatr Soc 24:529–533
Ferris SH, Crook T, Clark E, McCarthy M, Rae D (1980) Facial recognition memory deficits in normal aging and senile dementia. J Gerontol 35:707–714
Ferris SH, Crook T, Flicker C, Reisberg B, Bartus RT (to be published) Psychometric assessment of treatment effects. In: Poon LW (ed) The handbook of clinical memory assessment of older adults. American Psychological Association, Washington
Flicker C, Bartus RT, Crook T, Ferris SH (1984) Effects of aging and dementia upon recent visuospatial memory. Neurobiol Aging 5:275–283
Fozard JL (1980) The time for remembering. In: Poon LW (ed) Aging in the 1980s. American Psychological Association, Washington
Fozard JL (to be published) Normal and pathological age differences in memory. In: Brocklehurst JC (ed) Textbook of geriatrics and gerontology. Livingstone, Edinburgh
Fozard JL, Wolf E, Bell B, McFarland RA, Podolsky S (1977) Visual perception and communication. In: Birren JE, Schaie KW (eds) Handbook of the psychology of aging. Van Nostrand, New York
Fuld PA, Katzman R, Davies P, Terry RD (1982) Intrusions as a sign of Alzheimer dementia: Chemical and pathological verification. Ann Neurol 11:155–159
Goodin DS, Squires KC, Starr A (1978) Long latency event-related components of the auditory evoked potential in dementia. Brain 101:635–648
Horenstein S (1971) The clinical use of psychological testing. In: Wells CE (ed) Dementia. Davis, Philadelphia
Inglis J, Caird WK (1963) Age differences in successive responses to simultaneous stimulation. Can J Psychol 17:98–105
Inglis J, Sanderson RE (1961) Successive responses to simultaneous stimulation in elderly patients with memory disorder. J Abnorm Social Psychol 62:709–712
Kaplan E, Goodglass H, Weintraub S (1983) Boston naming test scoring booklet. Lea and Febiger, Philadelphia
Kenshalo DR (1977) Age changes in touch, vibration, temperature, kinesthesis, and pain sensitivity. In: Birren JE, Schaie KW (eds) Handbook of the psychology of aging. Van Nostrand, New York
Kirshner HS, Webb WG, Kelly MP (1984) The naming disorder of dementia. Neuropsychologia 22:23–30
Levy R, Isaacs A, Hawks G (1970) Neurophysiological correlates of senile dementia: I. Motor and sensory nerve conduction velocity. Psychol Med 1:40–47
Levy R, Isaacs A, Behrman J (1971) Neurophysiological correlates of senile dementia. II. The somatosensory evoked response. Psychol Med 1:159–165
Martin A, Fedio P (1983) Word production and comprehension in Alzheimer's disease: The breakdown of semantic knowledge. Brain Lang 19:124–141
McCarthy M, Ferris SH, Clark E, Crook T (1981) Acquisition and retention of categorized material in normal aging and senile dementia. Exp Aging Res 7:127–135
Michalewski HJ, Thompson LW, Saul RE (1980) Use of the EEG and evoked potentials in the investigation of age-related clinical disorders. In: Birren JE, Sloane RB (eds) Handbook of mental health and aging. Prentice-Hall, Englewood Cliffs
Miller E (1977) Abnormal ageing. Wiley, New York

Miller E, Hague F (1975) Some characteristics of verbal behavior in presenile dementia. Psychol Med 5:255–259

Moscovitch M (1982) A neuropsychological approach to perception and memory in normal and pathological aging. In: Craik FIM, Trehub S (eds) Aging and cognitive processes. Plenum, New York

Muramoto O, Sugishita M, Ando K (1984) Cholinergic system and constructional praxis: A further study of physostigmine in Alzheimer's disease. J Neurol Neurosurg Psychiatry 47:485–491

Norris AH, Shock NW, Wagman IH (1953) Age changes in the maximum conduction velocity of motor fibres in human ulnar nerves. J Appl Physiol 5:589–593

O'Neil PM, Calhoun KS (1975) Sensory deficits and behavioral deterioration in senescence. J Abnorm Psychol 84:579–582

Pfefferbaum A, Ford JM, Wenegrat B, Tinklenberg JR, Kopell BS (1982) Electrophysiological approaches to the study of aging and dementia. In Corkin S, Davis KL, Growdon JH, Usdin E, Wurtman RJ (eds) Alzheimer's disease: A report of progress in research. Raven, New York

Pirozzolo FJ, Hansch EC (1981) Oculomotor reaction time in dementia reflects degree of cerebral dysfunction. Science 214:349–351

Rabbitt P (1977) Changes in problem solving ability in old age. In: Birren JE, Schaie KW (eds) Handbook of the psychology of aging. Van Nostrand, New York

Reed HBC, Reitan RM (1963) A comparison of the effects of the normal aging process with the effects of organic brain damage on adaptive abilities. J Gerontol 18:177–179

Reisberg B, Ferris SH, de Leon MJ, Crook T (1982) The global deterioration scale for assessment of primary degenerative dementia. Am J Psychiatry 139:1136–1139

Rosen WG (1981) Effects of senile dementia of the Alzheimer's type on verbal fluency. Int J Neurosci 12:245–246

Rosen WG (1983) Neuropsychological investigation of memory, visuoconstructional, visuoperceptual, and language abilities in senile dementia of the Alzheimer type. In: Mayeux R, Rosen WG (eds) The dementias. Raven, New York

Schaie KW (1980) Intelligence and problem solving. In: Birren JE, Sloane RB (eds) Handbook of mental health and aging. Prentice-Hall, Englewood Cliffs

Schwartz MF, Marin OS, Saffran EM (1979) Dissociations of language function in dementia: A case study. Brain Lang 7:277–306

Sim A, Sussman I (1962) Alzheimer's disease: Its natural history and differential diagnosis. J Nerv Ment Dis 135:489–499

Smith A (1967) The serial sevens subtraction test. Arch Neurol 17:78–80

Spooner JW, Sakala SM, Baloh RW (1980) Effect of aging on eye tracking. Arch Neurol 37:575–576

Squire LR (1974) Remote memory as affected by aging. Neuropsychologia 12:429–435

Storandt M (1977) Age ability level and methods of administering and scoring the WAIS. J Gerontol 32:175–178

Strother CR, Schaie KW, Horst P (1957) The relationship between advanced age and mental abilities. J Abnorm Social Psychol 55:166–176

Thomas M, Ballantyne JP, Hansen S, Weir AI, Doyle D (1982) Anterior horn cell dysfunction in Alzheimer's disease. J Neurol Neurosurg Psychiatry 45:378–381

Thompson LW, Optin E, Cohen LD (1963) Effects of age, presentation speed, and sensory modality on performance of a vigilance task. J Gerontol 18:366–369

Vrtunski PB, Patterson MB, Mack SL, Hill GO (1983) Microbehavioral analysis of the choice reaction time response in senile dementia. Brain 106:929–947

Wagman IH, Lesse H (1952) Maximum conduction velocities of motor fibres of ulnar nerve in human subjects of various ages and sizes. J Neurophysiol 15:235–244

Wapner S, Werner H, Comalli PE Jr (1960) Perception of part-whole relations in middle and old age. J Gerontol 15:412–416

Warrington EK, Sanders HI (1971) The fate of old memories. Q J Exp Psychol 23:432–442

Wechsler AF (1977) Presenile dementia presenting as aphasia. J Neurol Neurosurg Psychiatry 40:303–305

Wechsler D (1981) Wechsler Adult Intelligence Scale–Revised. Harcourt Brace Jovanovich, New York

Welford AT (1977) Motor performance. In: Birren JE, Schaie KW (eds) Handbook of the psychology of aging. Van Nostrand, New York

Wilson RS, Kaszniak AW, Fox JH (1981) Remote memory in senile dementia. Cortex 17:41–48

Wilson RS, Kaszniak AW, Bacon LD, Fox JH, Kelly MP (1982) Facial recognition memory in dementia. Cortex 18:329–336

Senile Dementia of the Alzheimer Type: Diagnostic and Differential Diagnostic Features with Special Reference to Functional Assessment Staging

B. REISBERG, S. H. FERRIS, and M. J. DE LEON[1]

Describing Senile Dementia of the Alzheimer Type: Historical Review

At the time we embarked on our investigations into the clinical symptomatology of senile dementia of the Alzheimer type (SDAT) approximately 6 years ago, little was known about this disorder. Old age as a cause of dementia had been recognized by Aretaeus of Cappadocia and popularized by Galen in the second century A.D. (Adams 1861; Galen 1821–1833). This conception does not appear to have advanced further until Rush's seminal description of a patient with "the marks of second infancy" (Rush 1793). In 1838, Esquirol provided a more general definition of *"démence sénile"* as an illness: (a) in which there occurs a weakening of the memory for recent experiences and a loss of drive and willpower; (b) which appears gradually; and (c) which may be accompanied by emotional disturbances. At approximately the same time, Prichard (1837) described an entity he called "senile incoherence", which he divided into four successive stages: (a) impaired memory; (b) loss of reasoning power; (c) incomprehension; and (d) loss of instinctive action. In 1907, Alzheimer described the case of a woman who succumbed to the illness in her fifties.

Until 1980, knowledge of the clinical syndrome of SDAT was summed up in the American Psychiatric Association's definition of primary degenerative dementia:

"The essential feature is the presence of Dementia of insidious onset and gradual progressive course for which all other specific causes have been excluded by the history, physical examination and laboratory tests. The Dementia involves a multifaceted loss of intellectual abilities, such as memory, judgement, abstract thought, and other higher cortical functions, and changes in personality and behavior.

The onset is insidious, and the course is one of uniform, gradual progression. In the early stages memory impairment may be the only apparent cognitive deficit. There may also be subtle personality changes, such as the development of apathy, lack of spontaneity, and a quiet withdrawal from social interactions. Individuals usually remain neat and well-groomed and, aside from an occasional irritable outburst, are cooperative and behave in a socially appropriate way. With progression to the middle stage of the disease various cognitive disturbances become quite apparent, and behavior and personality are more obviously affected. By the late stage, the individual may be completely mute and inattentive. At this point he or she is totally incapable of caring for himself or herself. This stage leads

1 Department of Psychiatry, New York University Medical Center, New York, New York 10016, USA

Senile Dementia of the Alzheimer Type
Ed. by J. Traber and W. H. Gispen

inevitably to death. With senile onset, the average duration of symptoms, from onset to death, is about 5 years (American Psychiatric Association 1980).

Hence, 5 years ago, we were confronted with the following questions:

1. The foremost question was whether SDAT is a characteristic clinical entity, distinguishable from other dementing disorders. Clearly, the early stages of this illness process, in which "individuals usually remain neat and well-groomed and are cooperative and behave in a socially appropriate way," are very different from the late stage, in which "the individual may be completely mute and inattentive." The stages of this process needed to be described in detail, if indeed they are sufficiently homogeneous to be described.
2. The borderline between normal aging and SDAT needed to be defined, along with the prognosis associated with each stage of the illness process, if indeed stages can be demonstrated. Previous investigations had revealed that normal aged individuals who score relatively poorly on psychological test measures are more likely to be deceased at follow-up than cohorts (including twin cohorts) who achieved higher scores on these measures (Jarvik and Falek 1963). At the other end of the illness spectrum, studies had revealed that persons institutionalized with dementia of diverse etiology suffer an increase in mortality in comparison with cohort and control populations. Studies beginning to appear 5 years ago indicated that persons institutionalized with more specifically diagnosed SDAT are more likely to be deceased at follow-up than persons instituionalized with dementia of other etiology (Kaszniak et al. 1978; Go et al. 1978). Between these extremes of morbitidy and mortality, little was known with respect to the course of the disease for community residing persons with mild, moderate, and severe cognitive impairment either with regard to each other or with regard to unimpaired elderly controls.
3. Assessment measures capable of assessing the magnitude of dementia symptomatology, irrespective of etiology were available (Blessed et al. 1968; Kahn et al. 1960; Folstein et al. 1975; Reisberg et al. 1981). However, at a certain point in the evolution of the illness, subjects achieve uniform scores of zero on all mental status and psychometric assessments. Thus, the course of illness needed to be described as it evolves beyond this untestable phase.
4. If indeed the evolution of SDAT is sufficiently homogeneous to lend itself to description, criteria for managing each stage of the illness had to be elucidated. Disease management requirements fall into two distinct categories: those relating to the patient and those relating to the primary care giver who, of necessity, shoulders much of the burden of coping with the illness. If feasible, management advice should be formulated in terms appropriate to each stage of the illness, since, clearly, the needs of the patient who remains "neat and wellgroomed" and who behaves "in a socially appropriate way" are very different from those of the patient who is "mute and inattentive".

In the past 5 years, we have attempted in our laboratory to provide answers to each of the above questions. Initially, case histories describing three broad phases of the illness process were published (Reisberg 1981). Subsequently, seven global stages of the normal aging process and of progressive Alzheimer's disease were described (Reisberg et al. 1982). A clinically assessed symptomatology corresponding to each of these seven stages was also elaborated. Initially, five concordant axes representing seven phases of change in progressive SDAT were published (Reisberg et al. 1983 a). These initial five axes of the Brief Cognative Rating Scale measured progressive changes in concentration, recent memory, past memory, orientation, and functioning. Pearson correlations between ordinal clinical assessments on any two of these axes ranged from 0.83 to 0.94 ($n = 50$, $P < .001$) (Reisberg et al. 1984 a). Subsequently, three additional axes of progressive alterations relating to language, motor functioning, and mood and behavior in normal aging and SDAT were published (Reisberg et al. 1983). While assisting in the further description of progressive changes in the SDAT clinical syndrome, the latter were somewhat less in agreement with stage-specific global descriptions of the illness. Hence, Pearson correlations of each of these axes with global descriptions of change on the Global Deterioration Scale (Reisberg et al. 1982) were 0.88, 0.62, and 0.64 respectively ($n = 30$, $P < .001$) (Reisberg et al. 1984 a). We have recently completed a clinical description of the progression of SDAT which introduces two additional axes to assess deterioration of constructional praxis and calculation ability. Together with the axes measuring changes in language, motor functioning, and mood and behavior, the latter two comprise part 2 of the final version of the ten-axis Brief Cognitive Rating Scale (BCRS) in Table 1.

The Global Deterioration Scale (GDS) describes in global terms the clinical progression of Alzheimer's disease and is thus a useful instrument in the diagnosis and the differential diagnosis of SDAT. If a clinical syndrome differes markedly from the GDS staging and progression, the diagnosis of SDAT might be called into question. Other recent work has revealed the prognostic concomitants of the global stages and elaborated operational definitions of normal aging, normal aged senescent forgetfulness, and early Alzheimer's disease (Reisberg et al. 1984 b). These investigations are summarized in Table 2. Independent observations and investigations have made it possible to formulate stage-specific criteria for managing each global stage of the illness (Reisberg 1984).

The BCRS ordinal axes provide a means of assessing clinical symptomatology and change at all stages of the illness in a continuous and sensitive fashion. Unlike most psychological test measures and mental status assessments, the utility of this instrument does not "bottom out" until relatively late in the evolution of SDAT. It was hoped that BCRS axis concordance would also provide a useful tool in the differential diagnosis of SDAT as opposed to other senescent dementing and/or pseudodementing disorders. Although the BCRS continues to show promise in assisting clinicians in differential diagnosis, succinct, rapid, clinically useful rules have not readily emerged. Hence, this instrument is primarily used at present as a sensitive clinical instrument for gauging the magnitude of clinically assessed symptomatology in pharmacologic trials. In this context, the GDS is implemented as an initial staging and diagnostic instrument.

Functional Assessment Staging of SDAT

We have recently developed a new assessment instrument derived from axis 5 of the BCRS. This instrument, known as the FAST, an acronym for Functional As-

Table 1. Brief cognitive rating scale (BCRS)[a] – Part 1

Axis 1: Concentration

1. No objective or subjective evidence of deficits in concentration
2. Subjective decrement in concentration
3. Minor signs of poor concentration (e.g., difficulty in subtracting serial 7s from 100)
4. Definite concentration deficit given the patient's background (e.g., marked deficit in subtracting serial 7s; frequent deficits in subtraction of serial 4s from 40)
5. Marked concentration deficit (e.g., naming months backwards or subtracting serials 2s from 20)
6. Forgets the concentration task; frequently begins to count forward when asked to count backwards from 10 by 1s
7. Marked difficulty counting forward to 10 by 1s

Axis 2: Recent memory

1. No objective or subjective evidence of deficit in recent memory
2. Subjective impairment only (e.g., forgetting names more frequently)
3. Deficit in recall of specific events evident upon detailed questioning; no deficit in the recall of major recent events
4. Cannot recall major events of previous weekend or week; scanty knowledge (not detailed) of current events, favorite television shows, etc.
5. Unsure of wheather, may not know current president or current address
6. Occasional knowledge of some recent events; little or no idea of current address, weather, etc. Given the current president's first name, may recall his last name
7. No knowledge of recent events

Axis 3: Past memory

1. No subjective or objective impairment of past memory
2. Subjective impairment only: can recall two or more primary school teachers
3. Some gaps in past memory upon detailed questioning; able to recall at least one childhood teacher and/or one childhood friend
4. Clear-cut deficit: the spouse recalls more of the patient's past than the patient. Cannot recall childhood friends and/or teachers but knows the names of schools attended. Confuses chronology in reciting personal history
5. Major past event's sometimes not recalled (e.g., names of schools attended)
6. Some residual memory of past (e.g., may recall country of birth or former occupation; may or may not recall mother's name; may or may not recall father's name)
7. No memory of past (cannot recall country, state, or town of origin; cannot recall names of parents, etc.)

Avis 4: Orientation

1. No deficit in memory for time, place, identity of self or others
2. Subjective impairment only: knows time to nearest hour, location
3. Mistakes in time of 2 or more hours, in day of the week of 1 or more days, in date of 3 or more days
4. Mistakes day of the month by 10 days or more, confuses month of the year by 1 month or more
5. Unsure of month and/or year and/or season; unsure of locale
6. No idea of date; identifies spouse but may not recall name; knows own name
7. Cannot identify spouse; may be unsure of personal identity

Axis 5: Functioning and self care

1. No difficulty, either subjective or objective
2. Complains of forgetting location of objects; subjective work difficulties
3. Decreased job functioning evident to co-workers; difficulty in traveling to unfamiliar locations
4. Decreased ability to perform complex tasks (e.g., planning dinner for guests, handling finances, marketing)
5. Requires assistance in choosing proper clothing
6. Requires assistance in feeding, toileting, bathing, and/or ambulating
7. Requires constant assistance in all activities of daily life

Table 1 (continued)

Part 2

Axis 6: Speech
1. No subjective or objective speech deficit
2. Subjective deficits in recalling names of persons or objects
3. Overt word-finding difficulties which may result in intermittent interruptions of speech or mild stuttering
4. Decrease of verbalization evident to family members but generally not evident on clinical interview; patient becomes more reticent or, alternatively, tendency to ramble
5. Overt paucity of spontaneous speech (evident in the course of clinical interview); sentence-production abilities remain intact
6. Inability to speak in sentences; responses tend to be limited to one or a few words
7. Verbal abilities are lost; vocabulary may be limited to one or two words, if any. Patient may repeat words or phrases (verbigeration) or make up new words or phrases (neologisms). Patient's vocabulary may be limited to grunts or screams

Axis 7: Psychomotor
1. No subjective or objective motor deficits
2. Subjective decrement in complex motor or physical abilities; no objective decrement in performance
3. Decreased ability to perform complex psychomotor tasks, such as sailing or complex constructive tasks
4. Gait becomes slowed. The deficit is notable to family members familiar with the patient but not necessarily to clinicians who may not know the patient well. Patient becomes more cautious with respect to movements and activities in general, such as driving an automobile
5. Slowing of gait and movement is clearly evident, even to strangers. Driving ability is compromised or abandoned
6. Steps become small and movements are markedly slowed; difficulty in signing name properly may develop
7. Ability to ambulate is lost

Axis 8: Mood and behavior
1. No subjective or objective changes in mood or behavior
2. Subjective increase in anxiety or concern with respect to cognitive fonctioning
3. Overt anxiety evident to clinician and/or patient's family
4. Blunting of emotional responses evident to family
5. Flattened affect evident to physician; patient may have crying episodes
6. Overt agitation and/or formal thinking disorder (e.g., paranoia, hallucinations, delusions)
7. Nonverbal agitation alternating with pathologic passivity

Axis 9: Praxis
1. No subjective or objective changes
2. Can draw a cube
3. Difficulty drawing a cube with proper perspective
4. Can draw a rectangle
5. Can draw a circle inside a circle
6. (a) Can draw a circle
   (b) Can draw a line
   (c)–(e) Can draw a scribble
7. Will not write anything, but may grasp a writing implement in a useable fashion

Axis 10: Calculation ability
1. No subjective or objective changes
2. Can subtract 43 − 17
3. Can subtract 39 − 14
4. Can subtract 15 − 6
5. Can subtract 9 − 4
6. (a) Can add 8 + 7
   (b)–(e) Can add 3 + 1
7. (e) May sometimes be able to add 1 + 1
   (b)–(f) cannot add 1 + 1

Table 2. Baseline clinical status and outcome according to Global Deterioration Scale (GDS)

Clinical status at baseline	Magnitude of baseline impairment	n	Age at baseline (Years, mean ± S.D.)	Follow-up interval (Years, mean ± S.D.)	Follow-up status	Negative outcome[a] (%)
Subjective complaints of memory deficits. No objective deficit in employment or social situations	GDS 2: very mild	40	68.80 ± 5.29	3.43 ± 0.41	40 community residing 2 clinically worsened[b] 38 clinically unchanged	5
Decreased performance in demanding employment and social situations. Objective evidence of memory deficit obtained only with an intensive interview conducted by an experienced clinician	GDS 3: mild	32	71.09 ± 6.79	3.59 ± 0.50	30 community residing 3 clinically improved 3 clinically worsened 24 clinically unchanged 1 institutionalized 1 deceased	16
Clearly manifest deficits on clinical interview in knowledge of current and recent events. May also demonstrate some memory deficit for personal history. Concentration deficit elicited in serial subtraction task. Decreased ability to shop and handle finances.	GDS 4: moderate	22	72.32 ± 5.75	3.68 ± 0.58	10 community residing 4 clinically worsened 6 clinically unchanged 6 institutionalized 6 deceased	73
Patient can no longer survive without assistance. Requires no assistance toileting or eating, but may have some difficulty choosing the proper clothing to wear.	GDS 5: moderately severe	6	72.33 ± 7.37	4.12 ± 0.66	3 community residing 1 clinically worsened 2 clinically unchanged 2 institutionalized 1 deceased	67
Largely unaware of all recent events and experiences in their lives. May occasionally forget the name of the spouse on whom they are entirely dependent for survival. Requires assistance dressing and sometimes bathing and toileting.	GDS 6: Severe	6	72.50 ± 3.83	4.17 ± 0.55	0 community residing 4 institutional 2 deceased	100

[a] Negative outcome is defined as Δ GDS $\geqq 2$, institutionalization, or death
[b] Clinical change is defined as a change of 2 or greater in GDS scores from baseline

sessment Staging of SDAT (Reisberg et al. 1984c), enables clinicians to assess cognitive impairment in the aged patient and, similtaneously, to perform tasks that were previously difficult or impossible:

1. To determine rapidly whether the nature of the dementing process is consistent with uncomplicated SDAT, in terms of both present manifestation and evolution.
2. To classify in a relatively detailed fashion even patients who are in the later stages of SDAT.
3. To differentiate various complications of Alzheimer's disease from the natural evolution of the illness.
4. To accomplish all of the above with sufficient facility to allow the preliminary diagnosis, differential diagnosis, and determination of complicating factors to be made on the basis of information provided by family members or, in many cases, even over the telephone, prior to the actual examination of the patient.

These diagnostic advances are possible for several reasons: (a) Alzheimer's disease is a pervasive dementing process, the evolution of which invariably follows a definite consistent course; (b) dementing processes associated with other etiologies evolve differently; and (c) many functional activities in all twentieth-century societies are identical, making it possible to describe functional decrements in universal terms. The Functional Assessment Stages (FAST) of normal aging and of SDAT have been enumerated so as to be optimally concordant with the corresponding stages of the Global Deterioration Scale (GDS) and the BCRS axes. The FAST stages are described in Table 3.

Table 3. Functional Assessment Stages (FAST) in normal aging and in senile dementia of Alzheimer type[a]

Global deterioration scale stage	Clinical diagnosis	FAST characteristics	Commentary
1. No cognitive decline	Normal	No functional decrement, either subjective or objetive, manifest	The aged subject's ostensible and subjective functional abilities in occupational, social, and other settings remain intact in comparison with his performance 5–10 years previously.
2. Very mild cognitive decline	Normal for age	Complains of forgetting location of objects; subjective and word-finding difficulties	The most common age-related functional complaints are of forgetting names, the location of objects, and decreased ability to recall appointments. These subjective decrements generally go unnoticed by intimates or co-workers. Complex occupational and social functioning is not compromised by the subjectively observed decrements.

[a] Copyright 1984 Barry Reisberg

Table 3 (continued)

Global deterioration scale stage	Clinical diagnosis	FAST characteristics	Commentary
			These sujective symptoms are very common in elderly individuals. They may also be troubling and lead the individual to consult a physician. The symptoms may be associated with primary affective disorder or primary anxiety, and symptoms of these conditions should be looked for carefully. In many cases, no condition other than normal aging is found.
3. Mild cognitive decline	Borderline impairment	Decreased functioning in demanding employment settings evident to co-workers; difficulty in travelling to new locations	An individual may begin to forget important appointments for the first time in his life. Similarly, a professional who may have been able to write hundreds of articles or reports over the course of his or her adult years now finds him- or herself unable to finish a single report for the first time. Functional decrement may also become manifest in complex psychomotor tasks, such as ability to travel to unfamiliar locations. Individuals at this stage have no difficulty with routine tasks, such as shopping, handling finances, or travelling to familiar locations. They may retire from demanding occupational and social settings, whereupon their deficits may no longer be manifest. Although clinically these symptoms may appear subtle, they can be of sufficient magnitude to alter a patient's life-style considerably. They can be alarming enough to induce him to visit a physician or clinic.
4. Moderate cognitive decline	Mild Alzheimer's disease	Decreased ability to perform complex tasks such as planning dinner for guests, handling finances, and shopping.	Individuals have difficulty returning with the correct items and proper amounts when marketing. Unless supervised, they have difficulty balancing their check-books and may make significant financial errors. Functioning in other complex areas is also compromised. One patient at this stage scheduled a dinner party and instructed half the guests to arrive on the following day. Another patient ostensibly continued to function as an attorney, in partnership with her husband. Although she was able to travel independently to and from her office daily, she could not recall the names or details of any of the "cases" she was supposedly continuing to work on, when queried. In actuality, her husband had taken on her work.

Table 3 (continued)

Global deterioration scale stage	Clinical diagnosis	FAST characteristics	Commentary
			Patients can still function independently in the community since they can dress, bathe, choose their own clothing and travel to familiar locations. However, independent community functioning is compromised. One woman at this stage lived alone and continued to pay her own rent; however, when queried, she underestimated the amount of her rent by 50%. This same woman incorrectly stated she lived in a hotel, when, in actuality, she resided in an apartment house. Many of these patients continue to function independently in a community setting, although their symptoms may lead to financial and other difficulties. Family members may become alarmed by the symptomatology at this stage and bring the patient for the first time to the physician for diagnosis.
5. Moderately severe cognitive decline	Moderate Alzheimer's disease	Requires assistance in choosing clothing; may require coaxing to bathe properly	At this stage, patients can no longer function independently. The care giver must assist not only in managing financial affairs and in marketing, but must also assist the patient in choosing the proper clothing for the season and occasion. The patient frequently wears obviously incongruous clothing combinations, unless the care giver intervenes. The inability to choose proper clothing is virtually pathognomonic of this stage. Less characteristically, some patients begin to forget to bathe regularly unless reminded. Sometimes, coaxing as well as a reminder to bathe is necessary. Another functional deicit which frequently becomes manifest at this stage is difficulty in driving an automobile. The patient may speed up and slow down the vehicle inappropriately, mistakenly go through a stopsign or stoplight, or even collide with another vehicle for the first time in many years. Frequently, the patient is sufficiently alarmed to discontinue driving voluntarily. Occasionally, coersion on the part of the care giver is necessary.

Table 3 (continued)

Global deterioration scale stage	Clinical diagnosis	FAST characteristics	Commentary
			Patients are still capable of putting on their clothing properly, once it has been selected for them. They are also capable of bathing themselves and even of adjusting the bathwater properly, when washing, although, as mentioned, they may have to be cajoled or reminded to bathe. Crying episodes or other emotional disturbances, including hyperactively and sleep rhythm disturbances, frequently result in crises and physician intervention at this stage.
6. Severe cognitive decline	Moderately severe Alzheimer's disease	(a) Difficulty in putting on clothing properly	Initially in this substage, many patients begin to put their regular clothing on over their night clothes. Other patients, for the first time in their adult lives, experience difficulties in tying their shoelaces properly, buttoning or zipping their clothing, tying neckties properly, or putting their shoes on the proper feet. As the illness advances, care givers increasingly assist the patient in putting his clothes on properly.
		(b) Requires assistance in bathing; may develop fear of bathing	At this stage, the patient's ability to adjust the bathwater properly declines. Difficulties in getting in and out of the bath, washing properly, and completely drying oneself may also become manifest. As noted previously, fear or resistance to bathing sometimes precedes actual bathing deficits.
		(c) Decreased ability to handle the mechanics of toiletting	Patients at this stage begin to forget to flush the toilet. They may also begin to forget to wipe themselves properly when toileting and may experience difficulty in readjusting their clothing. The care giver begins to assist the patient in handling the mechanics of toileting.
		(d) Urinary incontinence	Occasionally, this occurs virtually simultaneously with stage 6(c), but more frequently, there is a discernable interval of several months between these substages. Urinary incontinence occurs at this stage in the absence of infection or other genitourinary tract pathology. It appears to be entirely the result of decreased cognitive capacity to respond to urinary urgency with appropriate toileting behavior.

Table 3 (continued)

Global deterioration scale stage	Clinical diagnosis	FAST characteristics	Commentary
		(e) Fecal incontinence	This substage may also appear simultaneously with the preceding substage (urinary incontinence) or even when difficulties with the mechanics of toileting first become evident to the care giver. More frequently, this substage is temporally discrete, The cause as with urinary incontinence, appears to be decreased cognitive capatity. Agitation and overt psychotic symptomatology frequently produce crises in the sixth stage which may result in medical contact. Other symptoms, such as the onset of incontinence may also produce crises. Violence and/or incontinence may lead the family to consider institutionalization of the patient.
7. Very severe cognitive decline	Severe Alzheimer's disease	(a) ability of speak limited to a maximum vocabulary of approximately six words	Decreasing vocabulary and speech abilities mark the progression of Alzheimer's disease. Reticence and paucity of speech are frequently noted in the fourth and fifth GDS stages. In the sixth GDS stage, the ability to speak in complete sentences is gradually lost. Subsequent to the development of incontinence, speech becomes restricted to single words or short phrases, and spoken vocabulary limited to only a few words.
		(b) Intelligible vocabulary limited to a single word	The final spoken word for the Alzheimer patient varies. For some patients, the spoken vocabularly becomes limited to the word "yes," while for others, it is "no." One woman's final word was "okay," which she repeated in response to all speach-eliciting phenomena. Hence, if she wanted to toilet, express anxiety, affirmation or negation, she said "okay." As the illness progresses, the ability to speak even this single word is lost. However, months afterwards, the patient may suddenly articulate the seemingly forgotten final word, only to return to a state of obliviousness. After the capacity for intelligible speech is lost, vocalization is limited to grunts or screams.
		(c) Loss of ambulatory ability	Neuropathologic studies indicate that the motor cortex is spared except in the most severe (late) stages of Alzheimer's disease.

Table 3 (continued)

Global deterioration scale stage	Clinical diagnosis	FAST characteristics	Commentary
			Perhaps this late cortical deterioration explains why the loss of ambulatory ability occurs at this late point in the evolution of the disease. Lesser forms of ambulatory disturbance, however, are sometimes observed at earlier stages of Alzheimer's disease. These milder locomotor disturbances may be the result of decreased cognitive capacities and resultant psychomotor changes, rather than destruction of the motor cortex per se. For example, inappropriate gait speed (the patient either walks too quickly or slowly) is not infrequently noted in the earlier stages of the disease. In the sixth GDS stage, patients may begin to ambulate more deliberately and to take smaller steps. Assistance in walking up and down staircases is generally required prior to the loss of all ambulatory ability. The onset of ambulatory loss is somewhat varied. Some patients simply take progressively smaller and slower steps. Others begin to tilt forwards, backwards, or laterally when walking. Twisted gaits have also been noted. After ambulatory abilities are lost, other voluntary motor abilities become compromised. After several months to years many surviving patients develop contractures, although it is not certain at this time whether these are in some instances preventable by aggressive physical therapy.
		(d) Loss of ability to sit	After patients have lost the ability to ambulate without and, subsequently, even with assistance, they are still capable of sitting in a chair unassisted. Several months after ambulatory ability is lost, the ability to sit unassisted is lost. At this point, they are still capable of smiling, chewing, grunting, and grasping.
		(e) Loss of ability to smile	Alzheimer's disease survivors can generally still move their eyes and may appear to show deliberate ocular movements in response to stimuli. Grasp-reflexive ability is also preserved in many patients, as is the ability to swallow.

Table 3 (continued)

Global deterioration scale stage	Clinical diagnosis	FAST characteristics	Commentary
		(f) Stupor and coma	Many symptoms of the earlier stages and substages of Alzheimer's disease appear to be the functionally definable end products of accumulative pathology, which are recognizable, albeit less distinct, at earlier stages of the illness. Similarly, the stuporous and comatose states in the final substage of Alzheimer's disease may be related to progressive electrophysiologic slowing and decrements in cerebral metabolism which are known concomitants of the illness. Pathologic passivity frequently replaces earlier agitation in the seventh stage. Nevertheless, some patients become agitated or psychotic for the first time. Not infrequently, family members consult physicians for the first time with respects to a crisis, which may or may not result in institutionalization.

The Hierarchy of Functions in SDAT and in Normal Human Development

In 1964, de Ajuriaguerra et al. hypothesized that deficits in degenerative dementia occur in an order that is approximately the reverse of Piaget's childhood developmental stages. Viewed retrospectively, our observations are in agreement with this hypothesis. These relationships are detailed in Table 4.

Interestingly, in normal human development functional stages can be distinguished in ways that are also paralleled in the evolution of SDAT (Table 4). Hence, just as functional stages merge and overlap at certain points of normal human development, the borderlines between the various FAST stages in Alzheimer's disease are subtle rather than abrupt. Also, the total duration of normal developmental stages does not differ strikingly from that of the degenerative stages of SDAT. In this regard, it is interesting to return to the APA's Diagnostic and Statistical Manual's definition cited earlier, which states "with senile onset, the average duration of symptoms, from onset to death, is about 5 years" (American Psychiatric Association 1980). Particularly if we take into consideration the fact that approximately 50% of SDAT cases do not present until the fifth or sixth stage, the temporal course of degeneration represents the converse of the normal course of development and does not markedly diverge from it in length. Also to be taken into consideration is the fact that the vast majority of Alzheimer patients do not survive the full course of the illness. Many succumb in the sixth stage, while others, perhaps the majority, succumb in the early part of the seventh stage. Some

Table 4. Correspondence between normal human development and FAST deficits in normal aging and SDAT

FAST stage of normal aging and SDAT	Estimated duration of FAST stage in normal aging and in SDAT[a]	Approximate age at which function is acquired in normal development
1	50 years	adult
2	15 years	aged adult
3	7 years	young adult
4	2 years	7 years to adolescence
5	18 months	5–7 years
6 (a)	5 months	approximately 5 years (Eisenberg 1975)
(b)	5 months	approximately 4 years (Eisenberg 1975)
(c)	5 months	approximately 48 months (Vaughn 1969)
(d)	4 months	approximately 36–54 months (Pierce 1975)
(e)	10 months	approximately 24–36 months (Eisenberg 1975, Vaughn 1969, Pierce 1975)
7 (a)	7 months	approximately 12 months (Eisenberg 1975, Vaughn 1969)
(b)	6 months	approximately 12 months (Eisenberg 1975, Vaughn 1969)
(c)	6 months	approximately 12 months (Eisenberg 1975, Vaughn 1969)
(d)	6 months	approximately 6–9 months (Eisenberg 1975, Vaughn 1969)
(e)	6 months	approximately 8–16 weeks (Eisenberg 1975, Vaughn 1969)
(f)	–	perinatal

[a] In subjects who survive and progress to the subsequent deterioration stage

Alzheimer's patients succumb relatively early in the course of the illness, in the fifth or even the fourth stage. Death in the fifth stage from such tragedies as traffic accidents is sometimes clearly traceable to Alzheimer's disease, while death in the fourth stage may be less readily related to the disease.

If we consider the relatively late presentation of many cases of Alzheimer's disease and the rate of premature death for many patients over the course of the illness, the APA's estimated survival time of 5 years is not very different from the estimated duration of each stage of the illness, as shown in Table 4. Indeed, if we assume that the average patient presents at the end of the fourth stage or the beginning of the fifth stage and dies at the end of stage 7(b) or the beginning of stage 7(c), the average duration of the illness according to Table 4 would be exactly 5 years.

It is also evident from the FAST that, in both normal human development and the degenerative change of SDAT, the ordinal hierarchy of functions is relative rather than absolute. That normal human development proceeds in a certain order is, of course, indisputable. However, individuals occasionally deviate from the normal developmental hierarchy. Hence, whereas very few if any infants speak many words before they can sit up, and no infants speak before they can smile, some are capable of saying a few words before they can walk without assistance. Similarly, some Alzheimer patients may still be able to utter intelligible words after having lost the ability to walk. Even more subtle is the distinction in Alzheimer's disease patients between loss of ability to put on clothing properly and loss of ability to bathe properly. Developmentally, of course, these distinctions may also be subtle. Hence, although functional degeneration in Alzheimer's disease, like that of normal aging is unquestionably ordinal, occasional minor deviations from the usual evolution of the disease occur, particularly between adjacent substages of the hierarchy. Major hierarchical violations, however, indicate other confounding pathology.

The Staging of Severe SDAT

At stage 6 (a), when Alzheimer victims lose the ability to put on their clothing properly, their behavioral disturbances and cognitive deficits may limit their achievements on most psychometric and mental status evaluations to baseline (zero) scores. Thus, by the early part of the seventh stage, when patients lose the ability to speak, test measures and mental status assessments are uniformly valueless in differentiating the severity of patients' symptoms. In contrast, the FAST staging procedure makes possible the rapid identification of at least 11 ordinal stages of Alzheimer's disease beyond the point at which other assessment procedures are no longer of value.

The importance of this development for Alzheimer's disease research cannot be overestimated. Since contemporary in vivo and postmortem studies of SDAT patients do not attempt to classify patients with "severe" Alzheimer type dementia, these procedures provide a mechanism for remedying such deficiencies.

The Differential Diagnosis of Dementia

In conjunction with information about the onset, course, and presentation of SDAT, the FAST staging procedure is useful in diagnosing and staging uncomplicated Alzheimer's disease. it is also of great value in identifying extraneous, treatable complications of Alzheimer's disease as well as in distinguishing Alzheimer's disease from other dementing disorders of later life (Table 5).

Illnesses that might complicate an otherwise consistent picture of Alzheimer's disease include the following:

1. Inability to shop or handle finances at a time when a person can still function adequately in a demanding employment setting should lead the clinician to consider the possibility of a focal cerebral process associated with, for example, acalculia, or a "pseudodementing" process such as depression.
2. Inability to put on clothing properly at a time when a patient can still choose the proper clothing to wear can occur in depression. It can also, of course, occur as a result of focal cerebral pathology, as in stroke or CNS metastasis. Arthritis, a fracture, or other physically debilitating processes are other underlying causes of a reversal in the ordinal pattern observed in uncomplicated SDAT.

Table 5. Differential diagnostic considerations in cases of deviations from FAST

Stage	Characteristics	Differential diagnostic considerations (particularly if FAST stage occurs prematurely in the evolution of dementia)
1.	No functional decrement manifest, either subjectively or objectively	
2.	Complains of forgetting location of objects; subjective work difficulties	2. Anxiety neurosis, depression
3.	Decreased functioning in demanding employment settings evident to co-workers; difficulty in traveling to unfamiliar locations	3. Depression, subtle manifestations of medical pathology
4.	Decreased ability to perform complex tasks such as planning dinner for guests, handling finances, and marketing	4. Depression; psychosis, focal cerebral process (e.g., Gerstmann's syndrome)
5.	Requires assistance in choosing proper clothing; may require coaxing to bathe properly	5. Depression
6.	(a) Difficulty in putting on clothing properly	6. (a) Arthritis, sensory deficit, stroke, depression
	(b) Requires assistance bathing; may develop fear of bathing	(b) Arthritis, sensory deficit, stroke, depression
	(c) Inability to handle mechanics of toileting	(c) Arthritis, sensory deficit, stroke, depression
	(d) Urinary incontinence	(d) Urinary tract infection, other causes of urinary incontinence
	(e) Fecal incontinence	(e) Infection, malabsorption syndrome, other causes of fecal incontinence
7.	(a) Ability to speak limited to one to five words	7. (a) Stroke, other dementing disorder (e.g., diffuse space-occupying lesions)
	(b) Intelligible vocabulary limited to a single word	(b) Stroke, other dementing disorder (e.g., diffuse space-occupying lesions)
	(c) Ambulatory ability lost	(c) Parkinsonism; neuroleptic-induced or other secondary extrapyramidal syndrome, Creutzfeldt-Jakob disease, normal pressure hydrocephalus, hyponatremic dementia, stroke, hip fracture, arthritis, overmedication
	(d) Ability to sit lost	(d) Arthritis, contractures
	(e) Ability to smile lost	(e) Stroke
	(f) Stupor or coma	(f) Head trauma, metabolic abnormality, other medical abnormality, overmedication, encephalitis, other causes

3. Inability to handle the mechanics of bathing when the SDAT patient is still capable of choosing clothing appropiate to the season and occasion commonly results from arthritis or other physical debilities.
4. The premature development of urinary incontinence might indicate that the patient has developed a urinary tract infection which might respond to appropriate intervention with antimicrobial agents.
5. The development of fecal incontinence prior to the anticipated ordinal stage might indicate either a gastrointestinal infection or any of numerous other possible causes of incontinence in the elderly and should be investigated in an appropriate fashion.
6. Premature loss of speech in what is otherwise an uncomplicated Alzheimer-type presentation should lead the clinician to suspect the possibility of focal cerebral pathology, in particular, cerebral infarction: either a primary multi-infarct dementia or a mixed pathology involving degenerative dementia and infarction.
7. Premature loss of ambulatory ability in otherwise uncomplicated Alzheimer's disease can have numerous causes: cerebral infarction, CNS metastatic disease, hip or leg fractures, arthritis, severe peripheral vascular disease, primary or secondary parkinsonism, overmedication, as well as other primary causes of dementia, including Creutzfeld-Jakob disease, normal pressure hydrocephalus, or metabolic dementias.
8. Premature development of a comatose state in an Alzheimer patient may arise from many causes: overmedication, intercurrent illness, cerebrovascular or head trauma. Aspiration should always be suspected in late stages of the illness. This can lead to unconsciousness and apparent "foaming at the mouth" which can be mistaken for a seizure.

Table 6. FAST[a] characteristics in a man with amentia. M.H., 27 years old, amentia (Down's syndrome), Stanford Binet I.Q. = 17, Leiter International Performance Scale I.O. = 24

1.	No functional decrement, either subjective or objective, manifest	NA
2.	Complains of forgetting location of objects; subjective work difficulties	NA
3.	Decreased functioning in demanding employment settings evident to co-workers; difficulty in traveling to new locations	o
4.	Decreased ability to perform complex tasks such as planning dinner for guests, handling finances, and marketing	o
5.	Requires assistance in choosing proper clothing; may require coaxing to bathe properly	o
6.	(a) Difficulty in putting on clothing properly	o (tying shoes)
	(b) Requires assistance bathing; may develop fear of bathing	o
	(c) Inability to handle mechanics of toileting	×
	(d) Urinary incontinence	×
	(e) Fecal incontinence	×
7.	(a) Ability to speak limited to vocabulary of one to five words	o
	(b) Intelligible vocabulary limited to a single word	×
	(c) Ambulatory ability lost	×
	(d) Ability to sit lost	×
	(e) Ability to smile lost	×
	(f) Stuporous or comatose	×

NA, not applicable; o, present; ×, absent

[a] Copyright 1984 Barry Reisberg

Deficits Distinguishing Amentia from Dementia

It should be noted that the nature of deficits in amentia secondary to developmental disabilities do not necessarily follow the FAST developmental hierarchy. Hence, Table 6 describes the functional deficits in a 27-year-old man with Down's syndrome, whose intelligence quotient is 17. Although his speech is limited to only a few words, he is not incontinent and can still handle the mechanics of toileting. His parents need to supervise his bathing and assist him in choosing his clothing. Apart from difficulty in tying his shoelaces, he is capable of putting his clothing on properly, once it has been selected for him.

These deficits are very different from those which occur in uncomplicated SDAT. An Alzheimer's disease patient capable of toileting and continence can still speak with some degree of fluency. Similarly, a normal toilet-trained child is capable of articulating numerous words. Hence, functional deficits of developmental amentia may be distinguished from both the pathology of SDAT and from normal human functional development.

Distinctions Between SDAT and Normal Human Development

It should be noted that, although functional losses in SDAT occur in the reverse order of the functional gains of normal human development, in many other ways, SDAT deficits are not comparable to the normal developmental process. Clearly, the somatic gains of human development are not paralleled by somatic losses in SDAT. In terms of CNS functions, the emotional changes arising in SDAT, as outlined in axis 8 (Table 1) and described elsewhere in greater detail (Reisberg 1983; Reisberg and Ferris 1985) are not in general analogous to human emotional growth. However, the cognitive changes of SDAT as outlined in axes 1–4, 9, and 10 (Table 1) do appear to occur in the reverse order to which these functions are acquired in normal human development. The most succinct explanation for these striking parallels is that the deficits of SDAT reflect bilateral cortical degeneration, just as the gains in normal human development are largely the result of cortical maturation.

Conclusion

Impressive strides have been made over the past few years in our understanding of SDAT. Notably, advances have been made in the clinician's ability to diagnose, differentially diagnose, and manage the illness. Perhaps the most important of these advances is the very recent development of Functional Assessment Staging of SDAT. This procedure and its utility for the medical profession in diagnosis and differential diagnosis have been outlined here. The hope for the future is that the improved ability to diagnose and stage SDAT will assist in the elucidation of the etiology and treatment of this major illness of later life. For the present, improved diagnosis, differential diagnosis, and management should be of immediate value to SDAT patients, their families, and to geriatric patients in general.

References

Adams F (ed) (1861) The extant works of Aretaeus, the Cappadocian. Sydenham, London, p 103

Alzheimer A (1907) Über eine eigenartige Erkrankung der Hirnrinde. Allg Z Psychiatr Psych Gericht Med 64:146–148

American Psychiatric Association (1980) Diagnostic and statistical manual of mental disorders, 3rd edn. American Psychiatric Association, Washington DC, pp 124–126

Blessed G, Tomlinson BE, Roth M (1968) The association between quantitative measures of dementia and of senile changes in the cerebral grey matter of elderly subjects. Br J Psychiatry 114:797–811

de Ajuriaguerra J, Rey M, Bellet-Muller M (1964) A propos de quelques problèmes posés par le déficit opératoire des vieilliards atteints de démence dégénérative en début d'évolution. Cortex I:232–256

Eisenberg L (1975) Normal child development. In: Freedman AM, Kaplan HR, Sadock BJ (eds) Comprehensive textbook of psychiatry II, vol 2. Williams and Wilkins, Baltimore, pp 2036–2054

Esquirol JED (1838) Des maladies mentales. Balliere, Paris

Folstein MF, Folstein SE, McHugh PR (1975) Mini-mental state. A practical method for grading the cognitive state of patients for the clinican. Psychiatr Res 12:189–198

Galen C (1821–1833) De symptomatum differentis liber. In: Kuhn CG (ed) Opera omnia. Knobloch, Leipzig, pp 200–201

Go RCP, Todovov AB, Elston RC, Constantinidis J (1978) The malignancy of dementias. Ann Neurol 3:559–561

Jarvik LF, Falek A (1963) Intellectual stability and survival in the aged. J Gerontol 18:173–176

Kahn RL, Goldfarb AI, Pollack M, Peck A (1960) Brief objective measures for the determination of mental status in the aged. Am J Psychiatry 117:326–328

Kaszniak AW, Fox J, Gandell DL, Garron DC, Huckman MS, Ramsey RG (1978) Predictors of mortality in presenile and senile dementia. Ann Neurol 3:246–252

Pierce CM (1975) Enuresis and encopresis. In: Freedman AM, Kaplan HR, Sadock BJ (eds) Comprehensive textbook of psychiatry II, vol 2. Williams and Wilkins, Baltimore, pp 2116–2125

Prichard JC (1837) A treatise on insanity and other disorders affecting the mind. Haswell, Barnington and Haswell, Philadelphia, pp 69–80

Reisberg B (1981) Brain failure: an introduction to current concepts of senility. Free Press/Macmillan, New York

Reisberg B (1983) Clinical presentation, diagnosis, and symptomatology of age-associated cognitive decline and Alzheimer's disease. In: Reisberg B (ed) Alzheimer's disease. Free Press/Macmillan, New York

Reisberg B (1984) Stages of cognitive decline. Am J Nurs 84:225–228

Reisberg B, Ferris SH (1985) A clinical rating scale for symptoms of psychosis in Alzheimer's disease. Psychopharmacol Bull 21:101–104

Reisberg B, Schneck MK, Ferris SH, Schwartz GE, de Leon MJ (1983 a) The brief cognitive rating scale (BCRS): findings in primary degenerative dementia (PDD). Psychopharmacol Bull 19:47–50

Reisberg B, Ferris SH, Schneck MK, de Leon MJ, Crook T, Gershon S (1981) The relationship between psychiatric assessments and cognitive test measures in mild to moderately cognitively impaired elderly. Psychopharmacol Bull 17:99–101

Reisberg B, Ferris SH, de Leon MJ, Crook T (1982) The global deterioration scale for assessment of primary degenerative dementia. Am J Psychiatry 139:1136–1139

Reisberg B, London E, Ferris SH, Borenstein J, Scheier L, de Leon MJ (1983) The brief cognitive rating scale: language, motoric and mood concomitants in primary degenerative dementia. Psychopharmacol Bull 19:702–708

Reisberg B, Ferris SH, Anand R, Buttinger C, Borenstein J, Sinaiko E, de Leon MJ (1984a) Clinical assessments of cognition in the elderly. In: Shamoian CA (ed) Biology and treatment of dementia in the elderly. American Psychiatric, Washington DC, pp 15–37

Reisberg B, Ferris SH, Sinaiko E, Borenstein J, Anand R, Buttinger C, de Leon MJ (1984b) Aging and dementia of the Alzheimer's Type (DAT): longitudinal course of community residing subgroups. Collegium internationale neuro-psychiopharmacollegium, June 19–23. In: Book of Abstracts, p 164

Reisberg B, Ferris SH, Anand R, de Leon MJ, Schneck MK, Buttinger C, Borenstein J (1984c) Functional staging of dementia of the Alzheimer's type. Ann NY Acad Sci 435:481–483

Rush B (1793) An account of the state of mind and body in old age. In: Medical inquiries and observations, vol 2. Dobson, Philadelphia, p 311

Vaughn VC (1969) Growth and development. In: Nelson WE, Vaughn VC, McKay RJ (eds) Textbook of pediatrics. 9th edn. Saunders, Philadelphia, pp 15–57

Assessment of Cognition and Affective Symptoms in Dementia

R. C. Mohs[1], B. S. Greenwald[1], D. D. Dunn[1], and K. L. Davis[2]

Clinical Features of Dementia

The most prominent symptoms of dementing illnesses are a loss of various cognitive abilities, particularly memory, language, praxis, and judgment. For patients with dementia of the Alzheimer type (DAT), the clinical incidence of these symptoms has been documented in several series, some involving biopsy-proven cases (Coblentz et al. 1973; Sim and Sussman 1962) and other involving clinically diagnosed cases (Liston 1977). Clinical descriptions of patients with proven cases of multiinfarct dementia (MID) have not appeared in great detail, but what evidence is available suggests that there is considerable overlap in the symptoms of DAT and MID (Hachinski et al. 1975; Liston 1977). Thus, any assessment of symptom severity in patients with either of these two kinds of dementia must include measures of memory, language, praxis, and, if possible, judgment.

Although cognitive impairments are the most characteristic symptoms of the dementia syndromes, other symptoms, including agitation, psychosis (viz., delusions, hallucinations, neurologic signs, and affective abnormalities) may also be present (Sim and Sussman 1962; Liston 1977). Of these other symptoms, changes in affect have received the most attention for two reasons. First, the presence of depressive symptoms in patients with dementing illness increases the difficulty in differentiating patients with depression from those with dementia. This is particularly true for patients with early dementia, when cognitive impairments may be mild. Second, the fact that patients with biopsy-proven dementia may show prominent depressive symptoms (Sim and Sussman 1962) raises the possibility that there may be at least some biologic abnormalities which are shared by both patients with dementia and those with depression.

Our purpose is to review briefly recent work from the Clinical Research Center of the Bronx Veterans Administration Medical Center on the assessment of cognition and affective symptoms in patients with dementia. First, some traditional measures of cognition and affect which are unlikely to be very useful for dementia patients are reviewed. Secondly, the Alzheimer's Disease Assessment Scale (ADAS), an instrument developed specifically to assess symptoms of DAT is discussed. Finally, a study investigating the relationship of depressive symptoms to biological markers for depression is reviewed.

1 Psychiatry Service (116 A), VA Medical Center Bronx, NY 10468, USA
2 Department of Psychiatry, Mount Sinai School of Medicine New York, NY 10029, USA

Senile Dementia of the Alzheimer Type
Ed. by J. Traber and W. H. Gispen

Traditional Measures

Cognitive Function

The most widely used tests of cognitive function can be divided into at least two classes. One is the group of mental status exams, such as the test of Blessed et al. (1968) and the Mini-Mental State (MMS) Test devised by Folstein et al. (1975). Both of these tests were designed to provide an overall index of mental functioning in patients with dementia. They have the virtues of being short and relatively easy to administer, and the items generally have some face validity. In addition, scores on the test of Blessed et al. (1968) have been shown to correlate with the extent of neuropathologic changes in patients with DAT. However, some of the cognitive impairments typically seen in dementia, especially dysphasia and dyspraxia, are not specifically evaluated by the Blessed scale. While the MMS does evaluate memory loss, dysphasia, and dyspraxia, its brevity prevents it from measuring these functions in as much detail as might be desirable in a clinical drug trial. That is, small but clinically meaningful changes might go unrecognized with the MMS. Moreover, both the MMS and the Blessed text exist in only one form, so that repeated testing over time is difficult.

A second kind of traditional test used in the evaluation of dementia patients includes the psychometric tests, such as the Wechsler Adult Intelligence Scale (WAIS) (Wechsler 1958). The principal difficulty with these tests is that they are not designed to evaluate specific disease symptoms. Thus, it is often difficult to interpret scores on such tests in terms that are clinically meaningful. Also, many of the items on tests like the WAIS require that the patient be able to follow verbal instructions. Since the memory and language impairments of dementia often make this impossible, low scores by demented patients on such tests are difficult to interpret.

Thus, neither the standard mental status tests nor the standard psychometric tests are ideal for evaluating symptom severity in clinical trials with demented patients. Mental status exams are very useful as screening instruments but do not provide enough symptom detail for clinical trials. Most psychometric tests do not target disease symptoms and are often too difficult to give meaningful data in clinical populations.

Affect

Two general strategies have been used to evaluate affective changes in clinical populations. One is to have patients rate their own mood on a series of items, as is done in the Zung Self-Rating Scale for Depression (Zung 1965). A second strategy is to have a trained clinician rate various symptoms related to mood on a scale after interviewing and observing the behavior of the patient. The latter strategy is employed in scales such as the Hamilton (1960) Depression Rating Scale. For patients with dementia, it appears that the second strategy for evaluating depression has advantages over the first. As noted above, the cognitive impairments of demented patients often make it impossible for them to understand instructions necessary to complete self-rating instruments. Thus, self-rating instruments may give meaningless data.

When using an observer rating instrument, however, it is not intuitively obvious which symptoms should be rated. It is worth noting that symptoms on the Hamilton Scale are similar, but certainly not identical to, those used to make the diagnosis of major depression according to the Diagnostic and Statistical Manual III (1980) of the American Psychiatric Association. A minimal requirement would be to construct rating scale items so that they have both high reliability between raters and reasonably high retest reliability over short periods of time. Beyond that, it would be desirable to show that the symptoms rated have some biologic significance.

New Measures

Alzheimer's Disease Assessment Scale (ADAS)

Given the deficiencies described above in many of the traditional instruments used to assess cognition and affect, a series of studies were undertaken to develop an assessment instrument specifically for patients with dementia. Although the scale has been designed for patients with DAT, it is likely to be of use in evaluating symptom severity in patients whose dementia stems from some other cause. Much of the work done to validate this scale has been described in a previous publication (Rosen et al., 1984). Here, we present only a summary of the scale's principal characteristics. The ADAS was designed to have the following features: (a) it should assess all the principal cognitive and behavioral symptoms found in patients with DAT, (b) it should be simple enough to be administered in a short period of time (less than 1 h), (c) it should have high reliability between raters and between patients over short periods of time, and (d) it should be sensitive to changes in symptom severity, ranging from mild to severe, for a broad range of patients.

A total of 40 items were includes in the original version of the ADAS (Table 1). These items were selected to satisfy the first criterion listed above. Early on, it was determined that all of these items could be given to DAT patients in less than 1 h (criterion b). To maximize the sensitivity of the scale (criterion d, items of different degrees of difficulty were included to assess each major symptom area. As an example, tests of both word recall and word recognition were included to assess memory, since recall, as the more difficult test, is likely to be sensitive to early memory impairment, while word recognition can measure memory performance even in patients unable to recall words (Mohs et al. 1985). Similarly, to asses language naming, items of high, medium, and low frequency were included, since naming difficulty is known to be a function of word frequency (Barker and Lawson 1968).

Both the interrater and test–retest reliability of individual items were determined in a longitudinal study (Rosen et al. 1984). At baseline, all items were scored by two independent raters to determine interrater reliability. A follow-up

Table 1. Original version of the Alzheimer's Disease Assessment Scale (40 items)

1. Spoke language ability	21. Uncooperative: testing
2. Comprehension of spoken language	22. Uncooperative: home, unit
3. Recall test instructions	23. Aggressiveness: verbal
4. Word-finding difficulty	24. Aggressiveness: physical
5. Excessive talking	25. Lack of initiative
6. Poverty of speech	26. Socialization
7. Paraphasia: semantic	27. Delusions
8. Paraphasia: phonemic	28. Hallucinations
9. Palilalia	29. Pacing
10. Echolalia	30. Fidgeting
11. Following commands	31. Psychic anxiety
12. Naming: objects, fingers	32. Motor activity: increase
13. Construction: drawing	33. Motor activity: decrease
14. Ideational praxis	34. Tremors
15. Orientation	35. Insomnia: early
16. Word recall	36. Insomnia: middle
17. Word recognition	37. Insomnia: late
18. Tearful	38. Nocturnal confusion
19. Depressed mood	39. Daytime sleeping
20. Concentration/distractability	40. Appetite change

Table 2. Condensed version of the Alzheimer's Disease Assessment Scale (21 items)

1. Spoken language ability	11. Word recognition
2. Comprehension of spoken language	12. Tearful
3. Recall test instructions	13. Depressed mood
4. Word-finding difficulty	14. Concentration/distractability
5. Following commands	15. Uncooperative: testing
6. Naming: objects, fingers	16. Delusions
7. Constructions: drawing	17. Hallucinations
8. Ideational praxis	18. Pacing
9. Orientation	19. Motor activity: increase
10. Word recall	20. Tremors
	21. Appetite change

evaluation at 1 month was done to determine retest reliability. Table 2 presents the 21 ADAS items that were found we have both satisfactory interrater and retest reliabilities. As can be seen from the table, the shorter version of the ADAS still retains enough items to cover all of the principal symptoms common in dementia patients. In comparison to the original 40-item version, the shortened version contains a higher proportion of cognitive as opposed to behavioral and affective items. Nevertheless, several items related to depression are included in the final version, since they could be related reliably and were stable over time.

Depression in DAT

Although the study with the ADAS clearly demonstrates that some symptoms of depression in patients with DAT can be rated, a number of questions remain. One is whether depressive symptoms vary systematically with any other clinical characteristics of patients with dementia, and a second is whether there are distinct biologic characteristics associated with the appearance of depressive symptoms in patients with dementia. To investigate these questions, a study was recently completed in our laboratory involving patients with clinically diagnosed DAT. The majority of findings from this study have recently been reported (Greenwald et al. 1985). Each of a series of patients was evaluated by an experienced geriatric psychiatrist with regard to the presence of depressive symptoms. Since it was not clear exactly which symptoms might be most important, the entire list of major and minor symptoms compiled by Nelson and Charney (1981) was evaluated in each patient. Major symptoms were those consistently found to be associated with endogenous or biologic depression (e.g., agitation, retardation, severly depressed mood), while minor symptoms were those which often appeared even in patients not having endogenous depression (e.g., sleep disturbance, weight loss, poor appetite). The number of major and minor symptoms present in each DAT patient was recorded. Of interest to the present purpose was that the number of major depressive symptoms was greater in patients with senile (over age 65) onset and that the number of major symptoms correlated positively with the severity of dementia as measured by the Memory and Information Test (Roth and Hopkins 1953), a simple mental status exam. Minor symptoms of depression were unrelated to any clinical variables. These findings provide indirect support for the notion that depressive symptoms in DAT are a direct result of biologic factors and are not simply a psychological reaction to stress.

More direct data relevant to this point was obtained by administering the dexamethasone suppression test (DST) to 22 patients evaluated for depression. Previous investigators (e.g., Raskind et al. 1982; Spar and Gerner 1982) have demonstrated that patients with DAT often escape cortisol suppression by dexamethasone just as patients with endogenous depression do. However, the present study (Greenwald et al. 1985) was designed to determine whether escape is in any way related to depressive symptomatology. In all, 11 of 22 patients with DAT escaped suppression of dexamethasone at 8 a.m., 3 p.m., or 11 p.m. There was some tendency for senile onset cases to escape more frequently than presenile onset cases, although the trend was not statistically significant. Most interesting was the positive correlation between the level of cortisol at 8 a.m. and the number of major depressive symptoms. No correlation with minor symptoms was found. This result provides additional support for the notion that depressive symptoms in patients with DAT are the results of a biological abnormality. They also raise the possibility that there is at least some biochemical abnormality common to both dementia and endogenous depression.

References

American Psychiatric Association (1980) Diagnostic and statistical manual of mental disorders, 3rd edn. Washington DC

Barker MG, Lawson JS (1968) Nominal aphasia in dementia. Br J Psychiatry 114:1351–1356

Blessed G, Tomlinson BE, Roth M (1968) The association between quantitative measures of dementia and senile change in the cerebral gray matter of elderly subjects. Br J Psychiatry 114:797–811

Coblentz JM, Mattis S, Zingesser LH, Kasoff SS, Wisniewski H, Katzman R (1973) Presenile dementia: clinical aspects and evaluation of cerebrospinal fluid dynamics. Arch Neurol 29:299–308

Folstein MF, Folstein S, McHugh P (1975) "Mini-mental state: a practical method for grading the cognitive state of patients for the clinician. J Psychiatr Res 12:189–198

Greenwald BS, Davis BM, Mathé AA, Mohs RC, Levy MI, Johns CA, Davis KL (1985) Cortisol in Alzheimer's disease. Am J Psychiatry (to be published)

Hachinski VC, Iliff LD, Zilhka E, DuBoulay GH, McAllister VL, Marshall J, Russell RWR, Symon L (1975) Cerebral blood flow in dementia. Arch Neurol 32:632–637

Hamilton M (1960) A rating scale for depression. J Neurol Neurosurg Psychiatry 23:56–62

Liston EH (1977) Occult presenile dementia. J Nerv Ment Dis 164:263–267

Mohs RC, Greenwald BS, Dunn DD, Johns CA, Davis KL (1985) Assessing change in Alzheimer's disease: memory and language tasks. In: Poon LW (ed) Clinical assessment of older adults. American Psychological Association, Washington DC

Nelson JC, Charney DS (1981) The symptoms of major depressive illness. Am J Psychiatry 138:1–12

Raskind M, Peskind E, Rivard M (1982) Dexamethasone suppression test and cortisol and circadian rhythm in primary degenerative dementia. Am J Psychiatry 139:1478–1482

Rosen WG, Mohs RC, Davis KL (1984) A new rating scale for Alzheimer's disease. Am J Psychiatry 141:1356–1364

Roth M, Hopkins B (1953) Psychological test performance in patients over 60: Senile psychosis and affective disorders of old age. J Ment Sci 99:439–453

Sim M, Sussman I (1962) Alzheimer's disease: its natural history and differential diagnosis. J Nerv Ment Dis 135:489–499

Spar JR, Gerner R (1982) Does the dexamethasone suppression test distinguish dementia from depression? Am J Psychiatry 139:283–240

Wechsler D (1958) Wechsler's measurement and appraisal of adult intelligence. Williams and Wilkins, Baltimore

Zung WWK (1965) A self-rating scale for depression. Arch Gen Psychiatry 12:63–70

The AGP System: Assessment of Symptoms in Psychogeriatric Patients

S. Kanowski, H. Krüger, and K.-P. Kühl [1]

Development of the AGP System

The AGP system was developed by the Association for Gerontopsychiatry to facilitate the assessment of psychopathologic conditions in the elderly. This instrument permits the gathering of standardized data on psychiatric inpatients, outpatients, and partially hospitalized patients, usually aged 65 years and older. It was designed as a comprehensive assessment system suitable for the routine recording of clinical findings and for special research in gerontopsychiatry. However, for specific research problems it might be necessary to collect additional information by means of other instruments.

The first edition of the AGP system was elaborated by the Department for Gerontopsychiatry of the Free University of Berlin and the Psychiatric Clinic of the University of Lausanne (L. Ciompi and S. Kanowski, unpublished; Ciompi and Kanowski 1981). In working out the present, revised documentation system, the Departments of Gerontopsychiatry of the University of Düsseldorf and of the Psychiatric Clinic in Cologne-Mehrheim and the Department of Neurology of the University of Freiburg also collaborated (Ciompi et al. 1985).

The development of a special documentation system for gerontopsychiatry proved necessary because of the particularities of mental illness in the elderly.

Initial suggestions for an instrument of gerontopsychiatric documentation were published by Frost et al. (1971), based on the experience accumulated through the documentation system of the *Arbeitsgemeinschaft für Methodik und Dokumentation in der Psychiatrie* (the AMP system, Scharfetter 1972). The AMP system is a well-known psychiatric documentation system that has been in wide use in German-speaking countries for many years. Taking into account the proposals of Ciompi et al. (1972, 1973), the first edition of the AGP system was worked out by L. Ciompi and S. Kanowski (unpublished). For purposes of comparability, this AGP version relied heavily on the AMP. In particular, the section on psychopathologic assessment conformed to the AMP as closely as possible. To complement this instrument, documentation concentrating on social data was developed by Hermann (Hermann 1972 and U. Hermann, unpublished).

The entire AGP system, including the documentation of social data, was tested in a multicenter study (Bolm et al. 1973a, b; Junkers et al. 1976; Lieberz 1978) to evaluate its practicability. The results of this study and the development of new theoretical concepts led to a revision of the AGP system in the follwing years. In comparison with the first edition, more detailed information on specific

1 Abteilung für Gerontopsychiatrie, Psychiatrische Klinik der Freien Universität Berlin, Reichsstraße 15, 1000 Berlin 19, FRG

Senile Dementia of the Alzheimer Type
Ed. by J. Traber and W. H. Gispen

aspects of the socioeconomic status of elderly patients can now be recorded. The section on psychiatric history has also been reorganized and extended to improve its validity. Finally, the part dealing with neurologic disturbances was completely revised to allow for more accurate recording of the results of neurologic examinations.

In the meantime, a revised version of the AMP system , designated the AMDP system, had been published (AMDP 1981). The modifications of the AMDP system and the insights gained through experience with it were also taken over by the AGP in order to maintain comparability. To increase conformity, the scale graduations introduced in the AMDP system were adapted and the items of the revised AGP were constructed so as to correspond to them.

Organization of the AGP System

The AGP system consists of four integrated sections: anamnesis, psychopathologic symptoms, somatic signs, and diagnoses. Although the psychopathologic assessment section is identical to that of the AMDP system for such categories as mood, delusion, and drive other characteristics of geriatric conditions are analyzed much more extensively in the AGP system, including for example "disorders of attention and memory" and "social and nursing needs." Special attention is also devoted to the comprehensive assessment and gradation of organic brain syndrome (OBS), including operational definitions of its symptoms. Neurologic symptoms and somatic signs are also analyzed in more detail than in the AMDP system.

All items in the system are defined in a detailed glossary so as to permit the uniform practical application of the instrument. To ensure the comparability of the AMDP and the AGP systems, definitions of items belonging to both systems are identical and marked accordingly in the glossary. A thorough knowledge of the AGP system is essential to its proper use. In order to increase the reliability of the rating process, psychiatrists or clinical psychologists who are not familiar with this system are advised to undergo training supervised by an experienced examiner. Training should include actual or filmed psychiatric interviews, followed by independent ratings. Discussion of rating inconsistencies supplements training.

The entire AGP system consists of six forms, which can be read by an optical mark reader, as with the AMDP system. The first form (Fig. 1) elicits demographic data valid at the time of examination, e.g., "age," "marital status," "nationality," "household composition," "education," and "occupation." The second form (Fig. 2) comprises items which deal primarily with the psychiatric history of the patient and his family, including the patient's previous psychiatric and nonpsychiatric illnesses and the number of psychiatric admissions and suicide attempts. The current episode of illness and any treatment the patient may have received immediately prior to referral may be described in detail. Forms 3 and 4 (Figs. 3, 4) provide for a comprehensive assessment of psychopathology. A total of 176 items covering a broad range of psychopathologic behavior are divided

AGP Part 1. Demographic Data

CLINIC/HO. _____ STUDY_______ RATER_______ DATE EXAM____/____/____
M D Y

PT INITIALS_______ PT. NO._____ PERIOD______

STATUS IN___ OUT___ PART___ OTH_____________

SEX M__ F__ RACE W__ B__ I__ O__ OTH_____ ___________

BIRTHDATE ____/____/____
M D Y

---

1. SOURCE: Primary_____ Secondary____ Both____ NA____
2. AGE:_______ NA______
3. MARITAL STATUS: Single__ Mar'd__ Sep'd__ Div.__ Widw__ Cohab__ NA__
4. NATIONALITY: Citizen by birth___ Naturalized___ Alien___ Stateless___ NA___
5. CHILDREN: A. Number: 0___ 1___ 2___ 3___ 4___ 5___ >5___ NA___
   B. Presently Living: 0___ 1___ 2___ 3___ 4___ 5___ >5___ NA__
6. SIBLINGS: A. Number: 0___ 1___ 2___ 3___ 4___ 5___ >5___ NA__
   B. Presently Living: 0___ 1___ 2___ 3___ 4___ 5___ >5___ NA__
   C. Twin: Y____ N____ NA____
7. RELIGION: Protestant___ Roman Catholic___ Hebrew___ None___
   Other (Specify) ______________________ NA_____
8. RELIGIOUS CONVICTION: Weak___ Average___ Strong___ NA___
9. TRUSTEESHIP: Y___ N___ NA___
10. GUARDIANSHIP: Y___ N___ NA___
11. RESIDENTIAL SETTING: Urban___ Suburban___ Rural___ NA___
12. RESIDENTIAL STATUS: A. Present residence: Own Home___ Rental Accom.___
    Subtenant___ Indep. geriatric___ Supervised geriatric___ Nursing home___
    General/psychiatric hosp.___ No Fixed Address___ Other___ NA___
    B. Institutional residence: Pat.___ Spouse___ Pt/Spouse___ NA___
13. HOUSEHOLD COMPOSITION (excluding pt): Spouse___ Children___ Siblings___
    Parents___ Grandchildren___ Other___ NA___
14. HOUSEHOLD INCOME STATUS: A. Level: Dependent___ Marginal___ Adequate___ NA___
    B. Income Source: Pension___ Salary___ Capital Assets___
    Social Agency___ Other___ NA___
    C. Number Supported by Income: 1___ 2___ 3___ 4___ 5___ >5___ NA___
15. EDUCATION:

	Completed	Partial	NA
Special Education	______	______	______
Elementary (1-8)	______	______	______
High School (9-12)	______	______	______
College	______	______	______
Graduate School	______	______	______
NA	______	______	______

Fig. 1

AGP Part 1. Demographic Data *(continued)*

16. VOCATIONAL TRAINING:

	Completed	Partial	NA
Apprenticeship	___	___	___
Business/Technical School	___	___	___
Other: ___	___	___	___

17. OCCUPATION

A. Level

	Patient		Spouse	
	Highest Attained	Last Job	Highest Attained	Last Job
Homemaker	___	___	___	___
Homemaker-2nd job	___	___	___	___
Student	___	___	___	___
Self-employed Worker	___	___	___	___
Self-employed Entrepreneur	___	___	___	___
Major Professional	___	___	___	___
Minor Professional	___	___	___	___
Skilled Worker	___	___	___	___
Semiskilled Worker	___	___	___	___
Unskilled Worker	___	___	___	___
NA	___	___	___	___

B. Presently unemployed: Y___ N___ NA___

18. RETIREMENT: A. Not retired___ Retired usual___ early___ late___ NA___

B. Voluntary___ Involuntary___ No job___ NA___

19. FREETIME ACTIVITIES: Y___ N___ NA___

20. SOCIAL RELATIONSHIPS:

A. Objective: Frequent___ Seldom___ None___ NA___

B. Subjective: Satisfying___ Unsatisfying___ NA___

21. PREVIOUS CARE: None___ Spouse___ Family___ Friend___

Charitable Religious Agency___ Health Facility___ Other Gov/t Agency___

Other (specify)___ NA___

22. REFERRAL SOURCE: Self___ Spouse/Family___ Physician___ Clinic/hosp___

Service Agency___ Other (specify)___ NA___

23. TYPE OF ADMISSION: Voluntary___ Involuntary___ NA___

24. REASON FOR ADMISSION: Suicidal attempt___ Dangerous/self___

Dangerous/others___ Other (specify)___ NA___

Fig. 1 (cont.)

into 20 major categories corresponding to conventional classifications of psychomental functions, such as disorders of consciousness, perception, or affect and disturbances of drive and psychomotility.

Special attention has been given to providing careful operational definitions of OBS. Assessment of OBS proceeds in two ways. First the examiner makes a generalized assessment of the severity of the symptoms exhibited by the patient using a scale of three (Fig. 4). The individual pattern of symptoms must then be evaluated on symptom by symptom basis. These symptoms are categorized under

AGP Part 2. Psychiatric History

CLINIC/HOSP_____ STUDY_____ RATER_____ DATE EXAM___/___/___
M D Y

PT. INITIALS_____ PT. NO._____ PERIOD_____

STATUS IN__ OUT__ PART__ OTH_________

SEX M__ F__ RACE W__ B__ I__ O__ OTH_________________

BIRTHDATE___/___/___
M D Y

---

25. FAMILY PSYCHIATRIC HISTORY:

A. 1st Degree Relatives: None___ Suspected___ Confirmed___ Hosp.___ NA___

B. Distant Relatives: None___ Suspected___ Confirmed___ Hosp.___ NA___

26. PREVIOUS NON-PSYCHIATRIC ILLNESS: No CNS___ Oth Org___ Diseases NA___

A. CNS Diseases	None	Suspected	Confirmed	Sequelae	NA
Inflammatory	_	_	_	_	_
Trauma	_	_	_	_	_
Tumor	_	_	_	_	_
Constitutional	_	_	_	_	_
Intoxication	_	_	_	_	_
Epilepsy	_	_	_	_	_
Surgical	_	_	_	_	_

B. Other Organic	None	Suspected	Confirmed	Sequelae	NA
Inflammatory	_	_	_	_	_
Trauma	_	_	_	_	_
Tumor	_	_	_	_	_
Constitutional	_	_	_	_	_
Intoxication	_	_	_	_	_
Metabolic	_	_	_	_	_
Cardiovascular	_	_	_	_	_
Surgical	_	_	_	_	_

27. PREVIOUS PSYCHIATRIC ILLNESS:

None___	None	Suspected	Confirmed	Sequelae	NA
Constitutional/ childhood illness	___	___	___	___	___
Endogenous illness	___	___	___	___	___
Exogenous illness	___	___	___	___	___
Psychoneurotic reactions	___	___	___	___	___
Addiction	___	___	___	___	___

Alcohol___ Hypnotic/analgesic___ Opiate___ Other___ NA___

28. NUMBER OF PREVIOUS PSYCHIATRIC ADMISSIONS:

0___ 1___ 2___ 3___ 4___ 5___ >5___ Undetermined___ NA___

29. SUICIDAL ATTEMPTS:

A. Numbers: 0___ 1___ 2___ 3___ 4___ 5___ >5___ NA___

B. Most recent attempt: 1 mo___ <6 mo___ <1 yr___ <5 yr___ >5 yr___ NA___

30. PRESENT ILLNESS: (Items 31-36) Reliable__ Unreliable__

31. FIRST MANIFESTATION: <1 yr___ 1-<5 yr___ 5-<10 yr___ >10 yr___ NA___

32. NUMBER OF PREVIOUS EPISODES:

0___ 1___ 2___ 3___ 4___ 5___ >5___ Undertermined___ NA___

33. COURSE OF ILLNESS:

A. Type: Acute___ Intermittent___ Chronic___ NA___

B. Direction: Improving___ Static___ Worsening___ NA___

Fig. 2

AGP Part 2. Psychiatric History *(continued)*

34. PRESENT EPISODE:

A. Duration: >1 wk___ <1 mo___ <6 mo___ <1 yr___ <1 yr___ NA___

B. Symptoms during last week: Lessening___ Static___ Worsening___ NA___

C. Severity during last 3 mo.:

(1) Somatic: Mild___ Moderate___ Severe___ NA___

(2) Psychosocial: Mild___ Moderate___ Severe___ NA___

35. PRIOR TREATMENT (Present episode):

A. Status: Outpt___ Partial Hospitalization___ Inpt___ NA___

B. Psychopharmacological Rx: Neuroleptic___ Antidepressant___ Lithium___
Anxiolytic___ Hypnotic___ Anticonvulsant___ NA___

Other (specify):___________________________________

C. Pharmacological Rx: Digitalis___ Antihypertensive___ Antidiabetic___
Geriatric___ NA___

Other (specify):___________________________________

D. Nonpharmacological Rx: Psychotherapy___ Social Service___
ECT___ Other___________________________ NA___

36. TREATMENT PROVIDER (prior to present admission):

None___ GP___ Internist___ Psychiatrist___ NA___

Other (specify)___________________________________

Fig. 2 (cont.)

the following headings: "disturbances of orientation," "disorders of attention and memory," and "formal disturbances of thinking" (Fig. 3). Memory function, as a central feature of OBS, has been split into subitems reflecting disorders of recent and remote memory and memorization of specific subjects. Furthermore, hypermnesia of remote memory, ecmnesia, and forgetfulness can be recorded separately. Finally, localized brain dysfunctions, such as aphasias, agnosias, and apraxias can be documented either on a general level or in detail on Form 4 (Fig. 4). Further items included in this form deal with circadian disturbances and sleep and vigilance disturbances. Several items reflect social and nursing needs described in terms of activities of daily living. Somatic symptoms are specified on the fifth form (Fig. 5), which consists of two major parts, "general somatic disturbances," and "neurologic disturbances" and permits a detailed description of these disorders. Form 6 (Fig. 6) furnishes space for noting as many as three psychiatric and four somatic diagnoses, according to the International Classification of Diseases (ICD, 9th revision).

As stated above, special emphasis has been placed on documenting symptoms of OBS. With the AGP system, it is possible to record data on two levels, allowing for both standardized global assessment and individualized documentation of symptom profiles. We believe that both approaches are essential to advancing our knowledge of OBS by improving the comparability of research results. This seems of particular importance for the following research topics:

1. Evaluation of the basic symptoms of OBS, their variability and interaction and the elaboration of OBS subtypes. For instance, there is growing evidence in the literature that lability and shallowness of affect is not statistically correlated

AGP Part 3. Psychopathological Symptoms

CLINIC/HOSP_____ STUDY_____ RATER_____

PT INITIALS_____ PT NO._____ PERIOD____

DATE EXAM__/__/__ (M D Y) STATUS IN__OUT__PART__OTH__

SEX M__ F__ RACE W__ B__ I__ O__ OTH__________

BIRTHDATE__/__/__

TIME SPAN RATED TODAY__ <1 wk__ <1 mo__ >1 mo__

AB MI MO SV NA

DIS. CONSCIOUSNES __0

1. Lowered 0 1 2 3 9
2. Narrowed 0 1 2 3 9
3. Clouded 0 1 2 3 9
4. Hypnagogic 0 1 2 3 9
5. Parasomnia 0 1 2 3 9

DIS. ORIENTATION __0

6. Time 0 1 2 3 9
7. Place 0 1 2 3 9
8. Situation 0 1 2 3 9
9. Self 0 1 2 3 9

DIS. ATTENT/MEM. __0

10. Apperception 0 1 2 3 9
11. Concentration 0 1 2 3 9
12. Memorization 0 1 2 3 9
13. Mem. numbers 0 1 2 3 9
14. Mem. words 0 1 2 3 9
15. Mem. objects 0 1 2 3 9
16. Mem. forms 0 1 2 3 9
17. Mem. people 0 1 2 3 9
18. Mem. colors 0 1 2 3 9
19. Recent memory 0 1 2 3 9
20. Remote memory 0 1 2 3 9
21. Forgetfulness 0 1 2 3 9
22. Ecmesia 0 1 2 3 9
23. Hypermnesia 0 1 2 3 9

AB MI MO SV NA

24. Confabulat.. 0 1 2 3 9
25. Paramnesias 0 1 2 3 9
26. Suggestibility 0 1 2 3 9

DIS. THINKING __0

27. Inhibited 0 1 2 3 9
28. Retarded 0 1 2 3 9
29. Circumstantial 0 1 2 3 9
30. Restricted 0 1 2 3 9
31. Perseverative 0 1 2 3 9
32. Rumination 0 1 2 3 9
33. Pressured 0 1 2 3 9
34. Flight of ideas 0 1 2 3 9
35. Tangential 0 1 2 3 9
36. Blocking 0 1 2 3 9
37. Incoherence 0 1 2 3 9
38. Neologisms 0 1 2 3 9
39. Accelerated 0 1 2 3 9
40. Impaired abstraction 0 1 2 3 9
41. Conceptual impairment 0 1 2 3 9
42. Impaired judgment 0 1 2 3 9

FEARS, COMPULSIONS __0

43. Suspiciousness 0 1 2 3 9
44. Hypochondriasis 0 1 2 3 9
45. Phobias 0 1 2 3 9
46. Obsess. thoughts 0 1 2 3 9

Fig. 3

AGP Part 3. Psychopathological Symptoms *(continued)*

AB MI MO SV NA

47. Compul. impulses
 0 1 2 3 9
48. Compul. actions
 0 1 2 3 9

DELUSIONS __0

49. Delusional mood
 0 1 2 3 9
50. Del. perceptions
 0 1 2 3 9
51. Sud. del. thoughts
 0 1 2 3 9
52. Delusional idea
 0 1 2 3 9
53. System. del
 0 1 2 3 9
54. Del. dynamics
 0 1 2 3 9
55. Del. reference
 0 1 2 3 9
56. Del. persecution
 0 1 2 3 9
57. Del. Jealousy
 0 1 2 3 9
58. Del. guilt
 0 1 2 3 9
59. Del. impoverish
 0 1 2 3 9
60. Hypochond. del.
 0 1 2 3 9
61. Del. grandeur
 0 1 2 3 9
62. Other del
 0 1 2 3 9

DIS. PERCEPTION __0

63. Illusions
 0 1 2 3 9
64. Verbal halluc.
 0 1 2 3 9
65. Other auditory
 0 1 2 3 9
66. Visual halluc.
 0 1 2 3 9
67. Bodily halluc.
 0 1 2 3 9
68. Olfact/gust. halluc.
 0 1 2 3 9

DIS. EGO __0

69. Derealization
 0 1 2 3 9
70. Depersonalization
 0 1 2 3 9
71. Broadcasting
 0 1 2 3 9
72. Withdrawal
 0 1 2 3 9
73. Insertion
 0 1 2 3 9
74. Other influences
 0 1 2 3 9

DIS. AFFECT __0

75. Perplexity
 0 1 2 3 9

AB MI MO SV NA

76. Loss feeling
 0 1 2 3 9
77. Blunted
 0 1 2 3 9
78. Loss vitality
 0 1 2 3 9
79. Depression
 0 1 2 3 9
80. Hopelessness
 0 1 2 3 9
81. Anxiety
 0 1 2 3 9
82. Euphoria
 0 1 2 3 9
83. Dysphoria
 0 1 2 3 9
84. Irritability
 0 1 2 3 9
85. Inner restless.
 0 1 2 3 9
86. Complaintative
 0 1 2 3 9
87. Inadequacy
 0 1 2 3 9
88. Exag. self-esteem
 0 1 2 3 9
89. Feelings of guilt
 0 1 2 3 9
90. Impoverishment
 0 1 2 3 9
91. Ambivalence
 0 1 2 3 9
92. Parathymia
 0 1 2 3 9
93. Lability
 0 1 2 3 9
94. Incontinence
 0 1 2 3 9
95. Rigidity
 0 1 2 3 9

DIS. DRIVE/MOTILITY __0

96. Lack drive
 0 1 2 3 9
97. Inhibit. drive
 0 1 2 3 9
98. Stuporous
 0 1 2 3 9
99. Inc. drive
 0 1 2 3 9
100. Motor restless.
 0 1 2 3 9
101. Parakinesia
 0 1 2 3 9
102. Mannerisms
 0 1 2 3 9
103. Histrionics
 0 1 2 3 9
104. Mutism
 0 1 2 3 9
105. Logorrhea
 0 1 2 3 9
106. Negativism
 0 1 2 3 9
107. Indecisiveness
 0 1 2 3 9

Fig. 3 (cont.)

AGP Part 4. Psychopathological Symptoms

CLINIC/HOSP_____ STUDY_____ RATER_____

PT INITIALS_____ PT NO._____ PERIOD_____

DATE EXAM___/___/_____ STATUS IN__OUT__PART__OTH__
M D Y

SEX M__ F__RACE W__ B__ I__ O__ OTH______________

BIRTHDATE____/____/_____
M D Y

TIME SPAN RATED TODAY___ <1 wk___ <1 mo___ >1 mo___

108. PSYCHOORGANIC SYNDROME __0
Site Local___ Diffuse___ NA___
Severity MI___ MO___ SV___ NA___
Duration (yr) <1___ 1<2___ 3<4___ 4<5___ 5<6___
<10___ NA___

AB MI MO SV NA

GLOBAL PERFORMANCE DIS. __0

109. Aphasia
0 1 2 3 9

110. Agnosia
0 1 2 3 9

111. Apraxia
0 1 2 3 9

AB MI MO SV NA

LOCALIZED BRAIN DYSFUNCTION__0

FRONTOPARIETAL DIS. __0

112. Frontal aprax.
0 1 2 3 9

113. Facial aprax.
0 1 2 3 9

114. Prefront. I.S.
0 1 2 3 9

115. Frontobasal I.S.
0 1 2 3 9

116. Motor aphasia
0 1 2 3 9

OCCIPITAL DIS. __0

117. Color/recogn.
0 1 2 3 9

118. Color/naming
0 1 2 3 9

119. Color/visual.
0 1 2 3 9

120. Visual agnosia
0 1 2 3 9

121. Prosopagnosia
0 1 2 3 9

122. Dysmorphopsia
0 1 2 3 9

PARIETO-OCCIPITAL DIS. __0

123. Stereoagnosia
0 1 2 3 9

124. Somatagnosia
0 1 2 3 9

AB MI MO SV NA

125. Anosognosia
0 1 2 3 9

126. Conduction aphasia
0 1 2 3 9

127. Alexia
0 1 2 3 9

128. Agraphia
0 1 2 3 9

129. Acalculia
0 1 2 3 9

130. Ideomotor apraxia
0 1 2 3 9

131. Ideational apraxia
0 1 2 3 9

132. Construc. apraxia
0 1 2 3 9

TEMPORAL DIS. __0

133. Amnestic aphasia
0 1 2 3 9

134. Sensory aphasia
0 1 2 3 9

CIRCADIAN DIS. __0

135. Worse in AM
0 1 2 3 9

136. Worse in PM
0 1 2 3 9

137. Better in PM
0 1 2 3 9

138. Nighttime exacerb.
0 1 2 3 9

139. Symp. alternation
0 1 2 3 9

DIS. SLEEP/VIGILANCE __0

140. Diff. fall asleep
0 1 2 3 9

141. Interrupt. sleep
0 1 2 3 9

142. Early waking
0 1 2 3 9

Fig. 4

AGP Part 4. Psychopathological Symptoms *(continued)*

AB MI MO SV NA

143. Prolonged sleep
0 1 2 3 9
144. Shortened sleep
0 1 2 3 9
145. Night restless.
0 1 2 3 9
146. Night confusion
0 1 2 3 9
147. Drowsiness
0 1 2 3 9
148. Day-night reversal
0 1 2 3 9
149. Inc. dreaming
0 1 2 3 9

DIS. SOCIAL BEHAVIOR 0
150. Soc. withdrawal
0 1 2 3 9
151. Exces. soc. contact
0 1 2 3 9
152. Aggressiveness
0 1 2 3 9
153. Suicidal
0 1 2 3 9
154. Self-mutilation
0 1 2 3 9
155. Lack feel. ill
0 1 2 3 9
156. Lack insight
0 1 2 3 9
157. Uncooperativeness
0 1 2 3 9
158. Dissimulation
0 1 2 3 9
159. Self-neglect
0 1 2 3 9
160. Refuse nourish.
0 1 2 3 9
161. Dec. libido
0 1 2 3 9
162. Inc. libido
0 1 2 3 9

SOCIAL - NURSING 0
163. Financial needs
0 1 2 3 9
164. Housekeeping
0 1 2 3 9
165. Cont. med. care
0 1 2 3 9

AB MI MO SV NA

166. Walking
0 1 2 3 9
167. Dressing self
0 1 2 3 9
168. Pers. hygiene
0 1 2 3 9
169. Eating
0 1 2 3 9
170. Leisure activities
0 1 2 3 9
171. Transportation
0 1 2 3 9
172. Chewing disturb.
0 1 2 3 9
173. Bedridden
0 1 2 3 9
174. Urinary incontin.
0 1 2 3 9
175. Fecal incontin.
0 1 2 3 9
176. Smearing
0 1 2 3 9

RELIABILITY
0 1 2 3 9

ADDITIONAL EXAMINATIONS 0

EKG	Y
EEG	Y
Echoencephal-ography	Y
CAT	Y
Scintiscan	Y
Dopplersono-graphy	Y
Angiography	Y
ENG	Y
LP	Y
PEG	Y
EMG	Y
Psych. Tests	Y
RCBF	Y
Other (Specify)	

____

____

Fig. 4 (cont.)

with deficits of memory and orientation. Results of our own research using the AGP system for symptom evaluation underscore these findings (Gutzmann 1984).

2. The relationship between psychopathologic signs and morphological (as shown by CR or NMR) or functional changes (as evidenced by EEG, CBF, or PET) is presently neither sufficiently established nor well-elaborated. While the development of highly sophisticated technological approaches cannot be

AGP Part 5. Somatic Signs

CLINIC/HOSP______ STUDY_____ RATER_____

PT INITIALS______ PT NO._____ PERIOD____

DATE EXAM__/__/___ STATUS IN__OUT__PART__OTH__
M D Y

SEX M__ F__ RACE W__B__I__O__OTH______________

BIRTHDATE_____/_____/_____
M D Y

---

1. GLOBAL STATE OF HEALTH
   Good_____ Fair_____ Poor_____
   AB MI MO SV NA

AB MI MO SV NA
SOMATIC DISORDERS _0_

CARDIOVASCULAR DIS. _0_
2. Insufficiency
   0 1 2 3 9
3. Dysrhythmia
   0 1 2 3 9
4. Hypertension
   0 1 2 3 9
5. Other ____________
   0 1 2 3 9
6. RESPIRATORY DIS.
   0 1 2 3 9

GASTROINTESTINAL DIS. _0_
7. Hypersalivation
   0 1 2 3 9
8. Dry Mouth
   0 1 2 3 9
9. Nausea
   0 1 2 3 9
10. Constipation
    0 1 2 3 9
11. Diarrhea
    0 1 2 3 9
12. Other ____________
    0 1 2 3 9

UROGENITAL DIS. _0_
13. Renal Insuff.
    0 1 2 3 9
14. Micturition dist.
    0 1 2 3 9
15. Other ____________

SKELETOMUSCULAR DIS.
16. 0 1 2 3 9

METABOLIC DIS. _0_
17. Diabetes mellitus
    0 1 2 3 9
18. Other __________
    0 1 2 3 9
19. CHRONIC PAIN
    0 1 2 3 9
20. CHRONIC CONSUMPT. PROC.
    0 1 2 3 9

OTHER SOMATIC DIS. _0_
21. Blurred vision
    0 1 2 3 9
22. Excessive sweating
    0 1 2 3 9
23. Chills
    0 1 2 3 9
24. Excessive thirst
    0 1 2 3 9
25. Reduced thirst
    0 1 2 3 9
26. Excessive appetite
    0 1 2 3 9
27. Decreased appetite
    0 1 2 3 9
28. Headache
    0 1 2 3 9
29. Dizziness
    0 1 2 3 9
30. Other ____________
    0 1 2 3 9

NEUROLOGICAL DISORDERS _0_

AB LT BO RT NA
31. OLFACTORY DIS.
    0 1 2 3 9

VISION DIS. _0_
32. Central visual
    0 1 2 3 9
33. Peripheral visual
    0 1 2 3 9
34. Central gaze paresis
    0 1 2 3 9
35. Oculomotor paresis
    0 1 2 3 9
36. Optkinetic nystagmus
    0 1 2 3 9
37. Spontaneous nystagmus
    0 1 2 3 9

HEARING DIS. _0_
38. Middle ear
    0 1 2 3 9
39. Inner ear
    0 1 2 3 9

CENTRAL MOTOR DIS. _0_
40. Hemiparesis
    0 1 2 3 9
41. Paraparesis
    0 1 2 3 9

Fig. 5

AGP Part 5. Somatic Signs *(continued)*

AB LT BO RT NA

42. Quadriparesis
0 1 2 3 9

CENTRAL SENSORY DIS. 0

43. Hemihypesthesia
0 1 2 3 9
44. Tranverse
0 1 2 3 9

PERIPHERAL MOTOR DIS. 0

45. Distal
0 1 2 3 9
46. Proximal
0 1 2 3 9
47. PERIPHERAL SENSORY DIS:
0 1 2 3 9

SPINAL CORD LES 0

48. Cervical
0 1 2 3 9
49. Thoracic
0 1 2 3 9
50. Sacrolumbar
0 1 2 3 9

EXTRAPYRAMIDAL DIS. 0

51. Rigidity
0 1 2 3 9
52. Gross tremor
0 1 2 3 9
53. Fine tremor
0 1 2 3 9
54. Akinesia
0 1 2 3 9
55. Akathisia
0 1 2 3 9
56. Acute dyskinesia
0 1 2 3 9
57. Tardive dyskinesia
0 1 2 3 9

COORDINATION DIS. 0

58. Intention tremor
0 1 2 3 9

AB LT BO RT NA

59. Pointing ataxia
0 1 2 3 9
60. Postural ataxia
0 1 2 3 9
61. Gait ataxia
0 1 2 3 9

PRIMITIVE REFLEX 0

62. Perioral reflex
0 1 2 3 9
63. Grasp reflex
0 1 2 3 9
64. Palmomental reflex
0 1 2 3 9
65. Other ____________
0 1 2 3 9
66. EQUILIBRIUM DIS.
0 1 2 3 9

BULBAR DIS. 0

67. Speaking
0 1 2 3 9
68. Swallowing
0 1 2 3 9

CEREBRAL SEIZURES 0

69. Gen. primary
0 1 2 3 9
70. Gen. secondary
0 1 2 3 9
71. Focal
0 1 2 3 9
72. Unclassified
0 1 2 3 9

OTHER CNS 0

73. Peripheral
0 1 2 3 9
74. Central
0 1 2 3 9
75. Psychogenic
0 1 2 3 9
76. HANDEDNESS
0-4 5-9 10-14 9

Fig. 5 (cont.)

overlooked, there is still a lack of reliable instruments permitting the comprehensive and detailed recording of psychopathology. Our own research with the AGP data base including CT, EEG, and psychometric tests, has indeed revealed interrelationships which have proved to be of clinical importance (Gutzmann et al. 1982).

3. Evaluation of therapeutic and rehabilitative treatment. There is a growing interest in developing new pharmacologic and behavioral approaches to counteract the destructive and incapacitating consequences of dementia. However, most research on means of evaluating the efficacy of therapeutic interventions has not produced convincing results. Poor operationalization and standardization of psychopathology appears to be a main defect, which at present precludes the reliable and objective assessment of the efficacy of variuos therapeutic measures.

AGP Part 6. Diagnoses

CLINIC/HOSP____ STUDY____ RATER________________

PT INITIALS____ PT NO.____ PERIOD______

DATE EXAM__/__/__ STATUS IN__OUT__PT__OTH__
M D Y

SEX M__F__ RACE W__B__I__O__Oth__________

BIRTHDATE____/____/____
M D Y

CLINICAL EXPERIENCE (years)

<1__ 1-<3__ 3-<5__ >5__

PSYCHIATRIC DIAGNOSES

ICD-9__ DSM-III__

1. Name______________________
Code______________________
ICD-9 Section: E__ N__ Y__
Diagnostic Certitude: MI__ MO__ HI__
Age at First Manifestation:
0-20__ 21-30__ 31-40__ 41-50__
51-60__ 61-70__ 71-80__ >80__
Certitude (Age): MI__ MO__ HI__

2. Name______________________
Code______________________
ICD-9 Section: E__ N__ Y__
Diagnostic Certitude: MI__ MO__ HI__
Age at First Manifestation:
0-20__ 21-30__ 31-40__ 41-50__
51-60__ 61-70__ 71-80__ >80__
Certitude (Age): MI__ MO__ HI__

3. Name______________________
Code______________________
ICD-9 Section: E__ N__ Y__
Diagnostic Certitude: MI__ MO__ HI__
Age at First Manifestation:
0-20__ 21-30__ 31-40__ 41-50__
51-60__ 61-70__ 71-80__ >80__
Certitude (Age): MI__ MO__ HI__

SOMATIC DIAGNOSES None__

1. Name______________________
Code______________________
ICD-9 Section: E__ N__ Y__
Diagnostic Certitude: MI__ MO__ HI__
Age at First Manifestation:
0-20__ 21-30__ 31-40__ 41-50__
51-60__ 61-70__ 71-80__ >80
Certitude (Age): MI__ MO__ HI__

2. Name______________________
Code______________________
ICD-9 Section: E__ N__ Y__
Diagnostic Certitude: MI__ MO__ HI__
Age at First Manifestation
0-20__ 31-30__ 41-50__ 51-60__
51-60__ 61-70__ 71-80__ >80__
Certitude (Age): MI__ MO__ HI__

3. Name______________________
Code______________________
ICD-9 Section: E__ N__ Y__
Diagnostic Certitude: MI__ MO__ HI__
Age at First Manifestation
0-20__ 21-30__ 31-40__ 41-50__
51-60__ 61-70__ 71-80__ >80__
Certitude (Age): MI__ MO__HI__

4. Name______________________
Code______________________
ICD-9 Section: E__ N__ Y__
Diagnostic Certitude: MI__ MO__ HI__
Age at First Manifestation
0-20__ 21-30__ 31-40__ 41-50__
51-60__ 61-70__ 71-80__ >80__
Certitude (Age): MI__ MO__ HI__

Fig. 6

Evaluation of the AGP Documentation System

The first methodological study using the revised AGP documentation system was carried out to determine interrater reliability for the psychopathologic assessment section (Andrae 1979). Prior to the beginning of this study, several training sessions had been performed to increase the raters' awareness of psychogeriatric disorders. In the study, videotapes of preliminary examinations of 30 patients were shown to a group of four psychiatrists during their internship. After the ratings had been completed, no discussion among the raters was allowed. The videotapes which were rated consisted of interviews with patients of the Department of Gerontopsychiatry of the Free University of Berlin and includes three groups of ten patients each, with depressive, paranoid, or organic syndromes. Seven of the 30 patients were male, with a mean age of 69 years, 23 patients were female, with a mean age of 68 years.

For the purpose of data analysis, items rated mild, moderate, or severe were counted as present, whereas items marked "no answer," or "absent" were scored as "absent." For methodological reasons, only items that at least one rater had marked as present for 15% of the patients were included in the analysis. Following this criterion, 78 of the 183 items constituting the psychopathological section were analyzed.

Although interrater reliabilities were evaluated in different ways, we restrict ourselves here to the results obtained by calculating Cohen's kappa (Bartko and Carpenter 1976; Woggon et al. 1978). Kappa is a chance-corrected percent agreement measure making possible an estimate of the reliability of two or more raters by comparing the observed percent agreement with the percent agreement by chance. A test of significance of kappa (different from zero) is to divide kappa by its standard deviation. The resulting ratio is an approximate standard normal test statistic.

Kappa calculations were carried out in two ways, first, by taking pairs of the four raters and second, by pooling all the raters. We restrict ourselves here to the reliability scores obtained by considering all raters.

No assessment was available for 17 items because methodological difficulties prevented the interpretation of kappa. In all, 40 symptoms showed good or moderate interrater reliability, with a kappa coefficient greater than or equal to 0.4. Good or moderate agreement was noted in particular for the headings "disorders of attention and memory," "disorders of global performance," and "disturbances of orientation." Another 21 items had low reliability, with a kappa coefficient of less than 0.4. These critical items were concentrated under the heading "formal disturbances of thinking." This result might well be due to the fact that this heading mainly contains items which are nosological nonspecific, for example, "restriction" and "rumination." Apparently, pathologically specific symptoms are more clearly defined than pathologically nonspecific ones, which in turn allows a more precise evaluation. Another explanation might be that the raters were more adequately trained with regard to recognizing pathologically specific items.

At present, initial efforts are being made to reduce the number of items of the psychopathologic symptom section by using a factor-analytic technique. Calculations determining factors which can be used as a basis for describing psychopathologic syndromes are to be made. Classifying psychopathologic syndromes is important for several reasons. They can yield reliable data for the measurement of change over time in therapeutic studies. Furthermore, it may be of interest to determine whether the psychopathologic syndromes established on a factor-analytic basis correspond to the classic psychiatric diagnoses.

Psychopathologic findings of 204 patients admitted to the polyclinic of our department from July 1981 to December 1983 have been included in this ongoing study. For theoretical reasons, only those items which may contribute toward explaining variance are to be included in the calculations. This involves only 85 items of the psychopathologic symptom section which occur in the sampling of 204 patients with a frequency of at least 8 (4%). Two kinds of scales are to be employed for data analysis. The severity of the symptoms will be graded mild, moderate, severe, or not present. In addition, symptoms will be encoded as "present" or "absent." Principal component analysis (PCA) has been chosen as a method of statistical analysis. In the applied PCA method, the correlation matrix is not altered; i.e., the estimates of communality are equal to 1. This method does not require any assumptions about the general structure of the variables. By using Kaiser's criterion (i.e., eigenvalues greater than or equal to 1.0), this method yields 24 factors for the scale with four graduations and 25 factors for the scale with two graduations, explaining 75% and 72% of common variance respectively. Rotating the first-factor solutions by successively maximizing the variance (Varimax) yields about 6–12 interpretable factors. Further extensive calculations are required to obtain stable solutions for this factor analysis. Final results will be reported in the near future.

The revised AGP system is scheduled for publication in book form in 1985. The AGP manual includes detailed descriptions of all items occurring in the forms discussed here as well as advice on the use of this system. An English translation of the AGP system has already been prepared by Guy and Ban (1985) who have also published the English translation of the AMDP system (Guy and Ban 1982). Adjustment of certain headings of the AGP system to fit American conventions has been deemed necessary, however, especially for the sections canvassing demographic data. The English translation of the AGP system will be published by Springer-Verlag at the same time as the German edition.

References

Andrae W (1979) Zur Reliabilität des AGP-Systems. Erste Ergebnisse einer Interrater-Reliabilitätsstudie zu einer überarbeiteten Fassung des AGP-Dokumentationssystems anhand von 30 videogespeicherten Erstexplorationen. In: Oesterreich K (ed) Janssen Symposien Gerontopsychiatrie 8. Janssen, Düsseldorf, pp 162–179

Arbeitsgemeinschaft für Methodik und Dokumentation in der Psychiatrie (AMDP) (1981) Das AMDP-System. Manual zur Dokumentation psychiatrischer Befunde, 4th edn. Springer, Berlin Heidelberg New York

Bartko JJ, Carpenter WT (1976) On the methods and theory of reliability. J Nerv Ment Dis 163:307–317

Bolm H, Buckler R, Freudenthal K, Hermann U, Lieberz K, Schröter O, Werner V (1973a) Anwendungsmöglichkeiten einer gerontopsychiatrischen Sozialdokumentation bei unterschiedlichen Patientenpopulationen. In: Bergener M (ed) Janssen Symposien Gerontopsychiatrie 3. Janssen, Düsseldorf, pp 146–160

Bolm H, Buckler R, Freudenthal K, Kanowski S, Lieberz K, Schröter O, Werner V (1973b) Erste Erfahrungen und Ergebnisse einer vergleichenden Untersuchung verschiedener geriatrischer Populationen mit einer gerontopsychiatrischen Basisdokumentation. In: Bergener M (ed) Janssen Symposien Gerontopsychiatrie 3. Janssen, Düsseldorf, pp 161–187

Ciompi L, Kanowski S (1981) AGP, Dokumentationssystem der Arbeitsgemeinschaft für Gerontopsychiatrie. In: CIPS (Collegium Internationale Psychiatriae Scalarum) (ed) Internationale Skalen für Psychiatrie, 2nd edn. Beltz, Weinheim

Ciompi L, Lobrinus A, Müller C, Wertheimer J, Frost N, Helmchen H, Hermann U, Kanowski S (1972) Vorschlag für eine gerontopsychiatrische Basisdokumentation. In: Kanowski S (ed) Janssen Symposien Gerontopsychiatrie 2. Janssen, Düsseldorf, pp 211–232

Ciompi L, Lobrinus A, Müller C (1973) Basisdokumentation in der Gerontopsychiatrie: das „AGP-System". In: Bergener M (ed) Janssen Symposien Gerontopsychiatrie 3. Janssen, Düsseldorf, pp 130–145

Ciompi L, Kanowski S, Krüger H, Urban R (eds) (1985) Das AGP-System: Manual zur Dokumentation Psychiatrischer Befunde bei Alterskranken. 2. Fassung. (to be published)

Frost N, Helmchen H, Hermann U, Kanowski S (1971) Vorschläge für einen Merkmals-Katalog zur gerontopsychiatrischen Dokumentation. In: Bergener M, Kulenkampff C (eds) Janssen Symposien Gerontopsychiatrie 1. Janssen, Düsseldorf, pp 224–254

Gutzmann H (1984) Frontallappensyndrome bei (prä-)senilen Demenzen vom Alzheimer-Typ: eine korrelationsstatistische Untersuchung. Z Gerontol 17:128–131

Gutzmann H, Klimitz H, Avdaloff W (1982) Correlations between psychopathology, psychological test results and computerized tomography changes in senile dementia. Arch Gerontol Geriatr 1:241–259

Guy W, Ban TA (eds) (1982) The AMDP system. Manual for the assessment and documentation of psychopathology. Springer, Berlin, Heidelberg, New York

Guy W, Ban TA (eds) (1985) The AGP system. Translation of: Ciompi L, Kanowski S, Krüger H, Urban R (eds) (1985) Das AGP-System: Manual zur Dokumentation psychiatrischer Befunde bei Alterskranken, 2. Fassung. Springer, Berlin, Heidelberg, New York, Tokyo

Hermann U (1972) Möglichkeiten und Grenzen der Dokumentation gerontpsychiatrischer Sozialdaten. In: Kanowski S (ed) Janssen Symposien Gerontopsychiatrie 2. Janssen, Düsseldorf, pp 233–244

Junkers G, Kanowski S, Paur R (1976) Forschung, Lehre und Krankenversorgung aus der Sicht einer Abteilung für Gerontopsychiatrie. Z Gerontol 9:151–175

Lieberz K (1978) Ein Beitrag zur Weiterentwicklung eines Gerontopsychiatrischen Sozialdokumentationssystems – Ergebnisse einer Praktikabilitätsprüfung. Free University of Berlin, Berlin

Scharfetter C (1972) Das AMP-System, 2nd edn. Springer, Berlin Heidelberg New York

Woggon B, Baumann U, Angst J (1978) Interrater-Reliabilität von AMP-Symptomen. Arch Psychiatr Nervenkr 225:73–85

Cognitive Deficits in Parkinson's Disease

A. J. Lees[1]

Introduction

Motor abnormalities dominate the clinical picture of Parkinson's disease. Bradykinesia, caused by severe damage to the ascending nigrostriatal dopaminergic projection, leads to a slight hesitancy in initiating voluntary acts, a difficulty in performing repetitive movements with a progressive reduction in their amplitude, a poorly defined fatigue and possibly an additional defect of motor intention. Many patients also have an inability to attend to two motor commands simultaneously, and more complex perceptual-motor abnormalities have also been detected. Muscle rigidity, a coarse resting tremor and postural instability compound the patient's incapacities, all of which are exquisitely influenced by the emotions.

Minor cognitive abnormalities are also an invariable but, until recently, relatively neglected feature of the disease, which can be conveniently embraced under the descriptive term bradyphrenia. In the early stages of Parkinson's disease, most patients have little difficulty in perceiving, learning, remembering or understanding. Many continue in responsible, intellectually demanding jobs, and their ability to appreciate the finer nuances of life appears unaffected. Nevertheless, subtle changes in their behaviour may be apparent to their relatives and friends. A slight lack of spontaneity, increasing poverty of imagination, a blunting of emotions and a tendency to repetition may lead to difficulties in sustaining stimulating conversation. Other early complaints by the patient's family are of an increasing apathy, lack of initiative and sometimes mild word-finding difficulties. These sorts of problems are of course common to all of us with increasing age, but seem to be more severe and occur somewhat earlier in the parkinsonian patient.

In the last 10 years, there has also been an increasingly influential body of thought which considers that more severe intellectual deterioration and memory loss should be regarded as an integral feature of the disease process. It has been suggested that Parkinson's disease and Alheimer's disease should be looked on as two poles of a clinical spectrum of which the common feature is damage to the isodendritic core (Rossor 1981). Others have suggested that a specific type of dementia occurs in Parkinson's disease as a result of damage to certain ascending subcortical projections (Albert 1978).

In this paper, I will discuss the historical development of the term bradyphrenia and review some of the recent neuropsychological studies which have attempted to tease out the particular cognitive defects which compose it. I will also

1 The National Hospitals for Nervous Diseases, Maida Vale Hospital, London W9 1TL, UK

Senile Dementia of the Alzheimer Type
Ed. by J. Traber and W. H. Gispen

review the clinical and neuropathological data which have been marshalled to support the view that dementia of the Alzheimer type is common in Parkinson's disease.

Bradyphrenia

Clinical Observations

In 1882, Benjamin Ball described seven Parkinsonian patients, all of whom were admitted to a psychiatric hospital. He described their difficulties as follows:

"An invisible weight seems to crush the intellect and slow at the same time perception, movement and ideas... it is evidently a case of paralysis agitans accompanied by dementia; one cannot help in the presence of the observed symptoms but think of certain cases of melancholic stupor such as one sees in our mental hospitals."

In 1922, Naville reported what he believed to be a new psychiatric syndrome in some of the survivors of the pandemic of encephalitis lethargica. It comprised a diminution of voluntary attention, a lack of spontaneous interest, a loss of drive and initiative, fatigability and a mild amnesia. Intelligence was unaffected, but the capacity for intellectual activity was severely compromised. Those affected became uncommunicative and did nothing without constant prompting. In general, this remarkable mental slowing was mirrored by a coexisting motor retardation. Naville recognised that the distinction between a motor or mental cause fo these abnormalities was not easy to make. He devised a series of tests of increasing intellectual difficulty in which the motor component remained the same and on the basis of these studies concluded that, compared with controls, there was a slowing of intellectual processing and that this bore a direct relationship to the degree of motor slowing. Worster-Drought and Hardcastle (1924), however, using an electrical apparatus to measure psychomotor reaction and cerebration times, concluded that, although the former may be lengthened by 50%, the cerebration time was unaffected.

Steck (1931) examined all the survivors of encephalitis lethargica in Swiss mental hospitals and found bradyphrenia to be present in 43% of the 257 patients with coexisting parkinsonian features. He also found the same symptom in 38% of 197 postencephalitic parkinsonian patients living in the community or admitted to general hospitals and, after re-examining Naville's original cases, reported an incidence of 38% for these patients as well. He distinguished this mental state from dementia by the preservation of memory, judgment and orientation. Von Economo, L'Hermitte and Aubrun also studied bradyphrenia, and all concluded that it was a cerebral disorder. Kinner Wilson (1940) asserted that "slowness off the mark" was actually muscular in origin and that cerebration was not slowed, believing bradyphrenia to be psychogenically determined, caused by a depressive apathy. Mettler (1955), on the other hand, implicated the corpus striatum in mental function:

"With hypokinesia and rigidity appeared a slowed reaction time, a loss of mental speed and agility, a certain deliberateness and indecision or suspension of decision without any real evidence of impairment of intellectual capacity."

In 1965, Hassler described bradyphrenia in idiopathic Parkinson's disease, reporting a delay in emotional responses, failure of attention, slowness of thinking and indecisiveness. He speculated that these symptoms occurred as a result of cell loss in the nucleus basalis of Meynert. De Ajuriaguerra (1971) observed fully fledged bradyphrenia in only 9% of 204 patients, of whom 64 patients were institutionalised with Parkinson's disease or postencephalitic Parkinson's syndrome and 140 were L-dopa-treated patients. However, he noted apathy in 48% and drew attention to the links with depression.

Apparently unaware of this welter of literature, Albert and his colleagues (Albert et al. 1974; Albert 1978) described a subcortical dementia in the Steele-Richardson-Olszewski syndrome, in which the cardinal features are forgetfulness, slowness of thought, altered personality with apathy or depression and an inability to manifest acquired knowledge. McHugh and Folstein (1975) simultaneously reported a similar mental picture in Huntington's chorea and in depression (Folstein and McHugh 1978). The term subcortical dementia has subsequently been used to embrace the neuropsychological deficits seen in Parkinson's disease, lacunar states and retarded depression. The absence of language disorder, amnesia, agnosia and apraxia distinguishes it from the so-called cortical dementia of Alzheimer's disease. Albert speculated that the pathological substrate might lie in the connection between the basal ganglia and the limbic system and the frontal cortex.

Recently, Laplane and his colleagues (1984) reported three patients with profound psychic akinesia occurring after toxic encephalopathies and without associated bradykinesia. In two of these patients, stereotyped complex movements occurred, while in all three, computerised axial tomography revealed bilateral basal ganglia lesions principally affecting the globus pallidus.

After a review of the extensive descriptive literature, Todes and Lees (1985) have suggested that a particular behavioural syndrome including mental inflexibility, introspection, a withholding of emotions and a predisposition to depression may actually antecede the development of motor symptoms in Parkinson's disease by several decades. It is not clear however whether this constitutes an early symptom of the illness or a predisposing aetiological factor.

Neuropsychological Studies

The close similarity between bradyphrenia and some of the symptoms seen with frontal lobe syndromes has stimulated the use of psychological test batteries known to expose deficits in the latter group of disorders. A number of studies have demonstrated a particular difficulty in switching mental strategies for patients afflicted with Parkinson's disease. Barbeau (1973) was the first to point out that parkinsonian patients had great difficulty in changing from one mental concept to another. Using Goldstein's sorting test, parkinsonian patients were found to have great difficulty in sorting a number of common objects on the basis of their size, colour and various other physical characteristics. Bowen and her colleagues (1975) used the Wisconsin card-sorting test on 71 unselected patients with idiopathic Parkinson's disease and on 35 controls matched for age and WAIS verbal IQ. All but 18 were receiving L-dopa, and it is not stated whether the remainder were taking anticholinergic drugs or how many had had stereotactic surgery. The parkinsonian patients were found to have considerable difficulty in shifting sets and were frequently unable to attend to the completion of each category.

Lees and Smith (1983) studied 30 mildly disabled right-handed patients with Parkinson's disease. None of them had received any treatment, and all had normal CAT brain scans. Patients with high ischaemia scores or depression were excluded. Similar selection criteria were used in the age-matched controls. No impairment in general intellectual function or short-term verbal or visual memory was found in the patients, but they had significantly more difficulty than controls in switching from one concept to another and produced more perseverative errors on both the modified Wisconsin card-sorting test and Benton's word fluency test.

Cools and colleagues (1984) studied 18 relatively mildly disabled L-dopa-treated patients and 19 age- and intelligence-matched controls with a 3-h battery of tests which included the WAIS picture completion test, digit span and similarities test and the Stroop colour-word test. The selective tests employed included a variety of tasks: naming as many animals and then professions as possible in 1 min each; a block-sorting test comprising 27 blocks differing in form, colour and size; and an animal-sorting test consisting of two sets of 24 cards in which the patients had to distinguish between two categories, e.g. bird versus mammal, and then switch after several correct responses. A motor sequence test was also carried out. It was found that the patients produced fewer names of animals and professions, needed more trials for detecting a shift in a sorting criterion and exhibited fewer finger responses on a change of pushing sequences than controls. It was concluded that these deficits originate in a central programming deficit causing diminished shifting aptitude and that the disorder is due to dysfunction of the basal ganglia..

Matison and her colleagues (1982) administered the vocabulary subtest of the WAIS, the Boston Naming test and tests for word fluency to 22 parkinsonian patients, most of whom had received L-dopa therapy but had stable deficits. Impairment of confrontation naming which was capable of improvement by semantic or phonetic cues was demonstrated, and there were also impairments of category naming and sentence repetition. The authors suggested that a semantic retrieval deficit for confrontation naming may be present and that some of the observed difficulties might be due to problems in initiating a response set and in sequencing and shifting within it. In another study, motor planning deficits as measured by representational and nonrepresentational gestures has been reported in a group of patients who had no physical difficulty in carrying out the required motor act. Visuo-spatial deficits were also observed on the nonrepresentational gesture tests (Sharpe et al. 1983). Bowen (1976) also considered that most of the problems experienced by parkinsonian patients on a route-walking test occurred when the patients were not in the same orientation as the test requirements, which suggested to her that a failure to switch sets competently may have been a contributing factor.

Studies carried out in patients with severe L-dopa-induced oscillations in performance have shown that, compared with the striking swings in motor function, neuropsychological changes, although apparent, are modest. Delis and colleagues (1982) observed a general disinhibition of language, worsened memory and perseveration in off periods as compared with on, whereas Brown et al. (1984) found an adverse swing in affect/arousal state during the off period. Hardie et al. (1984) also commented on a striking swing in affect between on and off periods.

Wilson and colleagues (1980) compared 20 nondemented, drug-treated parkinsonian patients with 16 controls matched for age, education and verbal IQ on a measure of speed and accuracy in short-term memory scanning. They observed that the capacity to scan rapidly was impaired in the elderly patients and suggested that this deficit could not be totally explained by a motor abnormality but involved a cognitive slowing as well. Evarts and colleagues (1981), however, demonstrated a slight increase in simple reaction times in Parkinson's disease, as reported previously by many others, but no disproportionate or selective increase in choice reaction times. Nevertheless, they stressed that their results did not imply that there is no abnormality in call-up of motor programmes and emphasised that there is a need for further studies in which motor response is programmed to include other features. In 60 drug-treated patients, significant associations between psychomotor speed and timed and untimed visuo-spatial performance was found. In this study, the severity of limb bradykinesia was predictive of poor performance on the visuo-spatial tests not requiring motor speed or coordination, and the authors suggest that cognitive impairment in Parkinson's disease might be due to the same subcortical lesions as those responsible for motor symptoms (Mortimer et al. 1982). The neuropsychological deficits demonstrated in parkinsonian patients which may constitute the syndrome of bradyphrenia are listed as follows:

1. Clinical features:
   a) Slowness of thought
   b) Inattention
   c) Perseverative tendencies
   d) Apathy
   e) Forgetfulness
2. Neuropsychological deficits:
   a) Difficulty in switching conceptual sets
   b) Perseveration
   c) Attention/affect deficits
   d) Slowness in mnenomic scanning
   e) Perceptual-motor abnormalities

Relationship of Depression to Bradyphrenia

Depression and Parkinson's disease share many clinical features. Motor retardation, slowness of facial expression, a poverty of new ideas, weight loss, sleep disturbances and constipation are all common to both. About one-quarter of parkinsonian patients have a severe depressive illness long before the onset of their motor incapacities (Shaw et al. 1980), and depression has been claimed to be more common in Parkinson's disease than in any other chronically crippling physical illness (Robins 1976). When both conditions occur concurrently, electroshock therapy (Lebensohn and Jenkins 1975) can improve the mental and motor incapacities. Van Praag et al. (1975) have shown that cerebrospinal homovanillilc acid levels (HVA) are low in a subgroup of depressed patients with motor retardation and that L-dopa treatment alleviates this symptom restoring cerebrospinal HVA levels to normal. Other studies have also reported that L-dopa helps patients suffering depression with motor retardation (Goodwin et al. 1970) and sometimes has beneficial effects on depression occurring in Parkinson's disease. Bromocriptine has also been shown to alleviate both depression and parkinsonism in ten depressed patients, but no correlation between the two effects was noted (Jouvent et al. 1983). It seems possible, therefore, that Parkinson's disease and depression with motor retardation might also share some neurochemical abnormalities.

Steck (1931) discerned two postencephalitic depressive states: a neurasthenia, which often precedes the appearance of Parkinson's syndrome and leads to bradyphrenia, and a melancholia marked by tearfulness, hypochondriasis, suicidal thoughts and feelings of guilt and misery. De Ajuriaguerra (1971) noted that 62% of his 204 cases of Parkinson's disease had simple depressive states with neurasthenia, inertia and mild sadness. L-Dopa produced a parallel improvement in the bradykinetic and affective symptoms in these cases. A further 10% of them had severe melancholia which required tricyclic antidepressants. Agid and his colleagues (1984) have recently placed renewed emphasis on de Ajuriaguerra's view that retarded depression is an integral component of bradyphrenia. Support for this also comes from a study on 55 nondemented patients in which inattention and mild intellectual impairment were closely correlated with depressive symptomatology and independent of the severity of the motor symptoms (Mayeux et al. 1981).

Evidence for Considering Alzheimer-like Dementia as an Integral Component of Parkinson's Disease

According to the criteria of the Diagnostic and Statistical Manual of Mental Disorders (DSM III), dementia is defined as follows:

1. A loss of intellectual ability with resulting occupational and social handicaps
2. Memory impairment
3. One or more of the following:
   a) Impaired thinking
   b) Impaired judgement

c) Aphasia
d) Apraxia
e) Agnosia
f) Constructional difficulties
g) Personality change
4. Unclouded consciousness
5. No related organic cause or nonorganic mental illness

My own clinical experience suggests that, if this definition is rigidly adhered to, dementia is relatively uncommon even in the terminal stages of Parkinson's disease. Nevertheless, most recent reviews have uncritically reported dementia in about 30% of the patients in randomly selected groups attending hospital. In most of these reports, it is impossible to disentangle the relative contributions of depression, medical and surgical treatment, cerebrovascular disease and normal ageing from the effects of the diesase process itself. Nevertheless, generalised intellectual impairment has also been detected in groups of patients by the use of different neuropsychological tests (Warburton 1967; Loranger et al. 1972), and there appears to be some clinical (Pearce 1974), histological (Forno et al. 1978; Alvord et al. 1974; Whitehouse et al. 1981, 1983) and neurochemical overlap (Adolfsson et al. 1979; Dubois et al. 1983) between the terminal phases of Alzheimer's disease and Parkinson's disease. Cortical atrophy can also be demonstrated radiologically in some patients with Parkinson's disease (Selby 1968; Sroka et al. 1981), but it is still uncertain whether this is more than an age-related phenomenon (Pearce et al. 1981). Counting only those patients with unequivocal, severe dementia, a review of the available clinical studies (Tables 1 and 2) before and after the advent of L-dopa, reveals an average prevalence of about 10% at a mean age of 65 years. This is approximately twice the prevalence of Alzheimer type senile dementia at this age in the normal population (Kay 1972). Most of these reports, however, are based on selected hospital populations, although in Rajput's broad-based population study, (Rajput et al. 1984), a comparable figure of 9% was reported.

Loss of neurones in the locus ceruleus and the nucleus basalis of Meynert occur in both Parkinson's disease and Alzheimer's disease (Table 3). Lewy bodies are the histological hallmark of Parkinson's disease and occur in all the pigmented brain stem nuclei, the nucleus basalis, the adrenal medulla, the sympathetic ganglia and even in the cerebral cortex of demented patients (Yoshimura

Table 1. Prevalence of severe dementia in Parkinsonian patients without L-dopa treatment

Authors	Patients (*n*)	Mean age (years)	Mean duration of disease (years)	Patients with dementia (%)
Mjönes (1949)	194	67	–	3.2
Pollock and Hornabrook (1966)	84	67	8	5
University College Hospital, London (Shaw et al. 1980)	172	63	7.5	11

Table 2. Prevalence of severe dementia in L-dopa-treated patients with Parkinson's disease

Author	Patients (*n*)	Mean age (years)	Mean duration of disease (years)	Patients with dementia (%)
Celesia and Wanamaker (1972)	153	65.8	8	7
Sweet et al. (1976)	41	72.0	16	14
Martilla and Rinne (1976)	444	67.9	7	14
Lieberman et al. (1979)	520	67.0	6.5	32
University College Hospital, London, (Shaw et al. 1980)	48	74,0	18,5	32
Mindham et al. (1982)	37	61.9	9	5
Rajput et al. (1984)	119	76.0		9

Table 3. Characteristic markers of Parkinson's and Alzheimer's disease

	Nucleus basalis cell numbers	CHAT activity (cortex and nucleus basalis of Meynert	Cortical neuritic plaque count	Histologic marker in nucleus basalis of Meynert
Parkinson's disease	↓↓↓	→ or ↓	±	Lewy body
Parkinson's disease with dementia	↓↓↓	↓	++	Lewy body
Alzheimer's disease	↓↓	↓↓↓	+++	Neurofibrillary tangle
Senile dementia of Alzheimer type	↓	↓↓	++	Neurofibrillary tangle

→, same; ↓, slight decrease; ↓↓, moderate decrease; ↓↓↓, severe decrease; ±, possible increase; ++, possible increase; +++, marked increase

1983). About 10% of patients with Alzheimer's disease have been reported to have brain stem Lewy bodies (Forno et al. 1978). In contrast, cortical neurofibrillary tangles and neuritic placques are histological lesions characteristic of Alzheimer's disease, and tangles may also be found in certain brain stem areas such as the nucleus basalis.

A number of retrospective clinicopathological studies have now been conducted on highly selective groups of parkinsonian patients, some of which have reported extremely high incidences of severe Alzheimer type histological abnormalities in the cerebral cortex (Table 4). However, the most recent study by Tomlinson and his group from Newcastle emphasised that Parkinson's disease and Alzheimer's disease are in most cases morphologically quite distinct and rejects the extremely high incidences of Alzheimer's disease changes reported by Hakim and Mathieson (1979) and Boller and colleagues (1980). Nevertheless, Tomlinson and his co-workers conclude that the histological abnormalities which characterise Alzheimer's disease and Parkinson's disease seem to occur together too frequently to be explained by chance. They also found that neuritic plaques are more

Table 4. Postmortem studies of patients with Parkinson's disease

Authors	*n*	Mean age (years)	Clinical evidence of dementia		Alzheimer type histologie abnormalities	
			Patients (%)	Controls (%)	Patients (%)	Controls (%)
Hakim and Mathieson (1979)	34	75	56	6	50	3
Boller et al. (1980)	36	71	55	5	42	5
Jellinger and Grissold (1982)	100	73	58	9	33	24

numerous in some patients with Parkinson's disease than in controls, even when the total changes typical of Alzheimer's disease are absent, and that this increased plaque formation, which is often found in elderly people who are intellectually normal, increases the chances for dementia in Parkinson's disease.

Although a severe loss of neurones in the nucleus basalis of Meynert occurs in Parkinson's disease with dementia (Whitehouse et al. 1983), a considerable decrease in cells is frequently seen in the absence of any clinical history of dementia (Nakano and Hirano (1984). Loss of choline acetyltransferase, a chemical marker for cholinergic neurones in the nucleus basalis of Meynert and the cerebral cortex, correlates well with the severity of intellectual deterioration in Alzheimer's disease (Perry et al. 1978). Similar correlations have been found in Parkinson's disease (Dubois et al. 1983). Candy et al. (1983), however, noted a substantial loss of nerve cells in the nucleus basalis of Meynert without consistent evidence of choline acetyltransferase loss, suggesting that the surviving neurones might be able to maintain function. They also postulated that in Alzheimer-type senile dementia, there may be a specific reduction in choline acetyltransferase synthesis in the region supplying the cholinergic afferents to the cortex rather than any primary loss of nucleus basalis neurones. It seems possible, therefore, that the cholinergic and noradrenergic depletions which occur in the affected ascending forebrain structures may be more important in determining the degree of intellectual dysfunction than either the nerve cell loss from the nucleus basalis of Meynert or the cortical changes characteristic of Alzheimer's disease. A reduction in intrinsic cortical somatostatin in demented parkinsonian patients has also been reported recently, providing a further similarity between the neurochemical abnormalities in demented parkinsonian patients and those afflicted with Alzheimer's disease (Epelbaum et al. 1983).

References

Adolfsson R, Gottfries CG, Roos BE, Winblad B (1979) Changes in the brain catecholamines in patients with dementia of Alzheimer type. Br J psychiatry 135:216–223

Agid Y, Ruberg M, Dubois B, Javoy-Agid F (1984) Biochemical substrates of mental disturbances in Parkinson's disease. In: Hassler RG, Christ JF (eds) Advances in neurology, vol 40. Raven, New York, pp 22–218

Albert ML (1978) Subcortical dementia. In: Katzman R, Terry RD, Rick KL (eds) Alzheimer's disease. Senile dementia and related disorders. Raven, New York, pp 173–180
Albert ML, Feldman RG, Willis AL (1974) The "subcortical dementia" of progressive supranuclear palsy. J Neurol Neurosurg Psychiatry 37:121–130
Alvord EC, Forno LS, Kusske JA, Kauffman RJ, Rhodes JS, Goetowsky CR (1974) The pathology of Parkinsonism: a comparison of degenerations in cerebral cortex and brain-stem. In: McDowell FH, Barbeau A (eds) Advances in Neurology, vol 5. Raven, New York, pp 175–193
Ball B (1882) De l'insanité dans la paralysie agitante. Encephale 2:22–32
Barbeau A (1973) Biology of the striatum. In: Gall GE (ed) Biology and brain dysfunction, vol 2. Plenum, New York, pp 333–350
Boller F, Mizutani J, Roessman U, Gambetti P (1980) Parkinson's disease, dementia and Alzheimer's disease: clilnico-pathological correlations. Ann Neurol 7:329–335
Bowen FP (1976) Behavioural alterations in patients with basal ganglia lesions. In: Yahr MD (ed) The basal ganglia. Raven, New York, pp 169–180
Bowen FP, Kamienny RS, Burns MM, Yahr MD (1975) Parkinsonism: effects of levodopa on concept formation. Neurology 25:701–704
Brown RG, Marsden CD, Quinn N, Wyke MA (1984) Alterations in cognitive performance and affect-arousal state during fluctuations in motor function in Parkinson's disease. J Neurol Neurosurg Psychiatry 47:454–465
Candy JM, Perry RH, Perry EK, Irving D, Blessed G, Fairbairn AF, Tomlinson BE (1983) Pathological changes in the nucleus of Meynert in Alzheimer's and Parkinson's diseases. J Neurol Sci 54:59, 277–289
Celesia GC, Wanamaker WM (1972) Psychiatric disturbances in Parkinson's disease. Dis Nerv Syst 33:577–583
Cools AR, Van den Bercken JHL, Horstink MWI, Van Spaendonck KPM, Berger HJC (1984) Cognitive and motor shifting aptitude disorder in Parkinson's disease. J Neurol Neurosurg Psychiatry 47:443–453
De Ajuriaguerra J (1971) Etude psychopathologique des parkinsoniens. In: De Ajuriaguerra J, Gauthier R (eds) Monoamines, noyaux gris centraux et syndromes parkinsoniens. Masson, Paris, pp 327–351
Delis D, Direnfeld L, Alexander MP, Kaplan E (1982) Cognitive fluctuations associated with on-off phenomenon in Parkinson disease. Neurology 32:1049–1052
Dubois B, Ruberg M, Javoy-Agid F, Ploska A, Agid Y (1983) A subcortico-cortical cholinergic system is affected in Parkinson's disease. Brain Res 288:213–218
Epelbaum J, Ruberg M, Moyse E, Javoy-Agid F, Dubois B, Agid Y (1983) Somatostatin and dementia in Parkinson's disease. Brain Res 278:376–379
Evarts EV, Teravainen H, Calne DB (1981) Reaction time in Parkinson's disease. Brain 104:167–186
Folstein MF, McHugh PR (1978) Dementia syndrome of depression. In: Katzman R, Terry RD, Bick KL (eds) Alzheimer's disease, senile dementia and related disorders. Ageing vol 7. Raven, New York, pp 87–93
Forno LS, Barbour PJ, Norville RL (1978) Presenile dementia with Lewy bodies and neurofibrillary tangles. Arch Neurol 35:818–822
Goodwin FK, Brodie HK, Murphy DL, Bunney WE (1970) Administration of a peripheral decarboxylase inhibitor with L-dopa to depressed patients. Lancet I:908–911
Hakim AM, Mathieson G (1979) Dementia in Parkinson's disease: a neuropathologic study. Neurology 29:1209–1214
Hardie RJ, Lees AJ, Stern GM (1984) On-off fluctuations in Parkinson's disease: a clinical and pharmacological study. Brain 107:487–506
Hassler R (1965) Extrapyramidal control of the speed of behaviour and its change by primary age processes. In: Welford AT, Birrin JT (eds) Behaviour ageing and the nervous system. Thomas, Springfield, pp 284–306
Jellinger K, Grissold W (1982) Cerebral atrophy in Parkinson's syndrome. Exp. Brain Res [Suppl] 5:26–35
Jouvent R, Abensour P, Bonnet AM, Widlocher D, Agid Y, L'Hermitte F (1983) Antiparkinsonian and antidepressant effects of high doses of bromocriptine. J Affective Disord 5:141–145

Kay DWK (1972) Epidemiological aspects of organic brain disease in the aged. In: Galtz CM (ed) Ageing and the brain. Plenum, New York, pp 15–27
Laplane D, Bavlac M, Widlocher D, Dubois B (1984) Pure psychic akinesia with bilateral lesions of basal ganglia. J Neurol Neurosurg Psychiatry 47:377–385
Lebensohn ZM, Jenkins RB (1975) Improvement of Parkinsonism in depressed patients treated with ECT. Am J Psychiatry 132:283–285
Lees AJ, Smith E (1983) Cognitive deficits in the early stages of Parkinson's disease. Brain 106:257–270
Lieberman A, Dziatolowski M, Kupersmith M, Serby M, Goodgold A, Korein J, Goldstein M (1979) Dementia in Parkinson's disease. Ann Neurol 6:355–359
Loranger AW, Goodell H, McDowell FH, Lee JE, Sweet RD (1972) Intellectual impairment in Parkinson's syndrome. Brain 95:405–412
Marttilla RJ, Rinne UK (1976) Dementia in Parkinson's disease. Acta Neurol Scand 54:431–441
Matison R, Mayeux R, Rosen J, Fahn S (1982) "Tip of the tongue" phenomenon in Parkinson's disease. Neurology 32:567–570
Mayeux R, Stern Y, Rosen J, Leventhal J (1981) Depression, intellectual impairment and Parkinson's disease. Neurology 31:645–650
McHugh PR, Folstein MF (1975) Psychiatric syndromes of Huntington's chorea. A clinical and phenomenologic study. In: Benson DF, Blumer D (eds) Psychiatric aspects of neurologic disease. Grune and Stratton, New York, pp 267–288
Mettler FA (1955) Perceptual capacity, functions of the corpus striatum and schizophrenia. Psychiatr Q 29:89–111
Mjönes H (1949) Paralysis agitans, a clinical and genetic study. Acta Psychiatr Neurol Scand [Suppl] 54:1–195
Mortimer JA, Pirozzolo FJ, Hansch EC, Webster DD (1982) Relationship of motor symptoms to intellectual deficits in Parkinson disease. Neurology 32:133–137
Nakano I, Hirano A (1984) Parkinon's disease: neuron loss in the nucleus basalis without concomitant Alzheimer's disease. Ann Neurol 15:415–418
Naville F (1922) Etude sur les complications et les séquelles mentales de l'encephalite épidémique. La bradyphrénie. Encephalé 17:369–375, 424–436
Pearce J (1974) The extrapyramidal disorder of Alzheimer's disease. Eur Neurol 12:94–103
Pearce JMS, Flowers K, Pearce I, Pratt AE (1981) Clinical, psychometric and CAT scan correlations in Parkinson's disease. In: Rose FC, Capildeo R (eds) Research progress in Parkinson's disease. Pitman Medical, London, pp 43–52
Perry EK, Tomlinson BE, Blessed G, Bergmann K, Gibson PH, Perry RH (1978) Correlation of cholinergic abnormalities with senile plaques and mental test scores in senile dementia. Br Med J 2:1457–1459
Pollock M, Hornabrook RW (1966) The prevalence, natural history and dementia of Parkinson's disease. Brain 89:429–448
Rajput AH, Offord K, Beard CM, Kurland LT (1984) Epidemiological survey of dementia in parkinsonism and control population. In: Hassler RG, Christ JF (eds) Adv Neurol, vol 40. Raven, New York, pp 229–234
Robins AH (1976) Depression in patients with Parkinsonism. Br J Psychiatry 128:141–145
Rossor MN (1981) Parkinson's disease and Alzheimer's disease as disorders of the isodentritic core. Br Med J 283:1588–1590
Selby G (1968) Cerebral atrophy in parkinsonism. J Neurol Sci 6:517–559
Sharpe MH, Cermak SA, Sax DS (1983) Motor planning in Parkinsonian patients. Neuropsychologia 21:455–462
Shaw KM, Lees AJ, Stern GM (1980) The impact of treatment with levodopa on Parkinson's disease. Q J Med 49:283–293
Sroka H, Elizan TS, Yahr MD, Burger A, Mendoza MR (1981) Organic mental syndrome and confusional states in Parkinson's disease. Arch Neurol 38:339–342
Steck H (1931) Les syndromes mentaux postencéphalitiques. Schweiz Arch Neurol Psychiatry 27:137–173
Sweet RD, McDowell FH, Feigenson HS, Loranger AW, Goodell H (1976) Mental symptoms in Parkinson's disease during crhonig treatment with levodopa. Neurology 26:305–310

Todes CJ, Lees AJ (1985) The pre-morbid personality of patients with Parkinson's disease. J Neurol Neurosurg Psychiatry (J. Neurol. Neurosurg. Psychiat.)

Van Praag HMV, Korf J, Lakke JPWF, Schut T (1975) Dopamine metabolism in depressions, psychoses and Parkinson's disease: the problem of the specificity of biological variables in behaviour disorders. Psychol Med 5:138–146

Warburton JW (1967) Memory disturbance and the Parkinson syndrome. Br J Med Psychol 40:169–171

Whitehouse PJ, Price DL, Clark AW, Coyle JT, De Long MR (1981) Alzheimer's disease: evidence for selective loss of cholinergic neurons in the *nucleus basalis*. Ann Neurol 10:122–126

Whitehouse PJ, Hedreen JC, White CL, Price DL (1983) Basal forebrain neurons in the dementia of Parkinson's disease. Ann Neurol 13:243–248

Wilson RS, Kaszniak AW, Klawans HL, Garron DC (1980) High speed memory scanning in Parkinsonism. Cortex 16:67–72

Wilson SAK (1940) In: Bruce AN (ed) Neurology. Chapter VIII, epidemic encephalitis. Arnold, London, pp 120, 132

Worster-Drought C, Hardcastle DN (1924) A contribution to the psychopathology of residual encephalitis lethargica. J Neurol Psychopathol 5:146–150

Yoshimura M (1983) Cortical changes in the parkinsonian brain: a contribution to the delineation of diffuse Lewy body disease. J Neurol 229:17–32

Differential Diagnosis: Depression Versus Dementia*

J. R. M. Copeland and M. E. Dewey[1]

Introduction

Post (1951) and Roth and Morrisey (1952) drew attention to the importance of distinguishing between depressive illness and dementia in hospital samples of elderly persons aged over 65. They pointed to the difficulty of making the distinction and its important prognostic implications. Kramer (1961) had reported differences between the diagnostic frequencies for first admissions of the elderly to US state hospitals and Area mental hospitals in England and Wales. Organic disorders appeared to be almost twice as frequent among US admissions than UK admissions, in contrast to functional disorders, which comprised only about one-sixth of the proportion entering the UK hospitals. Kramer was concerned that numbers of functional disorders, particularly depression, were being diagnosed as organic disorders in American hospitals. The available statistics also showed that patients admitted to US hospitals were twice as likely to die in the hospital within 1 year of admission than those admitted to British hospitals, while British elderly patients appeard three times more likely than their US counterparts to be discharged within 1 year.

The US/UK Cross-national (Diagnostic) Project set out to explore this difference by examining consecutive series of admissions of elderly subjects from designated catchment areas to psychiatric hospitals serving New York and London, using standardised methods of psychiatric examination. The project found that, apart from a tendency for there to be more organic cases in the New York sample, the differences between the project diagnoses were not significant. However, the differences between the hospital diagnoses on the same patients were almost as great as those of the national statistics (Copeland et al. 1975). We were therefore able to conclude that differences in national statistics were not due to different illness characteristics of the patients but rather to descrepancies in the diagnostic criteria used by the psychiatrists.

When these patients were followed up with the same measures 3 months after the initial interview, the disputed cases in New York, i.e. those with hospital diagnoses of organic disorder but project diagnoses of affective disorder, had an outcome similar to those patients described by both hospital and project as having an affective disorder.

* The AGECAT system was developed with funds from the World Health Organization and the Mersey Regional Research Committee

1 University Department of Psychiatry Royal Liverpool Hospital, P.O. Box 147, Liverpool L69 3BX, UK

Senile Dementia of the Alzheimer Type
Ed. by J. Traber and W. H. Gispen

The method of examination included the Geriatric Mental State (GMS), which allowed for the calculation of symptom profiles. When the mean symptom profiles of the disputed cases were compared with those of the patients consistently diagnosed as having affective disorders, certain differences appeared. The disputed cases followed closely the profile for the undisputed cases except for high levels of "paranoid symptoms" and "observed belligerence", where patients were hostile, angry and sometimes abusive to the interviewer. The project was able to conclude that patients exhibiting these types of symptoms were likely to be misdiagnosed in the New York hospitals (Gurland et al. 1976). However, the outcome of these misdiagnosed patients was similar to that of the patients with undisputed diagnoses of affective disorders because the New York hospital psychiatrists, in spite of making the diagnosis of orgnaic disorder, treated these patients for depressive symptoms with antidepressants, and they recovered. Nevertheless, it is by no means certain that this treatment would always be given to such a misdiagnosed patient.

Our subsequent studies on community samples indicate that, given adequate examination of history and mental state, most cases of depression and dementia in this age group can be distinguished, but that, even with the greatest care, errors can still be made which are only revealed by outcome. At the same time, it is easy to understand why the distinction between depression and dementia may be a difficult one. It is well known that, in the elderly, physical and psychiatric illnesses tend to coexist. Depressive mood and even depressive illness are not infrequently reactions to physical illness. Patients with early chronic organic brain disease may be expected to react to failing cognitive ability by developing neurotic-type depression or dysthymic disorder. An organic illness also constitutes an unpleasant life event, and such events are known to precede cases of depressive psychosis or major affective disorder. Tumors directly invading brain tissue are also known to be associated with depressive illness. It is therefore not unreasonable that multi-infarct dementia, where small areas of the brain are destroyed, might also precipitate depression. Finally, depression itself, when accompanied by slowing of thought, may simulate dementia, resulting in so-called pseudodementia.

Geriatric Mental State Schedule

We have tried to tackle the task of differential diagnosis as part of the general problem of standardising the recording of mental state and diagnosis for research. For the hospital studies, the US/UK Cross-national Project developed the Geriatric Mental State referred to above (Copeland et al. 1976; Gurland et al. 1976). The project had already gained experience of standardised, semi-structured interviews to determine mental state by using the Present State Examination (Wing et al. 1974) and the Psychiatric Status Schedule (Spitzer et al. 1970). The GMS was constructed using items taken from both interviews to which a substantial number of new items dealing mainly with cognitive and other symptoms of organic disorders were added. Many existing items were simplified and rearranged for the elderly; new rating instructions were provided and a new manual prepared. A series of "boxed items" cover important areas of pathology early in the interview, thus allowing it to be discontinued if indicated by the patient's mental state.

For use with community samples, a shortened form of the GMS excluding many of the psychotic items and adding some minor symptoms was embedded in a more comprehensive interview, the CARE (Gurland et al. 1983), covering physical disorders, social problems and service needs and delivery. Reliability studies between medical interviewers were undertaken and shown to be satisfactory (Copeland et al. 1976).

Limited and Pervasive Depression and Dementia

To record mental state reliably is one thing, but to arrive at a reliable diagnosis based on these recordings is another. In our earlier studies, the medical interviewer made an intuitive diagnosis according to the guidelines of the World Health Orgnaization Glossary of Mental Disorders (World Health Organization 1978). However, for the project's comparative community studies of the prevalence of mental illness in New York and London, it was necessary to standardise the method of diagnosis used; this was done by constructing an algorithm for depression and dementia. This system, which it was possible to apply immediately after the interview, also provided for degrees of severity in the illnesses by incorporating behavioural items from the CARE interview. Through scoring based on five levels of severity, subjects are allotted to categories designated noncase, limited depression or dementia and pervasive depression or dementia. Pervasive dementia is assumed to follow a progressively declining course if intervention is not effective, while pervasive depression is assumed to warrant treatment for the psychiatric disturbance. Subjects with limited dementia and depression have symptoms which do not dominate their lives.

A subsequent comparison showed good agreement between this method and cases diagnosed as dementia and major affective disorder according to the criteria of the Diagnostic and Statistical Manual (DSM) III (American Psychiatric Association 1980). The terms and definitions are, however, more precise than those of DSM III, which we have found difficult to apply in practice. Using the pervasive/limited method, described in detail elsewhere (Gurland et al. 1983), we were able to demonstrate a clear distinction between dementia and depression, which was subsequently confirmed after 1 year. Levels of pervasive depression in New York reached 13% compared with a prevalence of 12.4% in London. However, with a prevalence of 4.9% pervasive dementia was shown to be twice as common in New York as in London, where it has a prevalence of 2.3%. A subsequent study of subjects in institutional care (Gurland et al. 1979) only served to confirm the higher proportion of organic disorders in New York. The pervasive/limited diagnosis can therefore be useful for research: however, it relies on the use of the CARE interview, which is more comprehensive than is generally required by studies concerned with achieving a psychiatric diagnosis for comparison with other measures.

AGECAT: A Computerised Diagnostic System

Recently, we have completed the first stage of a computerised diagnostic system, AGECAT, based on the items comprising the GMS, its shorter community version the GMSA and the CARE interview. Such a computerised system provides a reliable method for comparing the diagnostic composition of different study populations and for examining the consistency of individual diagnostic practice. However, it suffers from the disadvantage of not being usable until the data are entered into the computer. With new advances in portable computers, direct data entry will overcome this problem.

Computerised diagnostic systems for younger subjects, Catego (Wing et al. 1974) and Diagno (Spitzer et al. 1970), have existed for some time; AGECAT uses a somewhat different system. It condenses the 541 items of the GMS into approximately 150 symptoms, which are in turn condensed into 31 symptom groups, not simply on the basis of clinical clustering but according to the importance of their contribution in arriving at an overall diagnosis of a particular syndrome. These groups are then further combined to form levels of confidence in the diagnosis, ranging from 0 to 5 in most instances, for eight diagnostic clusters. The levels of confidence are then compared level for level according to a hierarchy of diagnoses extending from organic to anxiety, to produce a main diagnosis, subsidiary and alternative diagnoses if appropriate, as well as the levels of confidence for the eight diagnostic clusters. Clinical judgement only was used to develop each stage

Table 1. Items of Geriatric Mental State (GMS) forming the symptom components of the organic groups in AGECAT

Group A	Moderate memory disturbance and time disorientation
	Muddled thinking
	Memory for interviewer's name on second occasion
	Knowledge of current month
	Knowledge of current year
	Knowledge of prime minister's name
	Identification of objects
	Discrepancy between stated birthdate and age
	Bland about and indifferent to errors
	Perseveration
Group B	Mild memory disturbance
	Memory for interviewer's name on first occasion
	Rater's opinion of memory
	Knowledge of how long living at present address
	Evasive
Group C	Place and person disorientation and organic thought disorder
	Disorientation of person
	Confabulation
	Disorientation of place (only included if severe or if the items relating to prime minister's name or indifference to errors have already been positively scored)
	Rambling (only included if group A score is higher than 4 and group B score is higher than 1)

of AGECAT. When the AGECAT levels are compared with the psychiatrists' diagnoses of the same patients, levels 3 and above seem to accord well with the psychiatrists' concept of "a case." We have discussed the concept of "a case" elsewhere (Copeland 1981; Copeland et al. to be published). At this stage, we call cases "syndrome cases," implying no more than that the symptoms cluster in a

Table 2. Summary of items of Geriatric Mental State Schedule (GMS) forming the symptom components of the depressive groups in AGECAT

Group A	Mood
	Depressed mood admitted
	Crying
	Looks or sounds depressed
	Depression lasting longer than a few hours
Group B	Nonspecific symptoms
	Loss of concentration
	Loss of interest (3 items)
	Loss of enjoyment
	Tension, worries, irritability, headache (4 items)
	Subjective slowing of movement and thought (3 items)
	Guilt and morbid self-blame (2 items)
	Avoids people and feels upset by certain relationships (2 items)
	Lack of energy
	Mislays objects
	Indecisiveness
	Suicidal feelings
Group C	Characteristic of neurotic, reactive depression or dysthmic mood
	Feels worse, lack of energy in the evening (2 items)
	Difficulty getting to sleep
	Depersonalization
	Lonely
	Autonomic symptoms
Group D	Symptoms denoting severity
	Pessimistic about own future
	Wish to be dead
	Feeling worthless
	Suicidal plan or attempt
Group E	Characteristic of psychotic, endogenous depression or major affective disorder
	Severe appetite and weight loss
	Observed slowness of movement and speech (2 items)
	Mood and slowness worst in the morning (2 items)
	Early morning wakening
	Unable to cry
	Severely muddled thinking
	Monotonous voice
	Reduction in sexual interest
Group F	Delusions and hallucinations
	Depressive-type delusions (3 items)
	Mood-consistent auditory and visual hallucinations (2 items)
	Delusions and hallucinations believed to be deserved (3 items)

form recognised by the psychiatrist as similar to those of an illness. Syndrome cases would include, for example, bereavement reactions, although these would be recognised as such later in the procedure. The AGECAT system, whereby the symptoms of each subject are related to a level of confidence for the eight diagnostic clusters, allows for the recording of concurrent syndromes. For example, a patient may reach level 3 on the organic cluster and level 4 on the depressive cluster. This allows concurrent syndromes to be identified even though the overall AGECAT diagnosis may be one of depression. Table 1 lists symptoms forming the groups of the organic cluster while Table 2 shows symptoms constituting the depressive cluster. It is then possible to examine the degree of concordance between the psychiatrists' and AGECAT diagnoses of depression and dementia for the same patients.

Distinction Between Depression and Dementia on AGECAT Diagnosis

Three studies provide the data for the comparisons described below. The first examined a consecutive series of admissions to mental hospitals serving a designated area in London. Using the Geriatric Mental State, a standardised history and demographic schedule, 75 patients were interviewed within 72 h of admission. They were followed up in hospital or at home 3 months after the initial interview. For the second study, a random series of 75 patients entering a geriatric hospital serving the same area were similarly examined (Copeland et al. 1975). For the third study, 396 randomly selected community subjects living in Greater London were interviewed, using the CARE schedule. Of this group, 60% were reinterviewed 1 year later. The subjects had been located through a random sampling of general practitioners serving Greater London and through a further random sampling of their lists of patients over the age of 65. In all three studies, the subjects were over 65 years of age, and all interviews were conducted by psychiatrists employed full time on the Cross-national Project. For the community studies, a case of mental illness was defined as illness sufficiently severe to warrant professional intervention. The results have been reported in more detail elsewhere (Copeland et al. to be published).

Results

Table 3 shows the degree of accordance between psychiatrists' diagnoses and AGECAT for all 541 subjects in the hospital and community samples. Data on five subjects in the geriatric hospital were removed because these subjects were unfit to be interviewed using the GMS, due to physical illness.

It is apparent from this table that the psychiatrists agree with the AGECAT diagnosis in 91% of the organic cases and that AGECAT agrees with the psychiatrists in 82% of their cases. Five of the six psychiatrists' diagnoses designated noncases by AGECAT reached level 2 (borderline) on the AGECAT levels of confidence. Eight psychiatrists diagnoses of organic disorder are designated as depression by AGECAT; these are examined further.

Table 3. Concordance between diagnoses of psychiatrists and of AGECAT for 541 subjects in hospital and community samples (expressed as percentages)

Psychiatrists diagnosis	AGECAT diagnosis				
	Organic	Depression	Other	Noncase	
Organic	64 (91%)	8		6	78
Depression	1	94 (73%)		10	105
Other	1	7	17 (81%)	17	42
Noncase	4	19	4	289 (90%)	316
	70	128	21	322	541

With regard to the diagnosis of depression, the psychiatrists agree on 73% of the AGECAT cases. This lower level of agreement can be explained. Of the cases of depression diagnosed by AGECAT, the psychiatrists considered 19 to be noncases. Six of these are in the geriatric hospital. Five were found to be suffering from severe, crippling physical illness. A review of their case summaries and interview schedules revealed a substantial number of depressive symptoms for each. It is likely that the interviewing psychiatrists regarded these depressive symptoms as a normal or "justifiable" reaction to severe physical illness and consequently rated them as "not cases of mental illness requiring intervention." This is however an assumption which could be challenged. The remaining 13 cases are found in the community sample. They are not "justifiable depressions" but, in contrast, are physically healthy individuals who, on the evidence of their case summaries, had suffered severe mood swings over a number of years, each episode lasting from several hours to several days. The interviewing psychiatrists were probably correct in not designating these subjects as cases of mental illness, but the AGECAT system will have to await the incorporation of historical data before such subjects can be distinguished. In all, AGECAT agrees with 90% of the psychiatrists' diagnoses of depression. Of the ten psychiatrists' cases AGECAT describes as noncases, eight are in the community, all have depressive neurosis and all denied the presence of depressive mood. AGECAT has a mechanism for recording cases of depressive illness in which mood is denied, but these subjects did not reach the case threshold.

In order to illustrate the extent of disagreement for the disputed diagnoses of organic disorder, Table 4 shows the distribution of disputed psychiatrists' and

Table 4. Distribution of disputed cases of organic disorders on AGECAT levels for community and hospital samples ($n=541$)

	AGECAT levels of confidence (organic)						
	0	1	2	3	4	5	total sample
Disputed diagnoses of psychiatrists ($n=14$)	2		6	6			76
Disputed AGECAT diagnoses ($n=5$)			0	4	1		70

Table 5. Outcome of organic cases in community and psychiatric hospital sample ($n=471$)

	AGECAT levels				
	0–2	3–5	para-noid	depres-sion	too ill to be interviewed
Undisputed organic diagnoses					
dementia ($n=25$)	1	20	1		3
acute confusional state ($n=7$)	4	1	2		
Disputed psychiatrists' diagnoses					
dementia ($n=4$)	1	2		1	
acute confusional state ($n=2$)				2	
Disputed AGECAT diagnoses					
dementia ($n=2$)		2			
acute confusional state ($n=1$)	1				

Division into dementia and acute confusional state made on the basis of psychiatrists' diagnosis

AGECAT diagnoses on the AGECAT levels of confidence. Disputed diagnoses would be expected to cluster around the borderline levels, thus reflecting the difficult decision between case and noncase for some subjects. Table 4 shows this to hold true for the organic disorders, where most of the disputed diagnoses cluster in levels of confidence 2 and 3. Of the eight above-mentioned cases diagnosed by psychiatrists as organic disorder and by AGECAT as depression, six also achieved level 3 on the AGECAT organic cluster. Thus, these are patients with a substantial proportion of both severe depressive and organic symptoms. Unfortunately, it is not possible to examine the outcome of these disputed cases. Nearly all fell into the geriatric sample, where interviewers were faced with the additional problem of distinguishing psychiatric from normal cases. Nevertheless, Table 5 shows the outcome of the organic cases in the psychiatric hospital and community samples of 471 subjects. Although the data are not strictly comparable (the psychiatric hospital sample was followed up after 3 months, while the community sample was followed up after 1 year, they are grouped together for the sake of convenience. As AGECAT does not yet identify dementia and acute confusional states within the organic group, these subdivisions are made using the pschiatrists' diagnosis. As anticipated, the majority of cases of dementia still have AGECAT confidence levels of between three and five at follow-up and that six of seven acute confusional states no longer have AGECAT organic case levels at this time. As far as the disputed cases are concerned, both the psychiatrists and AGECAT can apparently claim to have made correct initial diagnoses in two cases each.

Table 6 shows a similar distribution on AGECAT levels of confidence for the disputed diagnoses of depression, where the disputed psychiatrists' diagnoses tend not to cluster around the borderline. All the disputed diagnoses of depression were designated to be depressive neurosis, except for one case of depressive psychosis. For the latter, no symptoms are recorded, and it must be assumed the illness was so severe that the interview had to be abandoned. It is likely that the interviewer forgot to make the appropriate explanatory rating. The rest are nearly all cases in which the patient denied his depressive mood and had few other

Table 6. Distribution of disputed cases of depression on AGECAT levels in community and hospital samples ($n=541$)

	AGECAT levels of confidence (depression)						
	0	1	2	3	4	5	total sample
Disputed psychiatrists' diagnoses ($n=11$)	4	3	3	1			105
Disputed AGECAT diagnoses ($n=34$)				31	2	1	128

Table 7. Outcome of depression cases in community and psychiatric hospital sample ($n=471$)

	AGECAT levels		Inconsistent diagnoses		Consistent diagnoses	
	0–2	3–5	organic	paranoid	manic	neurotic
Undisputed diagnoses ($n=53$)	35	11	3		1	3
Disputed psychiatrists' diagnoses ($n=6$)	5	1				
Disputed AGECAT diagnoses ($n=16$)	6	7	2	1		

recorded symptoms. Three of the patients attaining confidence level scores of 0 had summaries indicating that, while they suffered from mood changes, they were otherwise active people with a wide range of interests at the time of examination. It would thus seem likely that the psychiatrists were incorrect in designating these as cases. Of the 34 disputed AGECAT diagnoses, 31 are on the borderline, including patients with "justifiable" depression in the geriatric hospital and subjects with mood swings in the community. Here, AGECAT is capable of identifying syndrome cases of depression, though not yet of dividing them into those requiring or not requiring professional intervention. It should be emphasised that substantial numbers of depressive symptoms were recorded for all these subjects.

Table 7 shows the 3-month outcome for the depression cases included in the psychiatric hospital and community samples. It may be noted that almost three-quarters of the undisputed diagnoses are either no longer considered cases at follow-up or are judged to be unchanged with respect to the original diagnosis. Seven of the disputed AGECAT cases still achieve case levels of depression. AGECAT is probably correct in these diagnoses. At least three of the undisputed diagnoses of depression had become organic cases 3 months later. These cases were not identified by either the psychiatrists or AGECAT in the initial interview.

On the whole, the concordance between psychiatrists' and AGECAT diagnoses is probably higher than that reached in reliability studies comparing diagnoses made by psychiatrists among themselves. The majority of the remaining cases where there is a lack of agreement will not be resolved until historical information is incorporated into the AGECAT system. Measures for doing this are being tested at present.

In the total sample of 541 subjects, there were 24 cases in which AGECAT case levels of depression were accompanied by "borderline case" levels (levels 2 or 3) or organic disorder. AGECAT agreed reasonably well with the psychiatrists on whether to regard these as cases of depression or organic disorder. It is worth noting that, in the eight cases of dementia with high depression levels, all symptoms of depression had resolved at follow-up, leaving only organic levels.

Case-Finding Interview for Depression and Dementia (GMSA)

We are currently developing a case-finding measure of depression, dementia and other psychiatric disorders in elderly subjects. This instrument, called the GMSA, was developed from the data on the 396 randomly selected community subjects in London over the age of 65 interviewed by psychiatrists. A series of linear discriminant function analyses were undertaken between diagnoses of depression, dementia and other disorders and between these and noncases. Items selected by the discriminant scores as well as those considered important for diagnosis were used to construct the case-finding interview, which was then applied to a random community sample of 1,077 subjects aged over 65 in Liverpool, who were interviewed by trained, nonpsychiatric interviewers. Depression and dementia scores based on the London community sample were developed. Cases of depression were designated as those scoring 18 or above, while cases involving organic disorders were those attaining scores of four or above. Using these scores, 192 subjects diagnosed as cases of depression and dementia and a proportion of noncases; have so far been reinterviewed "blind" by psychiatrists. Table 8 summarizes data for the 192 subjects to compare case level scores achieved on the GMSA as given by psychiatrists; with their diagnoses after having administered the GMSA, an interview for historical and onset data and an interview for early behavioural change. Table 8 makes clear that sensitivity and specificity reached satisfactory

Table 8. GMSA case finding based on preliminary analysis of 192 interviews by psychiatrists in subjects' own homes[a]

Category	Sensitivity (%)	Specificity (%)
Depression score $\geqq 18$	96	88
Dementia score $\geqq 4$		
Cases	100	72
Borderline cases	90	72

[a] Includes cases of depression, organic disorders and a random selection of noncases interviewed blind. Cutting scores on the GMSA compared with the diagnoses made by psychiatrists at the time of interview using GMSA, history interview and behaviour-change interview with informant

levels. Borderline dementia cases are also included, as investigators may wish to identify these. Further analyses will match psychiatrists' diagnoses against the selection of cases on the basis of scores achieved on the initial interviews given by the trained nonpsychiatrists. The lowest level of specificity, 72%, would be acceptable for a two-stage case identification procedure, where the inclusion of some noncases (false-positives) would be acceptable. Further refinement of this procedure is being undertaken on urban and rural samples.

Acknowledgements. We wish to acknowledge the help of H. Griffiths-Jones with the analysis.

References

American Psychiatric Association (1980) Diagnostic and statistical manual of mental disorders (DSM III) 3rd edn. American Psychiatric Association, Washington DC

Copeland JRM (1981) What is a case, a case for what? In: Wing JK, Bebbington P, Robbins LN (eds) What is a case, the problems of definition in psychiatric community surveys. Grant McIntyre, London

Copeland JRM, Kelleher MJ, Kellett JM, Gourlay AJ, Barron G, Cowan DW, De Gruchy J, Gurland BJ, Sharpe L, Simon R, Kuriansky J, Stiller P (1975) Cross-national study of diagnosis of the mental disorders: a comparison of the diagnosis of elderly psychiatric patients admitted to mental hospitals serving Queens County in New York and the Old Borough of Camberwell, London. Br J Psychiatry 126:11–20

Copeland JRM, Kelleher MJ, Kellett JM, Gourlay AJ, Gurland BJ, Fleiss JL, Sharpe L (1976) A semistructured clinical interview for the assessment of diagnosis and mental state in the elderly. The Geriatric Mental State Schedule 1. Development and reliability. Psychol Med 6:439–449

Copeland JRM, Dewey ME, Griffiths-Jones H (to be published) The development and preliminary assessment of a computerised psychiatric diagnostic system for elderly subjects: GMS and AGECAT

Gurland BJ, Fleiss JL, Goldberg K, Sharpe L, Copeland JRM, Kelleher MJ, Kellett JM (1976) A semistructured clinical interview for the assessment of diagnosis and mental state in the elderly. The Geriatric Mental State Schedule 2. A factor analysis. Psychol Med 6:451–459

Gurland BJ, Kuriansky JB, Sharpe L, Simon RJ, Stiller PR, Fleiss JL (US) with Copeland JRM, Kelleher MJ, Gourlay AJ, Cowan DW, Barron G (UK) (1976) A comparison of the outcome of hospitalisation of geriatric patients in public psychiatric words in New York and London. Can Psychiatr Assoc J 21:421–431

Gurland BJ, Cross P, Defiguerido J, Shannon M, Mann AM, Jenkin R, Bennett R, Wilder D, Wright H, Killeffer E, Godlove C (1979) A cross-national comparison of the institutionalized elderly in the cities of New York and London. Psychol Med 9:781–788

Gurland BJ, Copeland JRM, Kelleher MJ, Kuriansky J, Sharpe L, Dean L (1983) The mind and mood of ageing: the mental health problems of the community elderly in New York and London. Haworth, New York

Kramer M (1961) Some problems for international research suggested by observations on difference in first admission rates to the mental hospitals of England, Wales and the United States. In: Proceedings of the Third World Congress of Psychiatry, vol 3. Montreal, pp 153–160

Post F (1951) The outcome of mental breakdown in old age. Br Med J 1:436–448

Roth M, Morrissey JD (1952) Problems in the diagnosis and classification of mental disorders in old age. J Ment Sci 98:66–80

Spitzer RL, Endicott J, Fleiss JL, Cohen J (1970) Psychiatric status schedule: a technique for evaluating psychopathology and impairment in role functioning. Arch Gen Psychiatr 23:41–55

Wing JK, Cooper JE, Sartorios N (1974) The description and classification of psychiatric symptoms: an instruction manual for the PSE and Catego System. Cambridge University Press, London

World Health Organization (1978) Mental disorders: glossary and guide to their classification in accordance with the Ninth Revision of the International Classification of Disorders. WHO, Geneva

Early Diagnosis of Dementia: Possible Contributions of Neuropsychology

J. JOLLES[1]

Introduction

Assessment of the very early stages of senile dementia appears to be of relevance for several reasons. First, it is important to differentiate between "normal" aging and various psychiatric and neurologic diseases, with a view toward possible intervention in the disease process through biological (drugs) and nonbiological (training, psychotherapy) methods. Treatment in an earlier stage of the disease process can be expected to be more successful in view of the less pronounced structural changes. There is some evidence in favor of this hypothesis with respect to treatment with vasopressin-like neuropeptides (e.g., Jolles 1983). Secondly, in the very early stages of senile dementia, the profile of behavioral, emotional, and cognitive deficits the patient exhibits may give some clue as to the cause of the disease or diseases and their pathogenesis.

Unfortunately, diagnostic aids contributing to early assessment are scarce. This paper therefore aims at providing some information on paradigms and methods presently used in assessing dementia and on the kind of insight they may provide on the nature of the aging and dementing process. In addition, the current understanding of behavioral and cognitive dysfunctions in aging and dementia is reviewed.

Neuropsychology of Aging and Dementia

Aging

Recent reviews of cognitive functions in elderly subjects show that there is an age-associated decline in nearly all cognitive functions tested (Jolles and Hijman 1983; Botwinnick 1981), The "normal" aging subject is characterized by a decrease in intellectual functioning, memory, language functions, problem-solving ability, and perception. However, it appears that certain behavioral functions are more affected than others. For instance, old people are not inferior in tasks in which they can rely on well-stored skills and knowledge. Characteristically, aspects of motor performance which have been trained for many years and which have become automatic do not deteriorate as much as the ability to learn new movement patterns. In addition, expressive language does not seem to decline with age. With respect to memory functions, recall memory is affected more than recognition

1 Psychiatric University Clinic; Nicolaas Beetsstraat 24; 3511 HG Utrecht; The Netherlands

Senile Dementia of the Alzheimer Type
Ed. by J. Traber and W. H. Gispen

memory, indicating that active encoding and retrieval processes are affected more than passive recognition.

Old people perform worse on tasks that require the processing of new information. This is especially the case in situations in which the planning of new activities is important or the active use of coding strategies (e.g., "memory aids") in working memory. The term "mild senescent forgetfulness" is used to describe the developing inefficiency in the consolidation of new information. Characteristic complaints are difficulties in remembering names and recent events and the increasing effort required to remember things which happened many years ago. In addition to this sometimes handicapping memory deficit, there is a tendency towards inflexibility, cautiousness, and conservatism; more effort is needed to change an opinion. With respect to perceptual processes, incoming sensory input seems to persist for a longer period of time and sometimes results in an increased "iconic memory." This "stimulus persistence" interferes with the consolidation of new information: this is a case of the proactive inhibition often seen in elderly people (Botwinnick 1981). The general rate of information processing decreases. This slowness in perception, thinking, and response planning can manifest itself as a memory deficit; when environmental stimuli change rapidly in time, only a limited number can be held in the working memory long enough to be consolidated into long-term memory.

Neuropsychologically, a clear pattern is visible in the cognitive deficits of normal aging. One common element is a link between aspects of cognitive functioning and frontal-lobe functioning. In this view, stimulus persistence, proactive interference, lack of behavioral planning, deficient memory search, and other deficits can all indicate less efficient frontal-lobe functioning (Luria 1973, 1980; Fuster 1980). Interestingly, there is morphological evidence that areas in the frontal lobes degenerate already in people aged 40–50 (Haug this volume). With respect to memory consolidation, limbic areas on the hippocampal and diencephalic levels must be involved (Newcombe 1980; Luria 1980). It remains to be seen whether a general decrease in the rate of information processing is specifically related to the ascending fiber system, according to a hypothesis based on Luria's model of brain-behavior relationships (1973, 1980).

Senile Dementia

No evidence has been found until now that the pattern of cognitive deficits typical of senile dementia of the Alzheimer type (SDAT) is different from that seen in "normal" aging (see Jolles and Hijman 1983), especially with respect to the earlier stages of the dementia. The performance of demented subjects is significantly inferior to that of age-matched controls on all functions tested, but the deficits of the former exhibit no distinct pattern. Thus, more or less profound deterioration is found with respect to perception, memory, language, higher cognitive functions, planning, rate of information processing, and other cognitive functions (Jolles and Hijman 1983; Miller 1981). Along with the deficits seen in normal subjects, SDAT patients also reveal diminished capabilities with respect to recognition memory and verbal IQ measures, which stay at a fairly constant level in normal aging. Interestingly, clear differences seem to exist in the pattern of cognitive deficits seen in other types of dementia. For instance, the (pre) senile dementia of the Pick type shows especially pronounced behavioral disturbances and deficits in the planning and organisation of behavior. These deficits are characteristic of dysfunctions of the frontal lobe. Incidentally, these frontal signs are much more pronounced than in the normal aging process which was discussed in the preceding section. This neuropsychological interpretation is in line with current knowledge on the cerebral substrate of Pick's disease, which appears to be a fairly specific degeneration of frontal lobe areas (see Strub and Black 1981). In addition, those dementias arising primarily from vascular disorders (multi-infarct dementia) can in principle be differentiated from SDAT because there is more evidence for focal deficits. (For example, a patient revealing modality-specific deficits for complex visual material and spatial disorientation, though no memory deficit for verbal material, almost certainly does not suffer from a primary degenerative dementia, but may have had an infarct confined to right-hemisphere structures).

It has been suggested that the behavior typical of the various SDAT stages may parallel comparable stages of neuroanatomical degeneration (Jolles and Hijman 1983). More specifically, the temporal sequence of the development of cognitive deficits in SDAT suggests that there might be a degeneration of association areas in the neocortex occurring as a result of the degeneration of ascending fibers projecting to the neocortex. This hypothesis is primarily based on the observation that subjects in the very early stages of dementia do not show neocortical – higher cognitive – deficits, but do show consolidation deficits (limbic system) and slowness (ascending fibers). After degeneration of the higer-order, non-modality-specific association areas (see also Luria 1973, 1980), a further degeneration affects the sensory association areas, whereas the primary sensory projection areas stay relatively intact until very late in the disease process. This appears from the fact that aphasia, apraxia, and agnosia (behavioral manifestations of cortical involvement) develop in later stages of the disease process. Furthermore, ability to perform simple motoracts is preserved (activity of the primary motor cortex and premotor area). Likewise, severely demented patients are still capable of the use of syllables and phonemes (but not words) in undirected babbling. Support for this neuropsychological hypothesis comes from histologic investigations providing evidence that several cortical areas remain relatively intact during the course of the disease (Brody and Vijashankar 1977; Hanley 1974) and from the correlation between the extent of cortical degeneration (number of senile plaques) and poor test performance (Blessed et al. 1968).

Methods of Early Assessment

Psychometry

Generally, standard tests have increased our knowledge of how deficits develop in normal aging and dementia. Unfortunately, although this knowledge has been applied to groups of elderly subjects and patients as a whole, no psychometric tests appear sensitive and reliable enough to be used in the early assessment of disorders in individuals. The advantages of psychometric tests are that they are standardized and that published norms are generally available. In addition, they are easy to administer and usually have good reliability.

A general drawback of the psychometric approach is that the use of test scores does not necessarily make it possible to identify the cognitive deficits that underlie the performance changes. Traditionally used tests allow only a fairly crude estimation of cognitive functions and, in addition, do not properly differentiate between different aspects of these functions. This is a consequence of the empirical, nontheoretical nature of these tests, which have been developed for purposes other than for use with brain-damaged subjects. For example, the Digit-Symbol subtest of the Wechsler Adult Intelligence Scale (WAIS) is the most sensitive among the 11 subtests, showing the greatest difference between the performance of young and old adults (Botwinnick 1981). However, it is not clear whether psychomotor slowing, poor learning or retrieval of the digit-symbol codes, poor visual motor coordination, or all of the above are responsible for the poor performance of aged subjects (Poon 1983).

The psychometric test measure thus gives a quantitative index of below-average performance, without any clue as to the nature of the cognitive deficit and the underlying cerebral substrate. In other words, psychometric tests generally measure performance and not cognitive functions. Consequently, they do not allow a proper differentiation of different aspects of these functions, and this limits their use both in the assessment of the early stages of senile dementia and in differential diagnosis.

A second drawback of the traditional psychometric tests is the relatively long time needed for test administration, when compared with the amount of data that the test or test battery yields. For instance, the administration of the WAIS takes several hours and yields only 11 (subtest) scores when the test are used in the classic way. These scores are usually converted into two scores for Verbal IQ and Performal IQ, which are often combined to yield the total IQ. Another test battery, the Halstead Reitan Neuropsychological test battery (HRNTB; administration in 5–6 h, has the drawback that standard norms are available for subjects up to 55 years of age, but not for older subjects.

Apart from the use of standardized test batteries (HRNTB, WAIS, the Nebraska battery), several more specific psychometric tests are used for the determination of deficits in aging and dementia, especially those concerning aspects of memory processes (see Jolles and Hijman 1983). Characteristically, the resulting quantitative data are used for the analysis of group differences (e.g., "young" versus "old" adults). Generally, the quantitative results do not lend themselves to use in individual diagnosis, especially in distinguishing early dementia from other syndromes. More recently, there has been some movement toward using psychometric tests and test batteries in a less rigid and more qualitative way (e.g., Lezak 1983; Goodglass and Kaplan 1979). Proponents of such an approach use quantitative results and more qualitative signs; however, no published data are available as yet on the use of this new approach in the early diagnosis of senile dementia (see "Behavioral and Cognitive Testing: An Integrated Approach" below).

Information Processing

Investigations of cognitive processes in the psychological laboratory have generally made use of an information-processing paradigm. The strength of this approach is the theoretical framework, which attempts to examine cognitive processes by analyzing behavior in terms of quantifiable components and qualitative patterns. Information-processing tasks are characteristically broken down into subtasks, and reaction time measurements are used to probe into the different stages of information processing (e.g., Brand and Jolles 1985).

The use of information-processing tasks developed in the psychological laboratory and later adapted for use in clinical testing is still in its infancy. The Sternberger Memory Comparison Task (Sternberg 1975) which has been used extensively in the laboratory, has been employed in group comparison studies and to determine the efficacy of drug trials but not in psychodiagnosis on an individual basis. However, a recently developed paper-and-pencil version appears to be a reliable and sensitive task which can be combined with clinical neuropsychological tests (Jolles and Gaillard 1985). Data obtained with this test suggest that the intercept of the Reaction-time – Set-size function increases with age. This suggests that aging is associated with a decreased rate of perception and motor performance (Jolles and Hijman 1983), but has no effect on the rate of memory search. However, an increased slope in demented subjects characterized by some aspects of frontal lobe dysfunctioning suggests a fairly specific effect on search processes.

Other information-processing paradigms have been recommended for use in geriatric psychopharmacology (Poon 1983). These methods might also be of importance in the clinical assessment of subjects suspected of suffering from incipient dementia. According to Poon, these paradigms assess common behavioral complaints both in community-dwelling elderly and in elderly patient populations. Large amounts of data have been obtained on speed, accuracy, and response patterns, expecially with respect to the following functions: ability to attend and concentrate, to make dexisions quickly, to acquire and retrieve new information, to retrieve familiar information (naming), and to manipulate spatial information. It is again important to note that inferences are made with respect to aspects of cognitive functioning through the use of reaction time measurements. Poon (1983) recommends and describes the following procedures for use in geriatric assessment: (a) measurement of the alerting function to assess attention/arousal; (b) measurement of choice reaction time to assess decision-making processes; (c) measurement of continuous recognition memory to assess retrieval from primary and secondary memory; (d) measurement of naming latency to assess retrieval from tertiary memory; (e) measurement of mental rotation to assess spatial processing. A detailed description and rationale of these prcedures can be found in Poon (1983).

It is of interest to note that several psychometric tests which have been in clinical use for several decades can be used as an information-processing task: One example is the Stroop test (see Lezak 1983), which consists of three subtasks measuring (a) the speed at which color names are read, (b) the speed at which colors are named, and (c) the speed at which the color of printing ink is named when there is interference from the printed color name. An interference score can be calculated by subtracting the time scores 3–2. This is a relatively pure index which is not contaminated by a perceptual or motor component. A similar procedure can be performed with the Trail-Making test (see Lezak 1983). The subtraction of time scores gives a timed measure for the ease with which a concept shift is made (here, shifting between letters and digits, Vink and Jolles, in preparation).

Behavioral Neurology

A different approach toward assessing cognitive functioning relevant to geriatry has been developed by the Russian neuropsychologist A. R. Luria, who has elaborated a model of brain-behavior relationships to serve as a basis for an extensive neuropsychological investigation. His approach consists of a set of procedures which systematically assess the different aspects of cognitive functioning. The method Luria developed, which has become known in the adapted version of Christensen (1975), is qualitative and flexible in nature:

1. Motor functions
   - simple movements, dynamic organization
   - oral praxis
   - speech regulation of the motor act
2. Acoustico-motor organization
   - perception and reproduction of pitch and of rhythmic structures
3. Higher cutaneous and kinesthetic functions
   - cutaneous, muscle, and joint sensation
   - stereognosis
4. Higher visual functions
   - visual perception
   - spatial orientation
   - intellectual operations in space
5. Impressive speech
   - phonemic hearing
   - word comprehension
   - simple and complex grammar
6. Expressive speech
   - articulation
   - reflective speech
   - nominative speech
   - narrative speech
7. Writing and reading
   - word analysis and synthesis
   - writing
   - reading
8. Arithmetic skills
   - comprehension of number structures
   - arithmetic operations

9. Mnestic processes
   learning processes
   retention and retrieval
   logical memorizing
10. Intellectual processes
   thematic pictures and texts
   concept formation
   discursive intellectual activity

According to this method, more than 250 simple tasks are given to the subject, ranging from tests for simple and complex motor acts and perceptual, language, and memory functions to tests for higher cognitive functions. Total administration time is 1–2 h. In essence, Luria's method aims at generating hypotheses concerning specific disabilities and testing these hypotheses by a proper choice of small tasks. For instance, with respect to memory functions, he discerns between memory for visual forms ("draw the figures that you saw") and verbal material ("write the words you saw"). Both the learning performance and the sensitivity to interference by homogenous or heterogenous material are measured (e.g., remembering three words after "interference" in the form of three other words or a visually presented scene). In addition, the formation of a stable intention to memorize or to associate is assessed in addition to several other aspects of memory (Luria 1976). Luria used his method originally in the examination of brain-injured subjects, and the tests have provided important information in assessing the location of brain injuries and in planning rehabilitation programs. More recently, it has appeared to be effective in determining "functional" psychiatric illness of "organic" patients (Purisch et al. 1978) as well as in the assessment of SDAT (Ernst et al. 1970; Sulkava and Amberla 1982; see "Stages in Dementia" below).

Luria's investigation is essentially an example of behavioral neurology. The administration of the tasks is systematic but nonstructured. Its main advantage is the fact that the assessment schedule is based on a theory of brain-behavior relationships, thus making it possible to offer an interpretation with respect to the aspect or part of a functional system affected. This approach gives rise to a wealth of data which has more coherence than the data derived from a battery of standard psychometric tests. A main disadvantage of the procedure is its qualitative nature, which necessitates extensive training and reduces interobserver reliability. In addition, the lack of quantifiable data prohibits the use of the paradigm in the assessment of treatment efficacy or of cognitive decline in individual subjects. However, used in combination with psychometric tests and information-processing tasks, it can provide important information on the selective nature of cognitive defects in elderly subjects and SDAT (see "Behavioral and Cognitive Testing: An Integrated Approach"). Recently, attempts have been directed at quantifying the results of Luria's neuropsychological investigation. Unfortunately, the Luria-Nebraska battery (Golden et al. 1979), a structured and semiquantitative test series, has lost the flexibility and richness of the original method, in addition to having several other shortcomings (Adams 1984 and several references cited there).

Behavioral and Cognitive Testing: An Integrated Approach

Because the psychometric, the information-processing, and the behavioral-neurological approaches all have their strengths and weaknesses, it may be more fruitful to use them in combination for the early assessment of SDAT and related disorders. The assessment procedure used for this purpose in our clinic is a combination of a qualitative behavioral-neurological examination and quantitative methods derived from psychometry and information-processing paradigms. The procedure is first to get a qualitative impression of the total range of cognitive functions (see p. 89). When signs indicating a possible deficit are revealed, a more detailed investigation is carried out to explore them further. Other qualitative tests are employed in order to determine whether there is indeed a deficit and to ascertain its specific nature. These tests are then followed by quantitative methods which "measure" the deficit and relate it to existing norms. This approach has several advantages. First, it is possible to make a profile of a broad range of cognitive functions. For instance, it is fairly easy to indicate the aspects of cognition which reveal no deficits. Second, the numerous observations increase the reliability of the eventual interpretation. Third, the duration of the neuropsychological investigation has been decreased as a result of the relatively shorter duration of the qualitative tests. Fourth, hypotheses based on a thorough knowledge of brain-behavior relationships are tested. Finally, much emphasis is given to pathognomonic signs, or clear signs of existing pathology. The psychometric tradition does not usually pay attention to these signs.

The test series used to assess early dementia in our clinic consists of the following tests and tasks: (1) the Luria-Christensen test battery described above; (b) a 15 word learning test giving information on the use of active coding strategies, consolidation versus retrieval, rate of retrieval, and sensitivity to interference (Luria 1976; Brand and Jolles 1985); (c) the Utrecht memory comparison task evaluating rates of perception, motor output, and memory comparison (Jolles and Gaillard 1985), (d) the Stroop Interference task (naming; retrieval of words, and color names, color-word interference; Lezak 1983); (e) the adapted version of the Trail-Making test (rate of perception, retrieval of letters, and flexibility in concept shifting; Lezak 1983); (f) the Road Map test (left-right discrimination, evaluation, mental rotation; Lezak 1983); and (g) the Symbol-Digit Modalities test of general speed of perception and motor output, Lezak 1983). In addition to this test series, a variety of other tests explore any specific deficits found more deeply. These tests are either chosen from standard batteries (e.g., tapping test from HRNTB or the block design test of the WAIS) or consist of experimental tasks used in an ad hoc fashion (e.g., experimental tasks designed to assess decision speed, tactile functions or the dichotic listening task).

Luria used syndrome analysis as a means of describing the profile of cognitive strengths and weaknesses in his subjects. Specifically, the syndrome he described appears to involve particular brain structures, for instance, the frontal areas, as seen in deficits relating to many different functional systems, such as perseveration in motor function, proactive memory interference, a flat learning curve on a word-learning test, and disabilities in shifting concepts among others. A similar syndrome analysis also appears to be important in conjunction with test methods such as those described here, enabling a profile of a subject's cognitive strengths and weaknesses at a given moment to emerge. A profile analysis of this type is an attempt to simplify a picture which might otherwise contain too much information to be intelligible. Examples of this approach are discussed in "Neuropsychological Contributions to Differential Diagnosis" below. Interestingly, the large amount of data gathered per individual subject appears to make possible a fairly reliable description of individual cases.

Neuropsychological Contributions to Differential Diagnosis

Reactive Depression Versus (Pre)senile Dementia: Case Studies

The approach described in the preceding paragraph is illustrated in the following description of a neuropsychological examination of two elderly patients. The first, a 63-year-old man, was referred to us for treatment of memory deficits and had been hospitalized for several years in a psychiatric clinic. He was diagnosed as suffering from a depression with "theatrical, hysteria-like character neurosis." He sometimes manifested bizarre behavior; both nurses and spouse complained about his tendency to "attract attention." The patient himself complained of occasional memory lapses for complex behavioral activities such as dish-washing and setting the table. He was afraid that he was suffering from incipient dementia and felt depressed about his decreasing capabilities. A neuropsychological examination provided the following information:

A normal conversation was possible, although the patient was fairly passive in his response towards instructions. Speech was adynamic and there was some inertia of movement. Intellect and consciousness were not overtly disturbed. Behavioral-neurologic investigation showed no particular deficits in simple or complex motor functions, except for a slight tendency to persevere on a movement pattern (for example, tapping four times when three times had been requested). Auditory, visual, and tactile perception were normal. However, he clearly manifested proactive interference suggestive a frontal cortex dysfunctioning according to Luria (see above discussion). A more clearcut perseveration was seen on the Luria Meander (Fig. 1, part A), a pattern capable of eliciting any tendency to persevere. The patient still manifested this perseveration several minutes later; the movement pattern of the meander appeared to interfere with the requested performance of a new motor pattern (Fig. 1, part B). Interestingly, another aspect of perseveration was seen on a higher cognitive level. The subject was requested to draw a simple figure from memory (Benton test; Fig. 1, part C). When similar tasks were set later (Fig. 1, parts D and E), there was a clear persistence of the movement and visual pattern belonging to the earlier task (Fig. 1, part C) that interfered with later stimuli. On quantitative tests such as the trail-making test, a fairly normal performance was seen on the first subtask, but the subject was much too slow on the second subtask and also made several errors. Consequently, there was a lack of flexibility without a general decrease in the rate of information processing. With respect to memory functions, imprinting appeared fairly normal

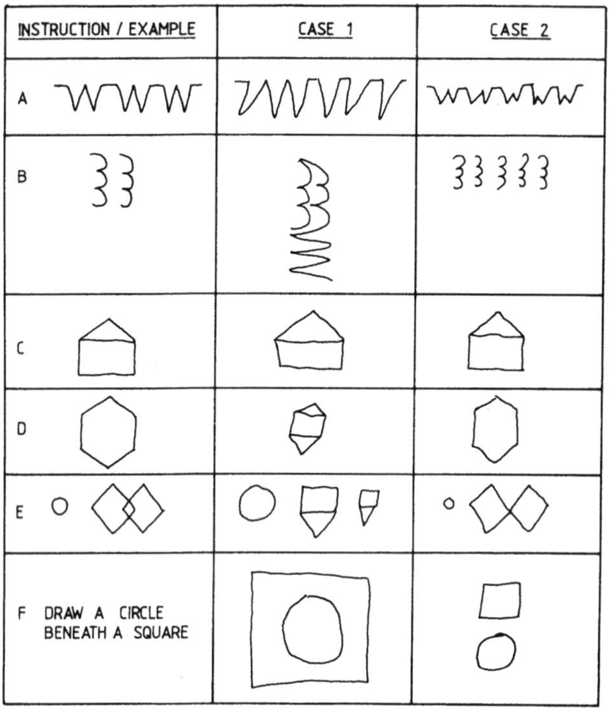

Fig. 1 A–F. Comparison of neuropsychological test results of two elderly subjects with depression, suspected of possible senile dementia

(recognition memory), but a flat learning curve was noted in a word-learning test: the subject encoded the material passively and in a fairly stereotyped manner, indicating that active encoding and active retrieval from memory was disturbed. Finally, with respect to language functions, vocabulary was normal, although one specific language disorder was present. Words used to describe relations in language (for instance, "because," "as," "if," "then," "greater than") appeared not to be understood. Part F of Fig. 1 shows how the instruction to "draw a circle beneath a square" was carried out in correctly. "Beneath" was interpreted in a concrete, three-dimensional fashion, whereas all normal elderly subjects would have drawn "beneath" according to a two-dimensional conception. The patient also failed on several other tasks in which similar logical relations in language had to be expressed. The performance of the other subject (case 2) was normal (Fig. 1).

Recapitulating, it appears that the subject had severe deficits in the planning and organization of complex behavioral acts. No clearcut disorder of perception, memory, and simple language functions and no general slowness were observed. It was concluded that the patient had a dysfunction of the frontal neocortex, particularly of the lateral surfaces, as indicated by the patients general inertia. A computerized tomography scan performed later has shown some central and peripheral atrophy, frontally more than posteriorly. The EEG was diffusely irregular. An early stage of Pick's disease was a possible diagnosis, although other causes of impaired frontal lobe functioning could not be excluded. A follow-up investigation will be undertaken at a later stage to asses whether there is further deterioration.

The other subject (male, 72 years of age) was referred to us because of persistent depression, failing memory, and possible early dementia. The subject was very sharp, with adequate responses and sometimes initiated the conversation. He complained of memory lapses and the fact that all his actions required so much energy. No pathognomonic signs appeared in the behavioral-neurological examination (Fig. 1), although he was very slow in performing complex acts of manual dexterity. His attention span appeared to be short, and automatic acts were performed in a controlled and time-consuming fashion slower than normal for his age. When given the time, his performance on many tests – including memory tests – was normal. No planning deficits and language deficits were seen, but there was a clear deficit in visuoconstruction and in performance on a test measuring mental rotation.

It was concluded that the scores of memory tests were not low enough to warrant a diagnosis of early dementia. In addition, there was no indication of specific frontal involvement. This profile of slowness and visuoconstructive deficits is often seen in certain subgroups of depressive patients. The neuropsychological examination of the two seemingly similar subjects thus gives rise to a strikingly different conclusion as to the nature of the underlying disorder and the cerebral substrate involved. The depression of the first subject is almost certainly secondary to some kind of dementia which is especially dependent on frontal cortex functioning. The second subject is depressed and not demented manifesting cognitive deficits more often seen in depression which might be mistaken for signs of dementia. The interpretations are based on a combined analysis of data obtained in the behavioral examination and the preliminary conversation (hypothesis generation). Indications of pathognomonic signs were discovered in the behavioral-neurological examination, while speed and other parameters were measured in psychometric and information-processing tasks. It is the combination of these modes of investigation which gives rise to the specific profile of deficits.

Stages in Dementia

A very important objective in the early assessment of dementia is the differentiation of "normal" aging from early dementia. The deficits accompanying normal aging are relatively mild; for instance, some mild frontal lobe signs corresponding to mild senescent forgetfulness develop, manifesting themselves as a deficit in active encoding and retrieval (see "Neuropsychology of Aging and Dementia"). However, a clear consolidation deficit is not seen in normal elderly people, in contrast to the early stages of dementia. A profile analysis of one individual illustrates this point (Fig. 2). The subject referred to here (female, 64 years of age) was normal in several different cognitive functions (higher language functions, arithmetic, simple perception, and simple motor functions). However, a very profound memory defect was evident, especially in the learning and retention of new material, resulting in a total inability to recall words learned 30 min earlier. In addition, passive recognition of words was also inferior to normal, indicating a consolidation deficit. The rate of information processing was moderately decreased. The dynamic organization of hand movements was much less efficient (e.g., the rapid alternation of movements between left and right hand or the smooth succession of different movement patterns with one hand, especially when hand movements had to be accompanied by speech acts). A very relevant finding was a gradual deterioration of memory functions and speed at a follow-up examination conducted 1 year later, while several other functions revealed no decreases. It appears that the various cognitive deficits may develop successively over time. The CT scan of this subject was normal (atrophy conforming to age), and she was tentatively diagnosed as suffering from DAT.

Figure 2 b shows the cognitive profile of a 59-year-old man whose memory deficits differ strikingly from those of the subject just described in that he exhibited more retrieval deficits than consolidation deficits and a degree of disordered memory secondary to planning disorganization. In addition, general slowness together with fairly good consolidation was evident, while impressive speech faculties and dynamic organization were far inferior to the performance of the female subject just discussed. Follow-up assessment after 0.5 and 1 year corroborated the first impression of primary degenerative dementia of the frontal type. A CT scan conducted 6 months later showed some sulcal enlargement and widened interhemispheric fissure, especially in the frontal lobe. The atrophy was more pro-

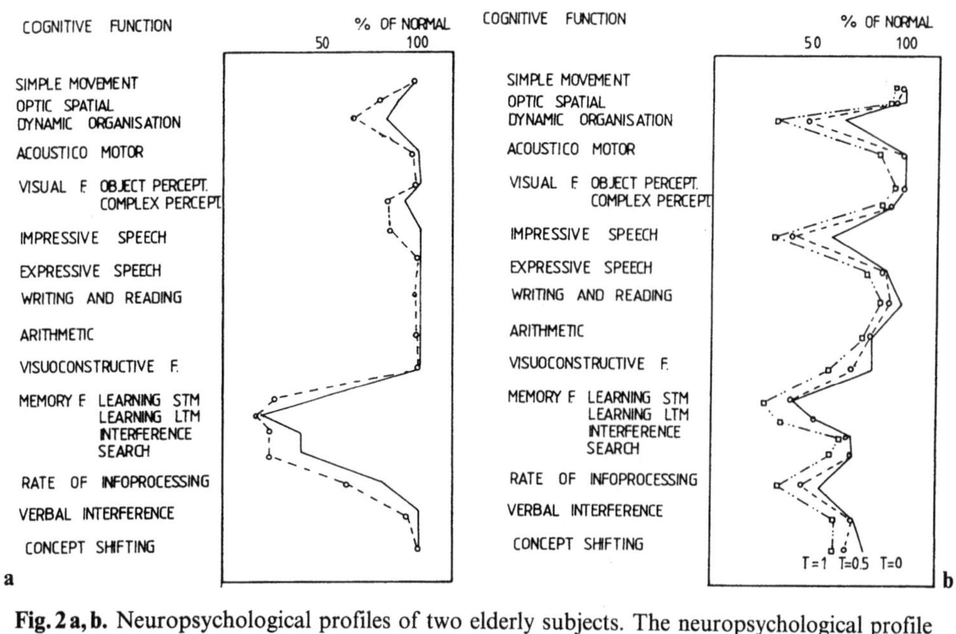

Fig. 2 a, b. Neuropsychological profiles of two elderly subjects. The neuropsychological profile is drawn for the cognitive functions measured by the test series described in the text. The individual qualitative tests were scored on an ordinal scale (0–2) and converted into mean scores for a specific function. Four functions (memory, rate, interference, and shifting) are based on quantitative data. The relative performance as compared with age-matched controls is given. **a** Subject (female, 64 years) was assessed two times; at $T=0$ (—) and $T=1$ year (---). **b** Subject (male, 59 years) was assessed three times, at $T=0$ (–), $T=0.5$ year (--), and $T=1$ year (..–..)

nounced 1 year after the first examination, which is in line with the interpretation based on the neuropsychological examination.

Further studies have been performed with larger groups of subjects who have, however, not been tested more than once. The general findings conform to those obtained by Sulkava andd Amberla (1982) in a study with the Luria-Christensen neuropsychological test battery. These investigators found that different phases in the development of dementia can be discriminated, even at the later stages. Both presenile and senile patients exhibited pronounced deterioration of orientation, memory and higher cognitive, visual, and motor functions. Impressive and expressive speech were relatively spared. All functions deteriorated gradually during the disease process, so that the differences between the various abilities and the slope of the performance profile were preserved. All neuropsychological abilities tested had disappeared by the final phase (Sulkava and Amberla 1982).

According to these authors, both the presenile and the senile form of DAT seem to follow a clearly definable course affecting different functions of the brain in a certain order. Symptoms such as a general diminishing of activity or deterioration of short-term memory and of awareness appear at an early stage of the disease. Consequent behavioral dysfunctions are disorientation and paranoid delusions. Theoretically, this may indicate that fibers ascending from the brainstem to the cortex are affected (see "Neuropsychology of Aging and Dementia"). In the next phase, apraxia, agnosia, and aphasia disorders appear, together with deterioration of logical reasoning and loss of control over behavior (i.e., indicating cortical involvement). In the advanced stages of the disease, only a few basic functions (e.g., automatisms) may still be preserved (Sulkava and Amberla 1982; Jolles and Hijman 1983). The data indicate that a neuropsychological examination based on Luria's brain-behavior model, coupled with a profile analysis, yields information of relevance both to early assessment of the disorder and to increasing knowledge not only of the succession of stages in DAT, but also – indirectly – of the cerebral substrate involved.

Dementia Versus Psychiatric Disorders

(Neuro)psychologists working in a psychiatric setting are frequently asked to assess whether a particular patient is demented or not, as it is very difficult to differentiate the early stages of senile dementia from depression. On the one hand, early stages of dementia are very frequently accompanied by a depressed mood (Jolles and Hijman, 1983; Strub and Black 1981), which is most probably a reaction to the subjective realization of suffering cognitive deterioration (cf. the first case study in "Reactive Depression versus (Pre)senile Dementia"). Incidentally, there is evidence that the major catecholaminergic pathways believed to be involved in depression (Van Praag 1982) play a similar role in the pathogenesis of SDAT (Rossor 1982), thus suggesting that there is – at least in part – a common cerebral substrate in both depression and dementia. On the other hand, profoundly depressed patients frequently display overt signs of dementia such as slowness, general inertia, disorientation, and memory disturbances. The differentiation of depression and dementia based on clinical observation alone thus appears very difficult. A thorough neuropsychological examination may be of importance in this respect.

Recently, a group of 29 depressive inpatients from the university psychiatric clinic were subjected to such an examination to determine whether any members of the group had been misclassified as demented (Jolles and Brand, in preparation). After neuropsychological analysis, it was possible to discern seven subgroups. Groups 1–6 had a fairly specific profile of cognitive deficits that could be used as a basis for making distinctions among them. Group 7 ("others") consisted of six different profiles which did not resemble those of any of the other subjects. Interestingly, these six subjects had had life events which were suggestive of some brain disease, thus explaining the specific pattern of deficits (two subjects with brain trauma; one with hysteric conversion, one with migraine, and two postanoxic subjects). Group 1 (two subjects) manifested only some nonspecific cognitive deterioration without any deficits relating to memory, motor functions, planning, or automaticity. Group 2 (six subjects) had similar nonspecific deficits as well as deficits in automatism and memory retrieval. Group 3 (six subjects) was very different, in that these subjects, in addition to the deficits characterizing group 2, were also very slow, manifesting some motor and higher cognitive perseverations or perceptual changes. Group 4 (three subjects) was similar to group 3, but also showed memory consolidation deficits. The extremely profound deficits of the patients in groups 3 and 4 suggest that they suffer from retarded depression. Groups 5 and 6 manifested clear-cut signs of brain dysfunctions. Group 5 ($n=2$) exhibited no slowing of actions but had especially pronounced motor dysfunctions suggestive of frontal cortex involvement. Group 6 ($n=3$) was characterized by subjects with profound cognitive and behavioral deficits in all cognitive functions measured. When these profiles are represented schematically, they suggest that group 6 consisted of demented subjects. One subject of this group later turned out to have multi-infarct dementia, while another subject suffered from lupus erythematosus. Long-term follow-up will make it possible to monitor groups 3 and 4. Until now, several subjects from groups 1–3 have evidenced some improvement of cognitive deficits, accompanied by an alleviation of their depression.

Besides depressive patients, another group of psychiatric patients can be distinguished from demented subjects only with difficulty. In view of the important role of the frontal lobe in behavioral planning and organization, dysfunctions of the frontal lobe or structures within it can easily manifest themselves as disorganized and bizarre behavior. This might thus be misinterpreted as a "functional" psychiatric disorder. The patients referred to in Figs. 1 and 2 and in group 5 are examples of such patients. It is interesting to note that most patients with Pick's disease die in a psychiatric hospital. It will be of more than scientific interest to explore how many psychiatric patients are in fact misclassified because they have deficits in behavioral planning and organization which – until now – have not frequently been recognized as an indication of frontal lobe involvement or as signs of a specific type of degenerative dementia.

Conclusion

Some evidence has been presented to show that most of the methods which have until now been used in the assessment of early stages of dementia have their drawbacks. It appears that the use of a *combination* of psychometric tests with techniques based upon information-processing paradigms and behavioral neurology may be the most fruitful approach. Future developments will almost certainly be in the direction of techniques that are more sensitive and capable of giving more insight into the nature of the cognitive deficits. Information-processing tasks such as those proposed by several authors (Poon 1983; Brand and Jolles 1985) will contribute, provided that some relation is made between cognitive functions and the underlying cerebral substrate, and provided that tasks are constructed which have ecological validity.

The neuropsychological profile analysis (Figs. 1, 2) illustrated here does no more than indicate a possible method for analyzing data. It is clear that a description purely in terms of test results is too crude to describe the complexity of an individual's pattern of cognitive strengths and weaknesses. Similar developments can be seen in psychiatric diagnosis. For example, the Present State Examination (Wing et al. 1972) and the Geriatric Mental Scale (Copeland, this volume) also use some kind of profile analysis in the description of psychiatric symptoms. The neuropsychological profile analysis proposed here is based on a model of brain-behavior relationships (i.e., the model of Luria). It is important to simplify the large amount of data into a smaller number of categories. A good brain-behavior model provides a rationale according to which this may be done.

With respect to the potential contributions of neuropsychology, several points are of interest. In the first place, modern neuropsychology is a neuroscience when it tries to relate behavioral and cognitive functions to the underlying cerebral substrate. A model such as that put forward by Luria presents a working hypothesis which is essential if aspects of behavior and cognition which would otherwise never have been suspected of containing common elements are to be related (see, for instance, the different aspects of frontal involvement). A model of DAT based on neuropsychological theory predicts that the evolution of behaviorally observable deficits in DAT may initially be a manifestation of an underlying degeneration of ascending fibers, followed by progressive atrophy of nonspecific hippocampal and sensory neocortical association areas and neocortical sensory association areas (see "Neuropsychology of Aging and Dementia" and Jolles and Hijman 1983).

Another theoretical contribution concerns the findings that – based on neuropsychological examination alone – there are no qualitative, but only quantitative differences between aging and DAT (Jolles and Hijman 1983) and between the presenile and the senile forms of DAT (Sulkava and Amberla 1982). Human neuropsychology may thus provide testable hypotheses which will deepen our insight into the nature of the underlying disease and its cerebral substrate.

A second relevance of neuropsychology concerns the implications which emerge from a better behavioral and cognitive description of the deficits. For instance, elderly individuals seem to lose the ability to retrieve information consolidated in the past. A consolildation deficit is especially evident in dementia. Might it not be the case that the real underlying deficit is a decreasing ability to cope with environmental stimuli and that mechanisms for handling new information are unused and thus atrophy? This notion could motivate changes in society allowing older people increased opportunities to engage in new activities and actively plan their own lives. Presently, there is a tendency in exactly the opposite direction, namely to take responsibility out of the hands of the elderly. This is especially true in psychiatric institutions. Patient rehabilitation and training based upon neuropsychological theory would prescribe training in order to compensate for lost capabilities. In this respect, much emphasis must be given to activating behavior planning as opposed to passive perception. The strategy of an "enriched" environment, which is known to have beneficial effect on cortical thickness and neuronal connections in animals, might have similar effects in man.

Analogous to the muscular atrophy that develops in a disused broken leg, brain atrophy may result from a lack of interaction between the organism and its environment. This atrophy might – theoretically – be reversible if noted in the very early stages. A stimulative therapy of the type suggested here, possibly in combination with newly developed drugs (e.g., neuropeptides), might be the treatment of choice in elderly people who are at risk of becoming demented.

References

Adams KM (1984) Luria left in the lurch: unfulfilled promises are not valid tests. J Clin Neuropsychol 6:455–458

Blessed G, Tomlinson BE, Roth M (1968) The association between quantitative measures of dementia and of senile changes in the cerebral grey matter of aged subjects. Br J Psychiatry 114:797–811

Botwinnick J (1981) Neuropsychology of aging. In: Filskov SB, Boll TJ (eds) Handbook of clinical neuropsychology. Wiley, New York, pp 135–171

Brand N, Jolles J (1985) Memory scanning and response requirements (to be published)

Brody H, Vijashankar N (1977) Anatomical changes in the nervous system. In: Finch CE, Hayflick L (eds) Handbook of the biology of aging. Van Nostrand, New York

Christensen AL (1975) Luria's neuropsychological investigation. Text, Munxgaard Copenhagen

Ernst B, Dalby MA, Dalby A (1970) Luria testing in demented patients. Acta Neurol Scand [Suppl] 43:97–98

Fuster JM (1980) The prefrontal cortex. Raven, New York

Golden CJ, Hammeke TA, Purish AD (1979) The Luria-Nebraska neuropsychological battery manual. Western Psychological Services, Los Angeles

Goodglass H, Kaplan E (1979) Assessment of cognitive deficit in the brain-injured patient. In: Gazzaniga M (ed) Handbook of behavioral neurobiology, vol 2. Neuropsychology. Plenum, New York

Hanley T (1974) Neuronal "fall-out" in the aging brain: a critical review of the quantitative data. Age Aging 3:133–151

Jolles J (1983) Vasopressin-like peptides and the treatment of memory disorders in man. Progr Brain Res 60:169–182

Jolles J, Gaillard AWK (1985) A paper and pencil version of the Sternberg memory Comparison Task (to be published)

Jolles J, Hijman R (1983) The neuropsychology of aging and dementia. Dev Neurol 7:227–250

Lezak MD (1983) Neuropsychological assessment, 2nd edn. Oxford University Press, New York
Luria AR (1973) The working brain. Penguin, Harmondsworth, UK
Luria AR (1976) The neuropsychology of memory. Winston, Washington DC
Luria AR (1980) Higher cortical functions in man, 2nd edn. Basic, New York
Miller E (1981) The nature of the cognitive deficit in dementia. In: Miller NE, Cohen GD (eds) Clinical aspects of Alzheimer's disease and senile dementia. Raven, New York, pp 103–120
Newcombe F (1980) Memory: a neuropsychological approach. Trends Neurosci 179–182
Poon LW (1983) Application of information-processing technology in psychological assessment. In: Crook T, Ferris S, Reisberg B (eds) Assessment in geriatric psychopharmacology. Powley, New Canaan, CT
Purish AD, Golden CJ, Hammeke TA (1978) Discrimination of schizophrenia and brain-injured patients by a standardised version of Luria's neuropsychological tests. J Consult Clin Psychol 46:1266–1273
Rossor MN (1982) Neurotransmitters and CNS disease: Dementia. Lancet II:1200-1204
Sternberg S (1966) High speed scanning in human memory. Science 153:652–654
Sternberg S (1975) Memory scanning: new findings and current controversies. Q J Exp Psychol 27:1–32
Strub RI, Black FW (1981) Alzheimer's/Senile dementia. In: Strub RI, Black FW (eds) Organic brain syndromes. Davis, Philadelphia, pp 119–164
Sulkava R, Amberla K (1982) Alzheimer's disease and senile dementia of Alzheimer type: a neuropsychological study. Acta Neurol Scand 65:541–552
Van Praag HM (1982) Depression. Lancet II:1259–1264
Vink M, Jolles J (1985) A new version of the trailmaking test as an information-processing task. J Clin Neuropsychol 7:162
Wing JK, Cooper JE, Sartorius N (1974) Measurement and classification of psychiatric symptoms. Cambridge University Press

Early Diagnosis of Senile Dementia of the Alzheimer Type
II. Brain Tissue Parameters

EEG and Evoked Potentials in the Diagnosis of Dementias

S. L. VISSER[1]

Electroencephalography

EEG in Normal Aged Persons

The EEG in normal adults is characterized by an occipitally dominant 10-Hz alpha rhythm (Fig. 1). The alpha rhythm is reactive, meaning it is attenuated when the eyes are open (Fig. 2) and reappears after eye closure. Even centenarians may have an EEG with a normal alpha rhythm. However, Busse et al. (1956) found that 51% of normal subjects over 60 years of age showed slight EEG abnormalities, mainly focal, in the anterior-temporal regions. The percentage of focal abnormalities increases with age from about 20% in the 40–59-year-old to about 30%–40% in the 60–79-year-old group (Busse and Obrist 1965). These findings have been confirmed by several other authors. The proportion of focal changes in normal aged subjects should not exceed 25% of the EEG record.

Other changes that have been described in EEGs of normal aged subjects are:

1. a decrease in the mean alpha rhythm frequency by 0.5 to 1.0 Hz (Obrist 1954, and many others)
2. an increase in the amount of the beta rhythm; the percentage of normal aged subjects with a slight excess of fast activity doubles from 12% in young adults to 24% in the aged (> 70 years) (Gibbs and Gibbs 1951)
3. an increase in slow activity; the percentage of normal subjects with a slight excess of slow activity doubles from about 7% in young adults to 15% in the aged (> 70 years) (Gibbs and Gibbs 1951).

It has been supposed that these anomalies, which occur in nearly 50% of the normal aged, should be regarded as without clinical significance. However, Obrist (1963) already found that other signs of general subclinical arteriosclerosis appear more often in normal aged individuals with these EEG abnormalities than in elderly subjects with quite normal EEGs. Moreover, Drachman and Hughes (1971) found a correlation between subclinical EEG abnormalities and decrease of memory function. Compared with normal adults, aged subjects (51–69 years) with an abnormal EEG scored lower on memory tests (67% of normal adult levels) than aged subjects with a normal EEG (96% of normal adult levels). It should thus be concluded that the slight EEG abnormalities found in about half of the aged

1 Department of Clinical Neurophysiology, Free University, Valeriuskliniek, Valeriusplein 9, 1075 BG Amsterdam, The Netherlands

Senile Dementia of the Alzheimer Type
Ed. by J. Traber and W. H. Gispen

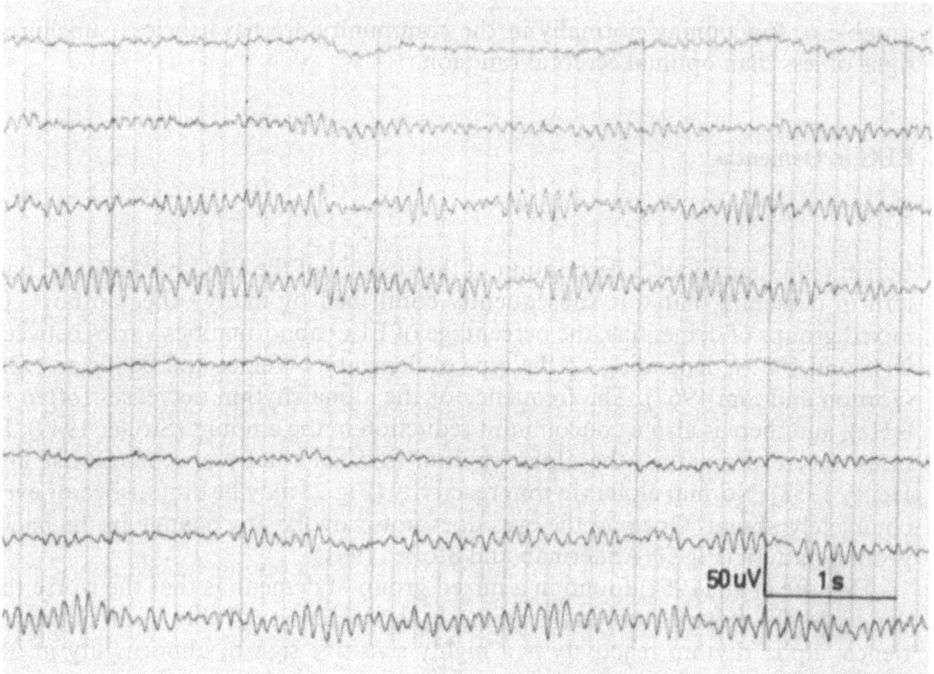

a

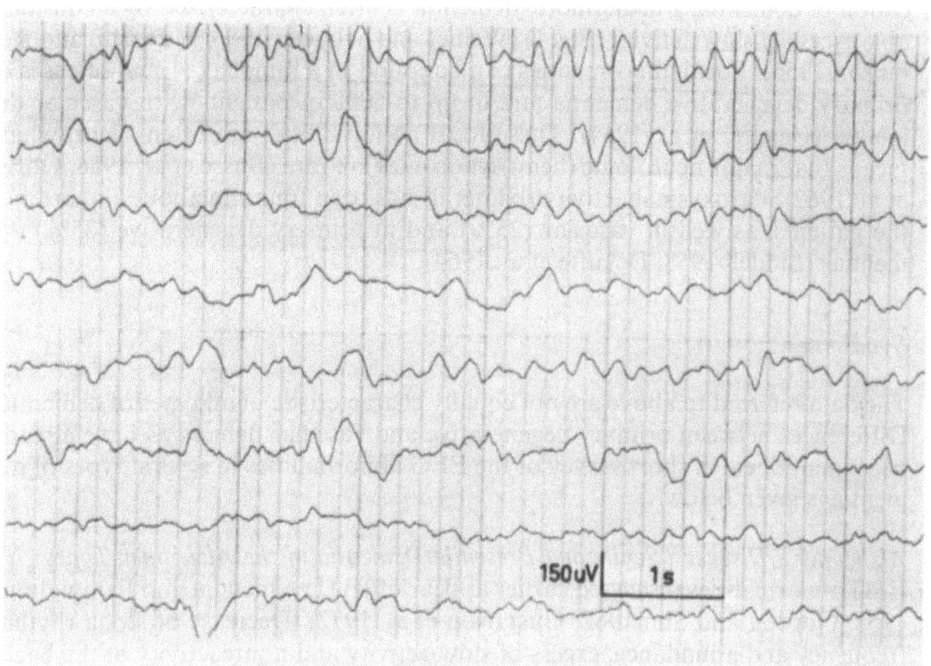

b

Fig. 1. a Normal adult EEG. **b** EEG with excess of slow activity

capable of functioning normally in the community are nevertheless subclinical signs of less than optimal cerebral function.

EEG in Dementia

General Aspects

Berger (1933) provided a description of the slowing of the EEG background pattern in dementia that was subsequently confirmed by many other authors. In mixed groups of dementias, the percentage of EEG abnormalities varies between 20% and 100%, depending on the type of dementia (Weiner and Schuster 1956; Gordon and Sim 1967). The frequency of the alpha rhythm decreases (often to 8 Hz), and there is also a concomitant reduction in the amount (Stoller 1949). In more severe dementias, the alpha rhythm is often totally absent (Obrist and Henry 1958). Normal alpha rhythm reactivity (Fig. 2) may be diminished or even completely absent. Opening the eyes does not provoke any change in the background pattern (Fig 2) (Anderman and Stoller 1961).

Dejaiffe et al. (1964) found in a mixed group of dementias that the worse the dementia, the more disturbed the alpha rhythm reactivity (Table 1). In our experience, alpha rhythm reactivity is a highly sensitive sign of abnormality in dementia diagnostics; i.e., nonreactivity of the background pattern is a strong indication of dementia. Furthermore, dementia is often characterized by a considerable excess of slow activity (Fig. 1) (Weiner and Schuster 1956; McAdam and Robinson 1956). Focal abnormalities can be found in a minority (13%) of cases of primary degenerative dementia and in up to 50% of patients with vascular dementia (Dejaiffe et al. 1964). These focal abnormalities are often silent, which means that major neurologic (hemi)syndromes are rare (Busse et al. 1956; Obrist et al. 1962). Paroxysmal activity (bilateral) has been found in about a quarter of the patients, as well in vascular (25%) and in primary degenerative (25%) dementias (Liddell 1958; Dejaiffe et al. 1964).

Syndromes

The data referred to above are not equally characteristic of all types of dementia. Differences between primary degenerative and vascular dementias have already been mentioned. A short survey of the EEG abnormalities in several types of dementia is given below.

Alzheimer's Disease (Senile and Presenile Dementia of the Alzheimer Type). All EEG abnormalities discussed earlier appear often (Letemendia and Pampiglione 1958; Gordon and Sim 1967; Gustafson et al. 1972). Decrease of alpha rhythm frequency and abundance, excess of slow activity and nonreactivity of the background pattern are almost always found and, often, focal and paroxysmal abnormalities are also evident. Because normal EEG is rare, a diagnosis of Alzheimer's disease should be doubted when the patient's EEG does not deviate from normal patterns.

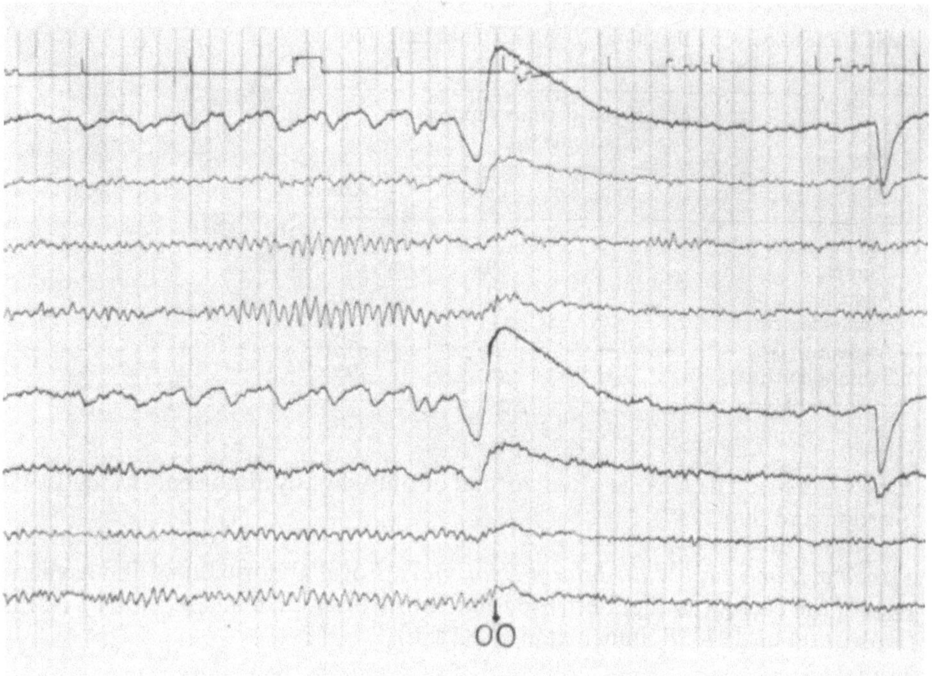

a

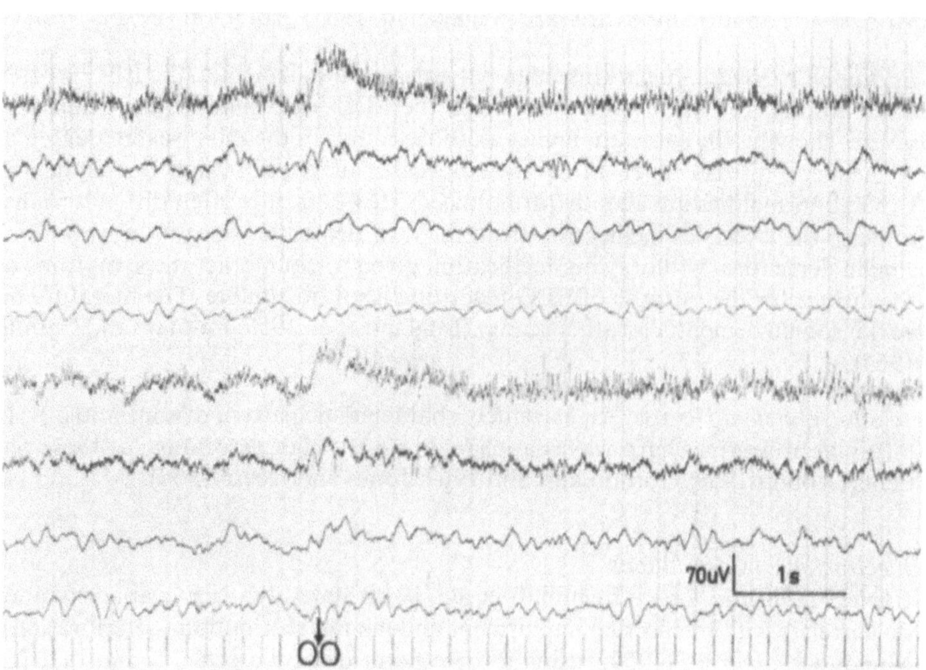

b

Fig. 2. a Normal reactivity of the background rhythm. **b** Nonreactivity of the background activity. (OO, opening of the eyes)

Table 1. Reactivity of the alpha rhythm in several types of dementia according to Dejaiffe et al. (1964)

	Alpha rhythm suppression in patients (*n*)		
	Complete	Partial	Absent
Senile dementia			
"Simple"	12	19	10
Alzheimer type	2	3	17
Presenile dementia			
Alzheimer type	0	1	4
Vascular dementia	7	18	19

Pick's Disease. The EEG is often normal or only slightly abnormal (Liddell 1958; Gordon and Sim 1967).

Vascular Dementia (Multi-Infarct Dementia). Focal abnormalities and asymmetries of the background pattern are found more often than in Alzheimer's disease (Roberts et al. 1978; Soininen et al. 1982a, b).

Huntington's Disease. The EEG often shows an irregular low-voltage fast pattern. More severe abnormalities are rare (Vogel et al. 1961; Scott et al. 1972).

Parkinson's Disease. In parkinsonian patients without dementia, the EEG is often quite normal. In parkinsonian dementia, the EEG abnormalities are often very severe, showing the same anomalies as those found in the most severe degree of Alzheimer's disease. Even in rather mild cases of parkinsonian dementia, the EEG abnormalities are already pronounced. However, it is often difficult to distinguish the effects of medication from those of dementia, since in most parkinsonian dementias, withdrawing medication given to counteract the symptoms of the disease for the purpose of EEG recording is not justifiable. The literature on parkinsonian dementia is rather scanty (England et al. 1959; Laidlaw and Catling 1964).

Jakob-Creutzfeld Disease. An extremely characteristic pattern of continous, 1-Hz bifrontal, repetitive sharp waves appears in a very high percentage of these patients (Abbott 1959; Gordon and Sim 1967; Jones and Nevin 1954).

Electroclinical Correlations

Clinical Dementia Rate. Greenblatt et al. (1945) stated that EEG abnormalities do correlate with intellectual impairment and mental retardation (deterioration). Mundy-Castle et al. (1954), using a three-point dementia scale, found that the EEG slow activity increase and the alpha rhythm decrease correlate with the degree of dementia. This has been confirmed by many authors. Especially in Alzheimer's disease, the correlation between EEG abnormalities and the severity of dementia is high.

Social Functioning. There is a correlation between social functioning and degree of EEG abnormalities, as has been found by Andermann and Stoller (1961). They compared three groups of dementias as summarized in Table 2. Lundervold et al. (1962) also compared three groups of patients with dementia who revealed different levels of social functioning (Table 3).

Rate of Disease Progress. Slowly evolving dementias show fewer abnormalities in the EEG than dementias which progress rapidly (Lundervold et al. 1962; Table 4).

Mortality Expectancy. Cahan and Yeager (1966) studied 233 aged psychiatric patients, of whom 65 had normal and 158, abnormal EEGs. The chances of dying within 1 year proved to be 2–3 times higher for the patients with an abnormal EEG than for those with a normal EEG.

Table 2. EEGs in three groups of dementia (Andermann and Stoller 1961)

	Abnormal EEG (%)	Alpha rhythm frequency (Hz)	Slow activity (%)
Social club ($n=50$)	17	11	2
Convalescent home ($n=50$)	39	9–9.5	31
Mental hospital ($n=50$)	38	9–10.5	34

Table 3. EEGs of demented patients with different levels of social functioning (Lundervold et al. 1962)

	Normal EEG (n)	Moderately or medium abnormal (n)	Markedly abnormal (n)
Patients who have partly retained capacity for work	15	11	0
Patients who have lost working capacity	9	20	2
Patients who have lost working capacity and are in need of care	9	22	11

Table 4. Percentage of abnormal EEGs in slowly as opposed to rapidly progressing dementia

	Abnormal EEGs (%)
Slowly progressing	35
Rapidly progressing	65

Cortical Metabolism Rate. Obrist (1963) found a correlation between cerebral blood flow (CBF), cerebral metabolism rate (CMR), and EEG abnormalities, as summarized in Table 5. This correlation has been confirmed for regional cerebral blood flow (rCBF) by Ingvar and Gustafson (1970) in 28 demented patients (Table 6). Other authors have confirmed these findings, as has the recent use of positron emission tomography (PET) (Friedland et al. 1983).

Neuroradiological Findings. The correlations of EEGs with neuroradiological findings are weaker. Diffuse slowing of the EEG background pattern correlates with cerebral atrophy. However, there are rather frequent discrepancies, as found by Sisson and Ellingson (1956) (Table 7). This lack of consistency had been observed earlier by Greenblatt et al. (1945). In 67 demented patients, EEG and pneumoencephalographic findings were compared. In patients with severe ventricular enlargement, 63% abnormal EEGs were found, while 33%–50% of those with slight or moderate enlargement had abnormal EEGs. The authors supposed

Table 5. Cortical metabolism rate and EEG (means ± standard deviation of mean) (Obrist 1963)

	Normal aged (n=26)	Dementia (n=10)
CBF (ml/100 g brain tissue/min)	57.8 ± 10.4	48.5 ± 11.5
CMR (O_2 ml/100 g brain tissue/min)	3.3 ± 0.4	2.7 ± 0.5
EEG peak frequency (Hz)	9.7 ± 0.6	7.5 ± 0.9
EEG % slow activity	11.0 ± 8.0	33.5 ± 18.3

CBF, cerebral blood flow; CMR, cortical metabolism rate

Table 6. Correlation rCBF and EEG (Ingvar and Gustafson 1970)

	EEG normal (n=10)	EEG slightly abnormal (n=14)	EEG markedly abnormal (n=14)
rCBF (ml/100 g/min)	46.0 ± 5.3	47.9 ± 12.6	37.3 ± 8.4

Table 7. Correlation of pneumoencephalogram and EEG in patients (n) (Sisson and Ellingson 1956)

	PEG	
	Slightly abnormal	Moderate to strong dilatation
EEG (normal)	5	2
EEG (abnormal)	6	12

PEG, pneumoencephalogram

Table 8. Classification of pathologic findings in patients (*n*) (Gloor et al. 1968)

Group I	affecting cortical gray matter	5
Group II	affecting cortical and subcortical gray matter	8
Group III	affecting white matter	8
Group IV	affecting cortical and subcortical gray and white matter	11

Table 9. Correlation of EEG and pathologic findings in patients (*n*) (Gloor et al. 1968)

EEG disturbances	Pathological classification			
	I (5)	II (8)	III (8)	IV (11)
Background activity	5	8	7	11
Unilateral paroxysmal	2	1	0	2
Bilateral paroxysmal	2	8	3	8
Periodicity	1	3	0	5
Polymorphous delta	3	0	8	9
Focal	2	5	1	2

For definitions of groups I, II, III, and IV, see Table 8

that normal EEGs in patients with ventricular dilatation might be a sign of a standstill in the dementing process. Again, the rate of disease progress is reflected more in EEG abnormalities and not primarily in the degree of cerebral atrophy. These findings have since been confirmed by many authors as well as by the recent use of computer-assisted tomography (CAT) (Roberts et al. 1978; Soininen et al. 1982a, b).

Neuropathologic Findings. The correlation between neuropathologic findings and EEG is also less strict, as can be illustrated by a well-documented study of Gloor et al. (1968). They distinguished four categories of neuropathologic abnormalities as shown in Table 8. This classification correlates with EEG abnormalities as shown in Table 9. It can be concluded from these data that: (a) EEG background activity abnormalities are found in all groups manifesting neuropathologic abnormalities; (b) bilateral paroxysmal activity and periodicity in EEGs are mainly observed in subjects with subcortical gray matter abnormalities; (c) polymorphic delta activity occurs mainly in patients suffering white matter abnormalities; and (d) EEG focal abnormalities correlate more or less with cortical and subcortical gray matter abnormalities.

Summary

EEG abnormalities are associated with dementia, often resulting in a decrease in alpha rhythm frequency, a decrease in or even a total suppression of alpha rhythm abundance and hypo- or nonreactivity of the background pattern. Less often, there are focal abnormalities and bilateral paroxysmal abnormalities. There is a high degree of correlation between EEG anomalies and the rate of clinical dementia, social functioning, the rate of disease progress, mortality expectancy, and decreases in cerebral blood flow and metabolism. EEG abnormalities correlate less well with cerebral atrophy, ventricular dilatation, and neuropathologic findings.

Evoked Potentials

Introduction

Evoked potentials are responses evoked by sensory stimulation of the peripheral and central nervous system. As these potentials have a small amplitude (0.5–20 μV), they are difficult to distinguish from the EEG background activity, which has a relatively large amplitude (25–100 μV). Consequently, special analyzing techniques (averaging) are needed to detect these potentials. The evoked potentials modalities most often used are (a) visual evoked potentials (VEP) resulting from retinal stimulation by flashes or pattern reversal; (b) auditory evoked potentials (AEP) elicited through cochlear stimulation by clicks; (c) somatosensory evoked potentials (SEP) resulting from electrical stimulation of peripheral nerves.

The response may be divided into three phases:

1. subcortical: of very small amplitude and short latency, located in the spinal cord or brain stem
2. specific cortical (primary complex): the earliest phase of the cortical response representing medium latency response of the specific cortical areas
3. cortical aspecific (secondary complex): the long latency phase of the response, which is dependent on task relevance and originates more diffusely, probably in the associative cortical areas.

Evoked potentials are specified by their peak parameters and nominated by their peak polarity (N is negative, P is positive) and mean normal peak latencies (in ms). P 100 means a positive peak with a mean latency of 100 ms in normal subjects.

Evoked Potentials in the Normal Aged

There is a slight, age-dependent increase in peak latencies. The data cannot be discussed in detail here.

Evoked Potentials in Dementia

Visual Evoked Potentials

Straumanis et al. (1965) examined 20 arteriosclerotic brain syndrome patients by means of VEP and found an increase in the amplitude of the medium-latency

Table 10. Flash VEP peak latencies in ms (mean ± standard deviation of mean) in normal subjects and SDAT patients

	Normal adults	SDAT patients
P70	73 ± 9	67 ± 10
N85	90 ± 17	100 ± 20*
P110	107 ± 23	151 ± 23*
N150	146 ± 26	211 ± 32*
P200	202 ± 18	269 ± 34*
N225	226 ± 16	331 ± 31

SDAT, senile dementia of the Alzheimer type
* significant latency increase

Table 11. Correlation of degree of dementia and VEP P100 latency (Cosi et al. 1982)

	P100 latency in ms (mean ± standard deviation of mean)
Normal adults (19–40 years)	117.5 ± 13.3
Aged subjects (41–81 years)	
no atrophy, no dementia ($n = 30$)	139.4 ± 27.0
atrophy, no dementia ($n = 30$)	150.0 ± 22.0
atrophy, dementia	193.3 ± 33.7

peaks and a latency increase in the long-latency peaks. Examining 19 patients with senile dementia of the Alzheimer type by flash VEP, Visser et al. (1976) also found for that type of dementia increased amplitudes for the medium-latency and increased latencies for the long-latency peaks (Table 10).

The degree of VEP latency increase correlates with the degree of dementia, as has been shown by Cosi et al. (1982) (Table 11).

Recently, our (Visser et al. 1976) findings of prolonged latencies of flash VEP in dementia were confirmed by Wright et al. (1984). However, Coben et al. (1983 b) were not able to confirm our data by using flash VEP; however, their patients were mild dements of the Alzheimer type, all of them outpatients. Our group consisted entirely of mental hospital inmates. The discrepancy may be explained by Cosi's findings (Cosi et al. 1982) that the degree of VEP abnormalities correlates with the severity of dementia. Coben et al. (1983 b) also used pattern reversal VEP in their group of mildly demented patients and demonstrated significant latency increases, again, especially for the late peaks. This was also confirmed in the mental hospital inmates with senile dementia of the Alzheimer type participating in our recent study using pattern reversal VEP (Visser et al. 1985; Table 12). Wright et al. (1984) were unable to confirm the findings of Coben and Visser for pattern reversal VEP. However, they mentioned only the major positive peak P 100, which indeed is not delayed, and they neglected the late peaks. Find-

Table 12. Pattern reversal VEP peak latencies in ms (mean ± standard deviation of mean)

	Normal adults	SDAT patients
P50	46 ± 18	48 ± 20
N60	60 ± 14	67 ± 17
P100	99 ± 11	103 ± 12
N140	149 ± 19	161 ± 21*
P200	203 ± 30	232 ± 35*
N250	269 ± 59	307 ± 49*

SDAT, senile dementia of the Alzheimer type
* significant latency increase

Table 13. Median nerve SEP peak latencies in ms (mean ± standard deviation of mean)

	Normal aged adults	Demented patients
N9	11 ± 1	11 ± 1
N14	14 ± 1	14 ± 1
N20	20 ± 1	19 ± 1
P25	30 ± 6	38 ± 9*
N35	35 ± 5	41 ± 4*
P45	44 ± 6	53 ± 5*
N60	65 ± 10	83 ± 13*
P100	93 ± 16	114 ± 23*
N140	156 ± 20	170 ± 24*

* significant latency increase

ings similar to those discussed here for senile dementia of the Alzheimer type have been published for Parkinson's disease and Jakob-Creutzfeldt disease.

Somatosensory Evoked Potentials

Levy et al. (1971) reported an SEP peak latency delay of the late components in a small group ($n = 9$) of dementia patients but were not able to confirm these findings in a later study (Hendrickson et al. 1979). Since literature on SEP in dementia is scanty, we performed a pilot study (Huisman et al. 1985). In ten dementia patients admitted to a mental hospital, we found an abnormal delay of the late complex peak latencies (Table 13).

Auditory Evoked Potentials

There are reports of late-peak latency increase in auditory evoked potentials (Laurian et al. 1977; Hendrickson et al. 1979) and even of increases in peak V of the short-latency (brain stem) AEP in dementia (McEvoy and Harkins 1981).

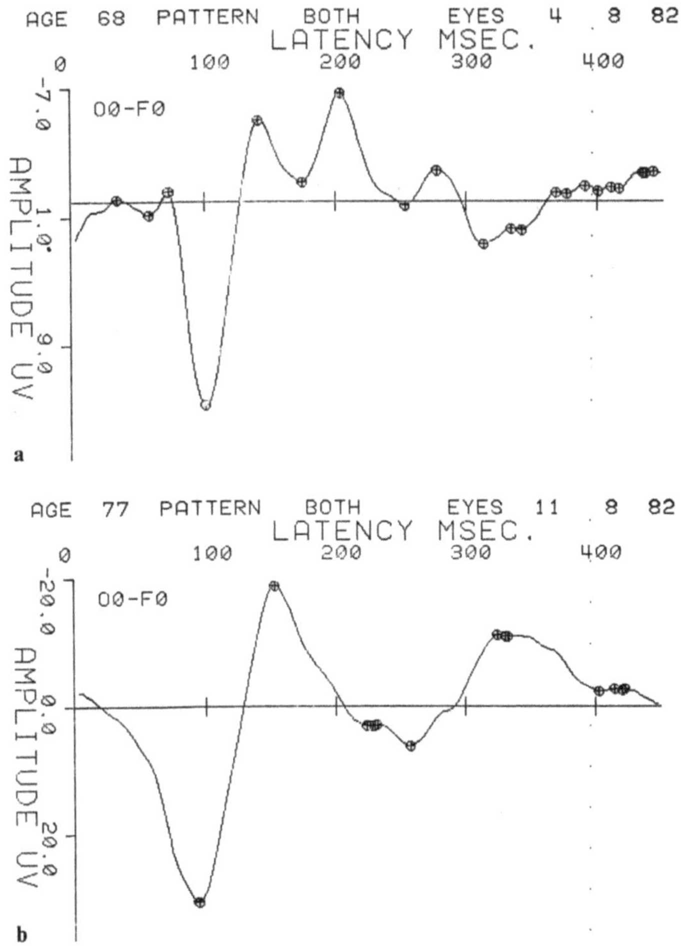

Fig. 3. a Latency increase of the VEP peaks. **b** Normal visual evoked potential

Summary

Both flash and pattern reversal VEPs show an abnormal latency increase in the late-component peaks in dementia, especially in SDAT (Fig. 3a, b). The same holds true for the late complex peaks of SEP and probably also for AEP.

Value of Evoked Potential Abnormalities in the Diagnosis of Dementia

Evoked potentials can help to differentiate between normal aged subjects and SDAT patients. However, they are of value in distinguishing normal subjects from demented patients only if it is possible to differentiate dementia from nonorganic depressive syndromes in the elderly. For that reason, Coben et al. (1983b) and Visser et al. (1985) included a group of elder patients with nonorganic psychiatric syndromes in their studies. In both studies, significant abnormalities of evoked potentials were found only in the dementia groups.

Coben et al. (1983 a) also described EEG abnormalities in the same group of demented patients but did not compare the VEP and EEG results. Our recent study (Visser et al. 1985) using both VEP and EEG proves that EEG detects dementia more often than VEP does. Because EEG sensitivity is higher than VEP sensitivity in the diagnostics of dementia, evoked potentials are not a substitute for EEG in the clinical diagnosis of dementia.

Evoked potentials, on the other hand, can give more specific information than EEG. In subcortical and brain stem disturbances, short-latency peaks are abnormal. In disorders involving demyelination of white matter, the primary complex latency peaks (for SEP N 20 and for VEP P 50, N 60, and P 100) are delayed. In primary degenerative dementia, only the late complex peaks are delayed. This type of differentiation is not possible with EEG alone.

Primary complex peaks are localized and originate in the primary specific cortical areas. Late complex long-latency peaks are more widely spread, probably originating in the associative cortical areas, and reflect the information-processing phase. From evoked potential studies, it can be concluded that the abnormalities in primary degenerative dementias are mainly localized in the associative cortex. This conclusion fits very well with neuropathologic findings (Brun and Gustafson 1978) and positron emission tomography (PET) data (Friedland et al. 1983), all of which demonstrate abnormalities, mainly localized in the parietotemporal associative cortical areas, in patients with senile dementia of the Alzheimer type.

References

Abbott J (1959) The EEG in Jakob-Creutzfeldt's disease. Electroencephalogr Clin Neurophysiol 11:184–185

Andermann K, Stoller A (1961) EEG patterns in hospitalized and non-hospitalized aged. Electroencephalogr Clin Neurophysiol 13:319

Berger H (1933) Über das Elektrencephalogramm des Menschen V. Arch Psychiatr Nervenkr 98:231–254

Brun A, Gustafson L (1978) Limbic lobe involvement in presenile dementia. Arch Psychiatr Nervenkr 226:79–93

Busse EW, Obrist WD (1965) Pre-senescent electroencephalographic changes in normal subjects. J Gerontol 20:315–320

Busse EW, Barnes RH, Friedman EL, Kelty EJ (1956) Aged individuals with normal and abnormal electroencephalograms. J Nerv Ment Dis 124:135–141

Cahan RB, Yeager CL (1966) Admission EEG as a predictor of mortality and discharge for aged hospital patients. J Gerontol 21:248–256

Coben LA, Danziger WL, Berg L (1983 a) Frequency analysis of the resting awake EEG in mild senile dementia of Alzheimer type. Electroencephalogr Clin Neurophysiol 55:372–380

Coben LA, Danziger WL, Hughes CP (1983 b) Visual evoked potentials in mild senile dementia of Alzheimer type. Electroencephalogr Clin Neurophysiol 55:121–130

Cosi V, Vitelli E, Gozzoli L, Corona A, Ceroni M, Callieco R (1982) Visual evoked potentials in aging of the brain. In: Courjon J, Mauguière F, Revol M (eds) Clinical applications of evoked potentials in neurology. Raven, New York, pp 109–115

Dejaiffe G, Constantinidis J, Rey-Bellet J, Tissot R (1964) Corrélations électrocliniques dans les démences de l'âge avancé. Acta Neurol Belg 64:677–707

Drachman DA, Hughes JR (1971) Memory and the hippocampal complexes. III Aging and temporal EEG abnormalities. Neurology (Minneapolis) 21:1–14

England AC, Schwab RS, Peterson E (1959) The electroencephalogram in Parkinson's syndrome. Electroencephalogr Clin Neurophysiol 11:723–731

Friedland RP, Budinger TF, Ganz E, Yano Y, Mathis CA, Koss B, Ober BA, Huesman RH, Derenzo SE (1983) Regional cerebral metabolic alterations in dementia of the Alzheimer type: positron emission tomography with [^{18}F]fluorodeoxyglucose. J Comput Assist Tomogr 7:590–598

Gibbs FA, Gibbs EL (1951) Changes with age, awake. In: Gibbs FA, Gibbs EL (eds) Atlas of electroencephalography, vol I. Methodology and methods. Addison-Wesley, Reading (Mass), pp 82–88

Gloor P, Kalabay O, Giard N (1968) The electroencephalogram in diffuse encephalopathies. Electroencephalographic correlates of grey and white matter lesions. Brain 91:779–802

Gordon EB, Sim M (1967) The EEG in presenile dementia. J Neurol Neurosurg Psychiatr 30:285–291

Greenblatt M, Levin S, Atwell C (1945) Comparative value of electroencephalogram and abstraction tests in diagnosis of brain damage. J Nerv Ment Dis 102:383–391

Gustafson L, Risberg J, Hagberg B, Hoigaard K, Nilssen L, Ingvar DH (1972) Cerebral blood flow, EEG and psychometric variables related to clinical findings in presenile dementia. Acta Neurol Scand [Suppl] 51:439–440

Hendrickson E, Levy R, Post F (1979) Averaged evoked responses in relation to cognitive and affective state of elderly psychiatric patients. Br J Psychiatry 134:494–501

Huisman UW, Posthuma J, Hooijer V, Visser SL, De Rijke W (1985) Somatosensory evoked potentials in healthy volunteers and patients with dementia. Clin Neurol Neurosurg 87:11–16

Ingvar DH, Gustafson L (1970) Regional cerebral blood flow in organic dementia with early onset. Acta Neurol Scand 46 [Suppl] 43:42–73

Jones DP, Nevin S (1954) Rapidly progressive cerebral degeneration (subacute vascular encephalopathy) with mental disorder, focal disturbances and myoclonic epilepsy. J Neurol Neurosurg Psychiatr 17:148–159

Laidlaw J, Catling J (1964) An EEG assessment of encephalopathy in Parkinsonism. J Neurol Neurosurg Psychiatr 27:232–236

Laurian S, Lobrinus S, Wertheimer J, Gaillard JM (1977) Evoked responses in dementia and the significance of the vertex potential. Electroencephalogr Clin Neurophysiol 43:525–526

Letemendia F, Pampiglione G (1958) Clinical and EEG observations in Alzheimer's disease. J Neurol Neurosurg Psychiatr 21:167–172

Levy E, Isaacs A, Behrman J (1971) Neurophysiological correlates of senile dementia. II The somatosensory evoked response. Psychol Med 1:159–165

Liddell DW (1958) Investigations of EEG findings in presenile dementia. J Neurol Neurosurg Psychiatr 21:173–176

Lundervold A, Engeset A, Lonnum A (1962) The EEG in cerebral atrophy. World Neurol 3:226–234

McAdam W, Robinson RA (1956) Senile intellectual deterioration and the EEG; quantitative correlation. J Ment Sci 102:819–825

McEvoy TM, Harkins SW (1981) Brainstem auditory evoked potentials in patients with presenile dementia. Abstracts XII Intern Congress Gerontology, Hamburg, vol 2, p 218

Mundy-Castle AC, Hurst LA, Beerstecher DM, Prinsloo T (1954) The electroencephalogram in senile psychoses. Electroencephalogr Clin Neurophysiol 6:245–252

Obrist WD (1954) The electroencephalogram of normal aged adults. Electroencephalogr Clin Neurophysiol 6:235–244

Obrist WD (1963) The EEG of healthy aged males. In: Birren JE, Butler RN, Greenhouse SW, Sokoloff L, Yarrow MR (eds) Human aging: a biological and behavioral study. US Govt Printing Office, Washington PHS Publ No 986, pp 79–93

Obrist WD, Henry CE (1958) Electroencephalographic frequency analysis of aged psychiatric patients. Electroencephalogr Clin Neurophysiol 10:621–632

Obrist WD, Busse EW, Eisdorfer C, Kleemeier RE (1962) Relation of the electroencephalogram to intellectual function in senescence. J Gerontol 17:197–206
Roberts MA, McGeorge AP, Caird FI (1978) EEG and computerized tomography in vascular and non-vascular dementia in old age. J Neurol Neurosurg Psychiatr 41:903–906
Scott DF, Heathfield KWG, Toone B, Margerison JH (1972) The EEG in Huntington's chorea: a clinical and neuropathological study. J Neurol Neurosurg Psychiatr 35:97–102
Sisson BD, Ellingson RJ (1956) The EEG in cerebral atrophy. J Nerv Ment Dis 123:244–248
Soininen H, Partanen VJ, Helkala EL, Riekkinen PJ (1982a) EEG findings in senile dementia and normal aging. Acta Neurol Scand 65:59–70
Soininen H, Partanen JV; Puranen M, Riekkinen PJ (1982b) EEG and computed tomography in the investigation of patients with senile dementia. J Neurol Neurosurg Psychiatry 45:711–714
Stoller A (1949) Slowing of the alpha rhythm on the EEG and its association with mental deterioration and epilepsy. J Ment Sci 95:972–984
Straumanis JJ, Shagass C, Schwartz M (1965) Visually evoked cerebral response changes associated with chronic brain syndromes and aging. J Gerontol 20:498–506
Visser SL, Stam FC, Van Tilburg W, Op den Velde W, Blom JL, De Rijke W (1976) Visual evoked response in senile and presenile dementia. Electroencephalogr Clin Neurophysiol 40:385–392
Visser SL, Van Tilburg W, Hooijer C, Jonker C, De Rijke W (1985) Visual evoked potentials (VEPs) in senile dementia (Alzheimer type) and in non-organic behavioural disorders in the elderly; comparison with EEG parameters. Electroencephalogr Clin Neurophysiol 60:115–121
Vogel F, Wendt GG, Oepen H (1961) Das EEG und das Problem einer Frühdiagnose der Chorea Huntington. Dtsch Z Nervenheilk 182::355–361
Weiner H, Schuster DB (1956) The electroencephalogram in dementia – some preliminary observations and correlations. Electroencephalogr Clin Neurophysiol 8:479–488
Wright CE, Harding GFA, Orwin A (1984) Presenile dementia – the use of the flash and pattern VEP in diagnosis. Electroencephalogr Clin Neurophysiol 57:405–415

Nuclear Magnetic Resonance and Early Diagnosis of Brain Pathology

W. L. CURATI and R. E. STEINER[1]

Introduction

For a variety of reasons, the initial efforts of many medical centres to put nuclear magnetic resonance (NMR) to clinical use have focussed on the brain:

1. A high level of grey-white matter contrast can be obtained with NMR, providing anatomical detail on a scale not available with other techniques.
2. Coronal and sagittal imaging are particularly useful in depicting areas of the brain.
3. The absence of bone artifacts is a major advantage over x-ray computerized tomography (CT).
4. Flow effects are well demonstrated using appropriate sequences.
5. NMR is sensitive to a variety of pathological changes within the brain.

In this paper, we review the normal appearance of the brain as well as a few examples of pathological change, such as vascular disease, white matter disease, cerebral tumours and paediatric neurological disease.

Methods

The NMR machine is based on a cryomagnet manufactured by Oxford Instruments Ltd. which provides a static magnetic field (Bo) of 0.15 tesla giving a resonant frequency of 6.5 MHz. Gradient coils are placed within the bore of the magnet to provide spatial encoding of the NMR signal and to select a slice. A radio-frequency transmitter coil surrounds the patient's head, and a smaller receiver coil detects the NMR signal (Young et al. 1982). Pulse sequences are summarised in Table 1. Contemporary x-ray CT scans are obtained in each case, either with a Siemens Somatom 2 whole-body scanner at Hammersmith Hospital or with an EMI CT 1010 head scanner. Some recent CT examinations have been performed with a GE 9800 whole-body scanner.

1 NMR Unit, Royal Postgraduate Medical School, Hammersmith Hospital, London W12 OHS, UK

Senile Dementia of the Alzheimer Type
Ed. by J. Traber and W. H. Gispen

Table 1. Pulse sequences used in Hammersmith NMR unit

Pulse sequence	Interpulse time (ms)		
	TR	TI	TE
SR 1000	1000		
IR 1500/500/44	1500	500	44
IR 1800/600/44	1800	600	44
SE 544/44	544		44
SE 1500/44	1500		44
SE 1500/80	1500		80
SE 1580/80	1580		80

TR, repetition time; TI, inversion time; TE, echo time; SR, saturation recovery; IR, inversion recovery; SE, spin echo

Results

Normal Appearance of the Brain

Inversion recovery (IR) scans (Fig. 1 a) display a high level of grey-white matter contrast, with white matter appearing white, grey matter appearing grey and CSF appearing black. The correspondence with classic anatomical sections is striking.

Spin-echo (SE) scans (Fig. 1 b) display a lesser degree of grey-white matter contrast, although the contrast becomes sharper as the echo time (TE) increases.

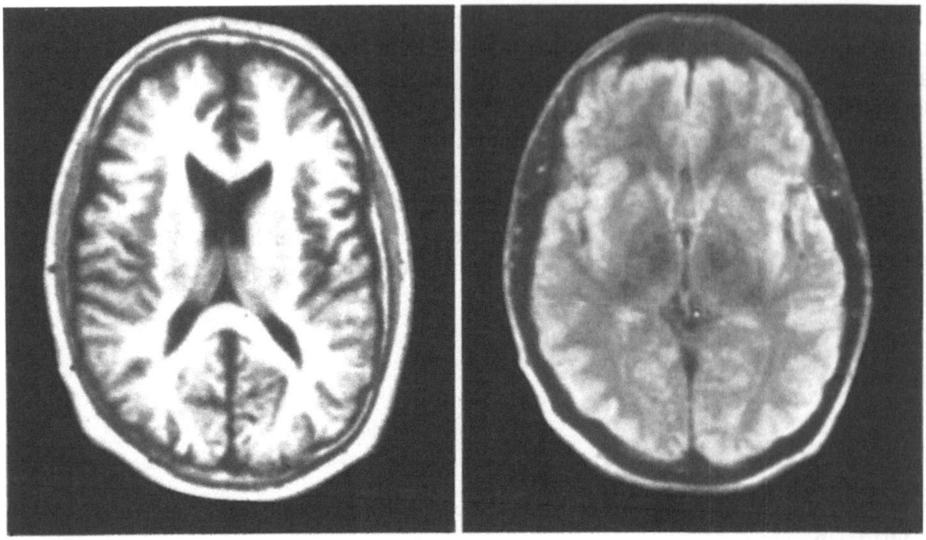

a b

Fig. 1 a, b. Normal brain. **a** (IR 1500/500) high level of grey-white matter contrast; **b** (SE 1580/80) poor grey-white matter contrast

As a result of the long longitudinal and transverse relaxation times (T_1 and T_2 respectively), CSF, which appears dark with a short TE, becomes light with a long TE. Cortical bone gives a low signal.

Vascular Disease of the Brain

Acute intracerebral haemorrhage frequently displays a short T_1 and a long T_2. In addition, central areas of liquefaction or clot dissolution may be seen (Fig. 2a, b). On both IR and SE sequences, acute haemorrhage appears light. When the haemorrhage resolves, it may eventually leave residual cysts. During this process, there is an increase in T_1 and T_2.

Cerebral infarction produces an increase in T_1 and T_2. On IR scans, grey-white matter contrast is lessened (Bydder et al. 1982). In addition, a mass effect is usually associated with large areas of infarction (Fig. 3a, b).

White Matter Disease of the Brain

The typical periventricular "plaques" of multiple sclerosis are well-demonstrated with NMR, and this was one of the first clinical applications of this technique (Young et al. 1981). The lesions are characterised by an increase in T_1 and T_2. Small lesions and those located in he posterior fossa are usually demonstrated with NMR, though not with CT (Fig. 4a, b). Leucodystrophy is also associated

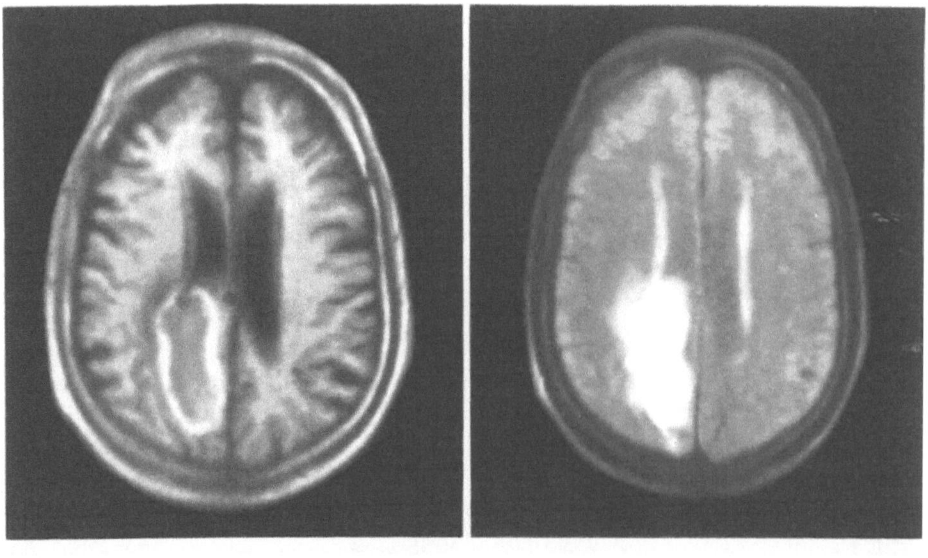

a b

Fig. 2a, b. Intracerebral haemorrhage appearing as light area. **a** (IR 1500/500) central liquefaction appears darker; **b** (SE 1580/80) both surrounding edema and periventricular edema are well-demonstrated as more extensive light areas

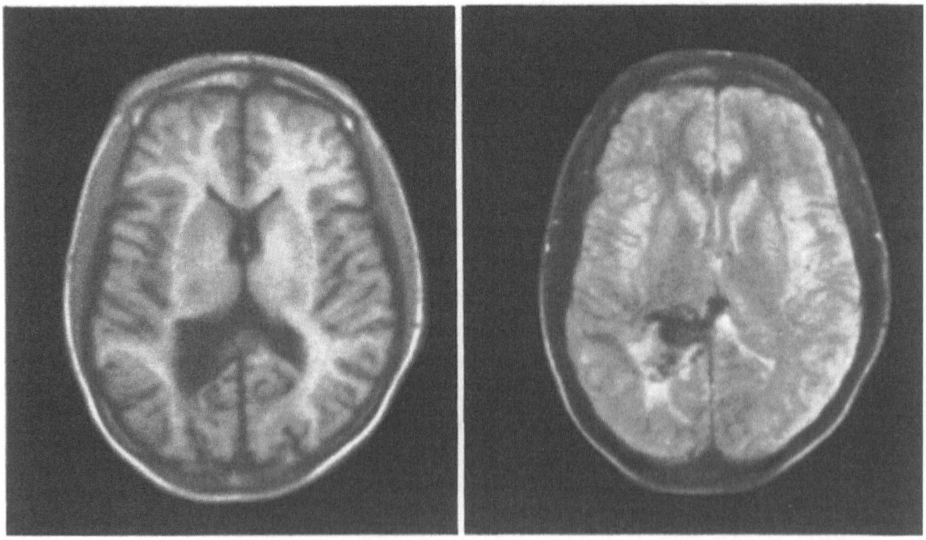

a b

Fig. 3 a, b. Infarction, showing increase in both T_1 and T_2. **a** (IR 1500/500) dark areas with dimination of grey-white matter contrast; **b** (SE 1580/80) appears as light area with some surrounding edema

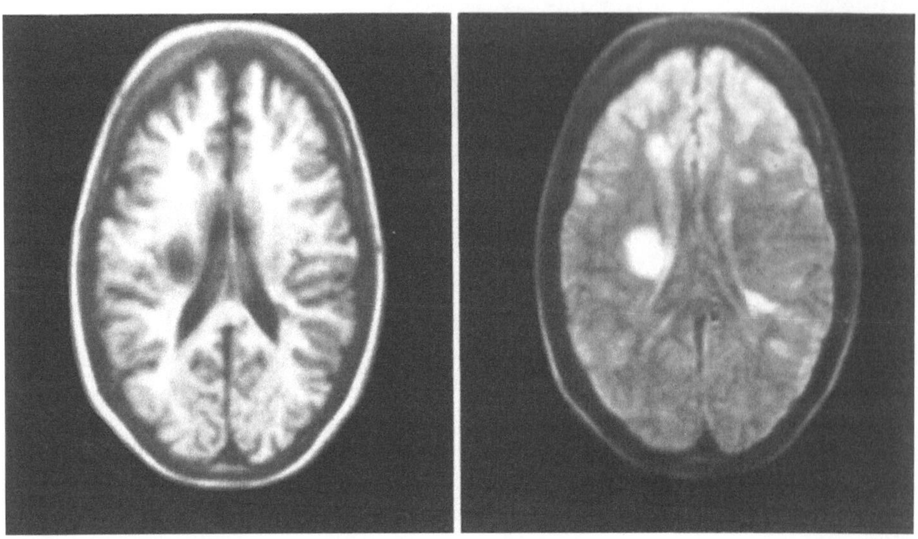

a b

Fig. 4 a, b. Multiple sclerosis affecting multiple areas showing an increase in both T_1 and T_2. **a** IR 1500/500; **b** SE 1500/80

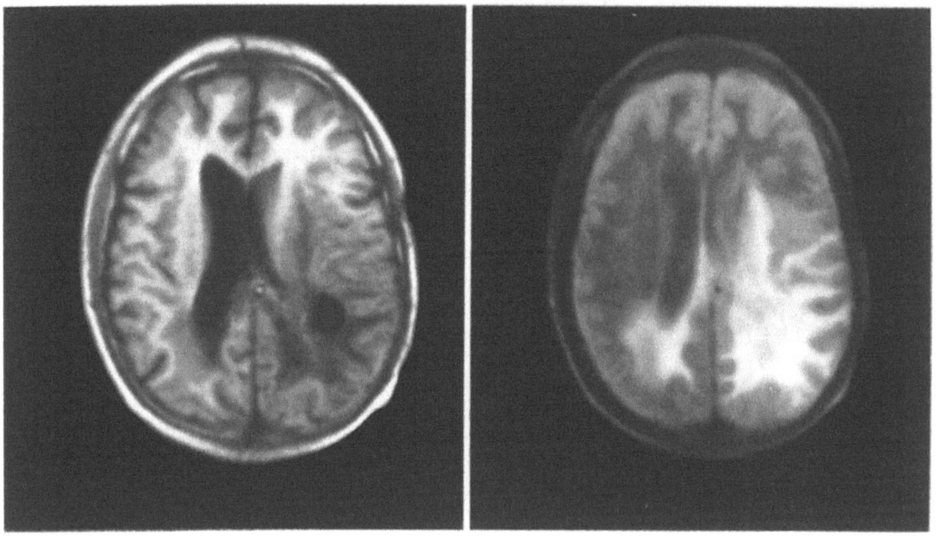

a b

Fig. 5 a, b. Temporoparietal ependymoma. **a** (IR 1500/500) good delineation and mass effect; **b** (SE 1500/80) extensive edema

with an increase in T_1 and T_2 relaxation times, with the abnormal white matter usually distributed as patchy periventricular areas.

Binswanger's disease and radiation damage are also characterised by abnormal white matter.

Cerebral Tumours

Tumours are usually characterised by a focal increase in T_1 and T_2. The increase in T_1, which appears as a dark region, is best seen with IR scans. Associated with the increase in T_1 is a diminution of grey-white matter contrast. The increase in T_2 appears as a light area relative to brain on SE scans. Since there is little contrast between white and grey matter, localization of the tumour is not as precise as with IR (Fig. 5 a, b) (Bydder et al. 1984).

Additional features associated with cerebral tumours include haemorrhage and calcifications, peritumoral edema (causing increases in T_1 and T_2, as with the tumour itself) and mass effects and displacement.

Paediatric Neurological Development and Diseases

Extensive postmortem study of normal brain development has established the normal pattern of maturation, including the degree of myelination (Johnson et al. 1983; see the extensive bibliography). For example, the IR scan of a 6-month-old infant shows white matter present in the posterior internal capsule and thalamo-occipital radiation (Fig. 6).

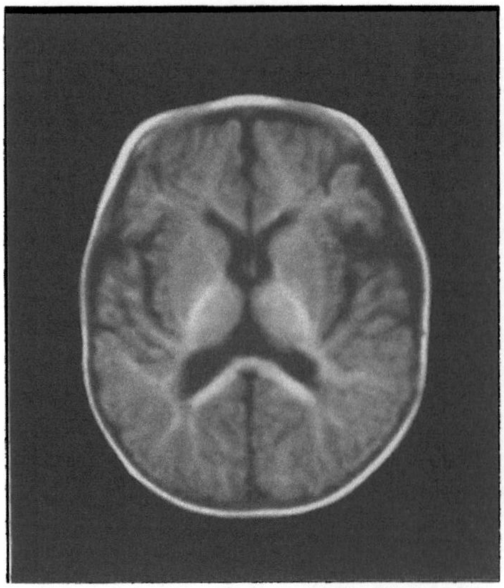

Fig. 6. Myelination in the brain of a normal 6-month-old child (IR 1800/600). This long TR-long TI sequence is normal, given the high water content of the brain at this age

A whole range of abnormal appearances is very well-demonstrated by NMR, from delayed myelination to tumours.

Conclusion

NMR imaging is sensitive to many different pathological changes. The fact that NMR has no known hazards is an advantage both in the examination of children as well as for repeated examinations. The lack of bone artifacts with NMR, in contrast to x-ray CT, results in better imaging of areas such as the posterior fossa, the base of the skull and the spinal cord. The potential clinical application of NMR contrast agents such as gadolinium-diethylene triamine penta-acetic acid is under investigation (Carr et al. 1984). Enhancement of cerebral tumours by means of this technique has so far proved to be very promising.

References

Bydder GM, Steiner RE, Young IR, Hall HS, Thomas DJ, Marshall J, Pallis CA, Legg NJ (1982) Clinical NMR imaging of the brain. Am J Roentgenol 139:215–236

Bydder GM, Pennock JM, Steiner RE, Orr JS, Bailes DR, Young IR (1984) The NMR diagnosis of Cerebral Tumors. Magnetic Resonance in Medicine 1:5–29

Carr DH, Brown J, Bydder GM, Steiner RE, Weinmann HJ, Spreck U, Hall AJ, Young IR (1984) Intravenous Gadolinium-DTPA as a Contrast Agent. Am J Roentgenol 143:215–224

Johnson MA, Pennock JM, Bydder GM, Steiner RE, Thomas DJ, Hayward R, Bryant DRT, Payne JA, Levene MMI, Whitelaw A, Dubowitz LMS, Dubowitz V (1983) Clinical NMR imaging of the brain in children: Normal and neurological disease. AJNR 4:1013–1026

Young IR, Bailes DR, Burl M, Collins AG, Smith DT, McDonnell MJ, Orr JS, Banks LM, Bydder GM, Greenspan RH, Steiner RE (1982) Initial clinical evaluation of a whole body NMR tomograph. J Comput Assist Tomogr 6:1–18

Young IR, Hall AS, Pallis CA, Legg NJ, Bydder GM, Steiner RE (1984) NMR imaging of the brain in multiple sclerosis. Lancet ii:1063–1066

Positron Tomography and the Differential Diagnosis and Pathophysiology of Alzheimer's Disease *

R. P. FRIEDLAND [1,2], T. F. BUDINGER [2,3], W. J. JAGUST [1,2], E. KOSS [1,2], S. DERENZO [2], R. H. HUESMAN [2], and Y. YANO [2]

The diagnosis of Alzheimer's disease (AD) remains a diagnosis of exclusion. While less frequent varieties of non-Alzheimer dementia are now diagnosed with relative ease using widely available laboratory tests, the definitive diagnosis of Alzheimer's disease still requires the examination of excised tissue. However, recently developed methods for the noninvasive in vivo quantitation of cerebral rates of glucose use have demonstrated regional abnormalities in Alzheimer subjects which are of diagnostic import and can offer us some insight into the pathophysiology of the disease.

Positron Emission Tomographic (PET) Studies with ^{18}F-labeled 2-fluoro-2-deoxy-D-glucose (FDG)

Glucose is the brain's main energy source, and with PET studies of the uptake of the glucose analogue FDG, we are able to measure regional rates of glucose use (Phelps et al. 1979; Reivich et al. 1979; Kuhl et al. 1985). This parameter is closely related to rates of neuronal activity and reflects neuronal processes in both health and disease. We performed PET studies with FDG using the Donner 280-crystal tomograph, which has a resolution of 8 mm full width at half maximum (Friedland et al. 1983 b). A bolus of 5–10 mCi of FDG was injected intravenously, and tomographic data were obtained dynamically from one transverse section of the head, initially at 2.5- to 5-s intervals, followed by progressively longer intervals, for a period of 45 min. Multiple adjacent transverse sections 1 cm thick were imaged using 5-min intervals for data acquisition after the initial 45 min of dynamic data acquisition. Venous blood collected from a warmed hand was used to determine the input function (Phelps et al. 1979). Subjects remained awake with eyes open and ears unoccluded during the study. Transmission data obtained from an external source automatically deployed in the tomograph were used to correct for attenuation.

Emission tomographic data obtained 40–70 min after injection were studied. Regions of interest containing 3.5–29 resolution elements were drawn in each individual image to sample activity in the anterior frontal (F), temporal-parietal

* Supported in part by the Medical Research Service of the Veterans Administration, U.S., and the U.S. Department of Energy under Contract No. DE-AC03-76SF00098

1 VA Medical Center, Martinez, California 94553 and Department of Neurology, University of California, Davis, USA
2 Donner Laboratory, University of California, Berkeley, CA 94720, USA
3 Dept. of Radiology, University of California, San Francisco, CA, USA

Senile Dementia of the Alzheimer Type
Ed. by J. Traber and W. H. Gispen

(TP), and entire cortex regions of both sides. Percentage differences were computed comparing mean counts per cm^2 per s in the different regions. Dynamically collected blood input and tomographic data were used to determine the three rate constants of the three-compartment model developed by Sokoloff and colleagues (1977). FDG utilization rates were calculated using the product of the ratio $k_1^* k_3^* / k_2^* + k_3^*$ and the plasma glucose concentration, without consideration of the essentially unknown lumped constant for diseased brain.

Thus far, 17 subjects with probable AD (McKhann et al. 1984) and seven healthy, aged controls have been studied. All the AD subjects met current criteria for the diagnosis, including progressive impairment of mental function and no evidence of other pathologic processes (Friedland et al. 1983 b; 1985 b). For the AD group, the mean age was 64 years (SD, 6.7 years), and the mean score on the Mattis Dementia Rating scale (Friedland et al. 1983 b) was 93.9 (SD, 23.1), with a range of 129–55 (normal range, 144–140). The healthy, aged controls (mean age, 63 years; SD, 3.0 years) had normal general medical, neurologic, and neuropsychological exams. A complete description of instrumentation, data collection and analysis, and patient selection has been previously published (Friedland et al. 1983 b; 1985 b).

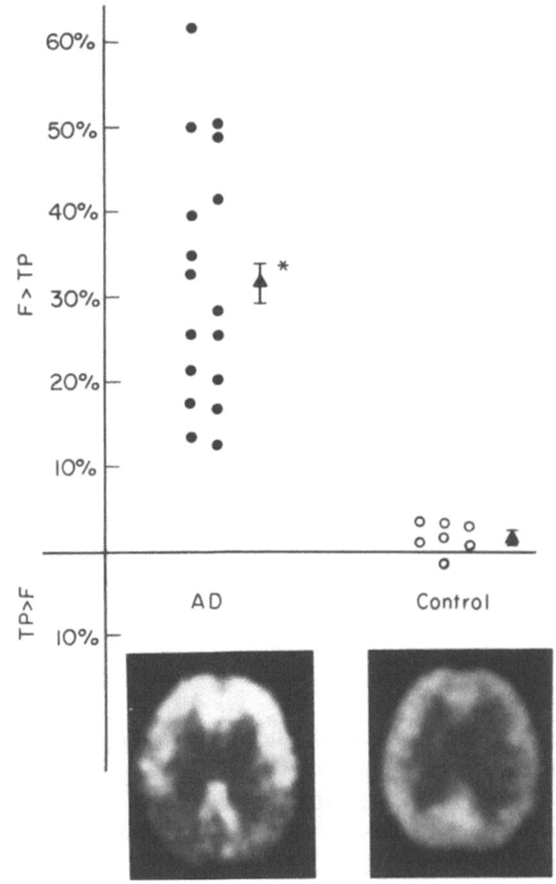

Fig. 1. (*Top*) Individual values for F-TP percentage difference of activity densities (mean of right and left cortices). ▲, mean and standard error of the mean for each group. $n = 17$ for AD patients (*filled circles*); $n = 7$ for controls (*open circles*). *, mean different from control group ($P < 0.0005$, one tailed). (*Bottom*) PET images of FDG accumulation, midventricular level. The subject's left hemisphere is on the *right side* of the image. Bilaterally diminished uptake in temporal-parietal cortex, right greater than left, is noted in the AD subject. (Adapted with permission from Friedland et al. 1985 b)

Table 1. FDG utilization rates

	Rate of cerebral metabolism of FDG (mg/100 g/min)		
	Frontal cortex	Temporal-parietal cortex	Entire cortex
Probable Alzheimers disease ($N=9$)	3.64[a] (1.40)	3.05[b] (1.26)	3.71[a] (1.40)
Healthy aged subjects ($n=6$)	4.32 (0.71)	4.19 (0.73)	4.23 (0.75)

Values expressed are means, with standard deviations in parentheses
[a] No significant difference from control group
[b] $p<0.025$, one-tailed

Figure 1 presents F-TP percentage difference values for the AD and healthy, aged subjects. These percentage differences reflect regional metabolic alterations because, by 40 min after FDG injection, ^{18}F concentrations are proportional in a linear fashion to regional rates of glucose use [Phelps et al. 1979; Sokoloff et al. 1977). All of the AD subjects demonstrated hypometabolism in the TP as compared with the F cortex (Fig. 1), while in the control group, there was no difference between F and TP activity levels. These F-TP differences are related to features of cognitive impairment (Friedland et al. 1983 b; 1985 b).

Metabolic rates for FDG are presented in Table 1, displaying TP hypometabolism in the AD group. Temporal hypometabolism was also noted at other levels in these subjects. The greater coefficient of variation for the CMR_{fdg} values as compared with the percentage differences is in accord with previous studies in healthy subjects. In our healthy subjects, the CMR_{fdg} was 1.54 mg/100 g/min (SD, 0.40; $n=2$) in white matter, producing a mean CMR_{fdg} of 2.88 mg/100 g/min, assuming a 50–50 gray-white composition (Phelps et al. 1979). Using the FDG lumped constant of 0.52 recently determined experimentally in normal young subjects by Reivich and colleagues (1984), we obtain a mean whole brain glucose utilization rate of 5.54 mg/100 g/min, which is similar to that reported by others using the arteriovenous extraction technique (5.38 mg/100 mg/min) (tabulated by Phelps et al. 1979).

Implications for Differential Diagnosis

A most important feature of our results is the finding of a decrease in the metabolism of the TP cortex relative to that of the F cortex in all of the 17 AD subjects studied. Similar findings of metabolic changes in these regions have been reported by others in studies of glucose use (Benson et al. 1983; Chase et al. 1984) and in studies of regional cerebral oxygen utilization ($rCMRO_2$) and regional cerebral blood flow (rCBF) rates (Frackowiak et al. 1981). Although these regional changes have not been detected in all reported PET-FDG studies of AD patients, this discrepancy is probably due to differences in spatial resolution, data analysis, and composition of subject populations. The lack of overlap between the F-TP percentage difference values of AD and healthy aged subjects (Fig. 1) suggests that metabolic imaging could be of value as a diagnostic test for AD. We cannot comment, however, on the presence of these metabolic changes in very "early" cases of AD, as all of our subjects were definitely demented (mild-moderate severity) at the time of testing.

We feel that the mapping of metabolism with PET provides a measure of disease processes on the microscopic level, as opposed to the gross structural measures provided by anatomical imaging. This is evident in the striking comparison to be made between the accentuated effects of the disease on FDG uptake in the TP region and the regional pathology of the disease (Brun 1984; Brun and Englund 1981). Histopathologic grading for senile plaques, neurofibrillary tangles, gliosis, spongiosis, and cytoarchitectural integrity performed by Brun and colleagues had demonstrated that the neocortical involvement in AD is most severe in the posterior temporal and parietal cortex (Brun 1984; Brun and Englund 1981) (Fig. 2). Thus, the cortical areas found to be most severely involved using PET-FDG studies of glucose use are the same regions found to be most severely affected by pathologic studies performed on a separate group.

The predilection of the metabolic and anatomical characteristics of AD for the TP area is not generally shared by other dementing illnesses. PET-FDG images typical of non-Alzheimer dementia are presented in Fig. 3. Most importantly, multi-infarct dementia (MID) produces diffuse lesions, and in PET-FDG studies of two MID subjects, we have not found the TP accentuation seen in AD. A more extensive series of PET-FDG studies of MID subjects by Kuhl and colleagues has demonstrated multiple deep and superficial lesions, with more lesions found by PET than by CT (Kuhl et al. 1985). Also, TP focality was not observed in studies of patients with presumed Pick's disease, communicating hydrocephalus (CH) (preshunt) (Jagust et al., to be published), and alcoholic dementia. Diffusely diminished CMR_{fdg} rates were observed, and other focal alterations were detected in these subjects. This is particularly important in the three cases of CH, all of whom improved following cerebrospinal fluid shunting procedures Hill. In one case of autopsy-confirmed Creutzfeldt-Jakob disease (CJD), however, bilateral and asymmetrical temporal-parietal hypometabolism was detected (Friedland et al. 1984b).

New developments in imaging instrumentation may be important in expanding the clinical availability of this diagnostic approach. While PET is limited at present to a few centers, single photon emission computed tomography (SPECT) with isotopes for relative cerebral blood flow measurement can provide regional physiologic data without the need for a local cyclotron, at a cost comparable to that of other clinical imaging modalities. Preliminary studies performed by Hill and colleagues (1984) and Cohen et al. (1984) indicate that SPECT studies may also be of value in the noninvasive identification of focal alterations of brain physiology in AD. These findings suggest that physiologic imaging could be used to develop a diagnostic test for AD.

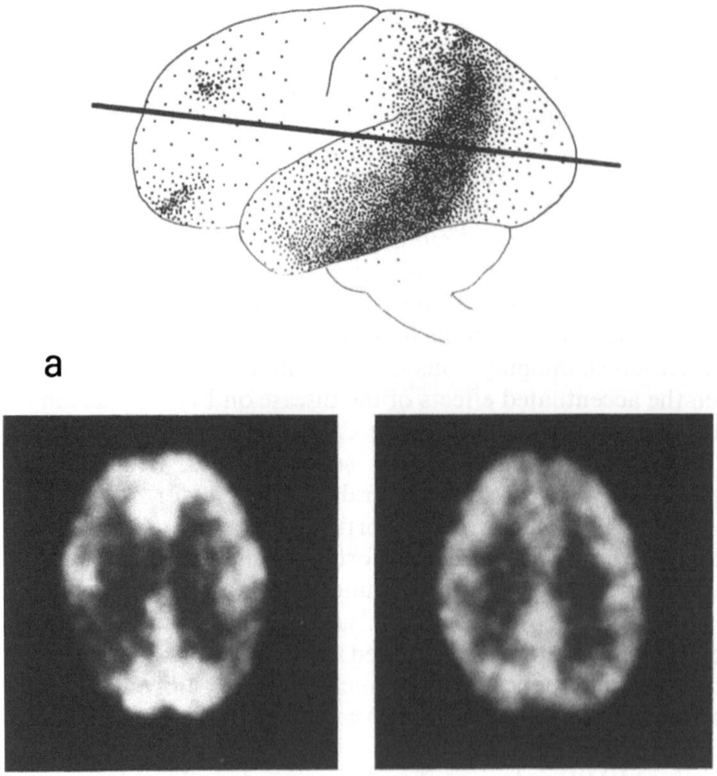

a

b c

Fig. 2. a Schematic representation of the distribution and severity of degeneration on the lateral brain surface in a representative Alzheimer case. The darker the area, the more pronounced the degeneration. (Brun 1984, reproduced with the permission of the Free Press, New York.) The *line* represents the plane of section (parallel to the canthomeatal line) of positron images of (^{18}F)-2-fluorodeoxyglucose accumulation in **b** an Alzheimer patient and **c** an healthy, aged control subject. Marked temporal-parietal hypometabolism is observed in **b**, more severe in the subject's right hemisphere. (The subject's left hemisphere is on the *right side* of the image). (Adapted from Friedland et al. 1985c)

The issue of diagnosis is an important one in dementia, as other noninvasive modalities have not detected *specific* brain changes in AD. While cortical atrophy and ventricular enlargement are often seen on X-ray computed tomography and nuclear magnetic resonance proton imaging of AD patients, they are also commonly seen in healthy elderly subjects. Also, our preliminary studies using NMR spin echo imaging have not disclosed any global or regional changes allowing for differentiation of AD patients from the healthy elderly (Friedland et al. 1984a).

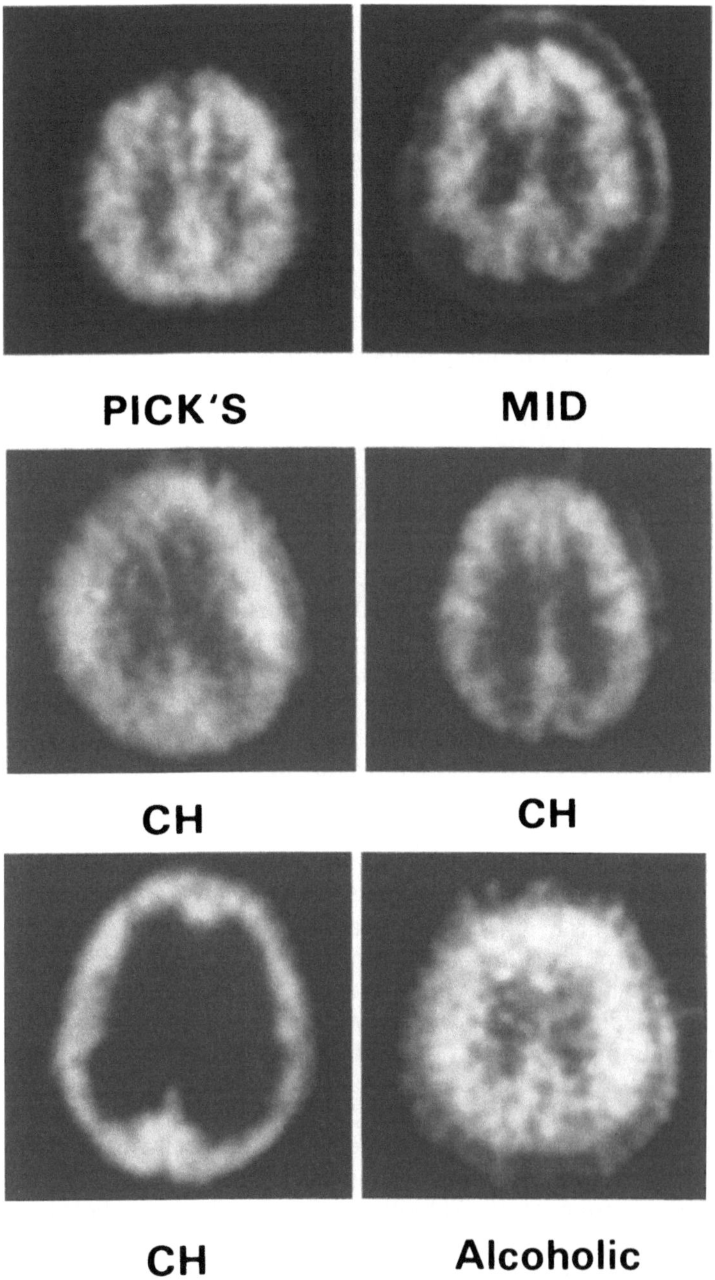

Fig. 3. Images of FDG uptake, midventricular level, in non-AD dementia subjects. (*MID*, multi-infarct dementia; *CH*, communicating hydrocephalus)

Implications for Pathophysiology

We cannot determine at present whether the diminished glucose use in the TP cortex characteristic of AD is caused by a decreased activity rate per neuron in a neuronal population of normal number, by a decreased neuronal number with normal or even increased metabolism in surviving neurons, or by a combination of these possibilities. We believe that areas of diminished cellular *viability* in disease are likely to be reflected by reduced uptake of *all* tracers, either through decrease in flow, metabolism, or receptor binding, as long as blood-brain barrier mechanisms remain intact. That is, reduced uptake of tracers such as FDG, ^{123}I-iodoamphetamine, ^{123}I-(R)-3-quinuclidinyl-4-iodobenzilate, or ^{11}C-methionine in AD may only be nonspecific markers of impaired neuronal function. Nevertheless, their behavior does provide a means of detection and evaluation of the precise brain regions most affected by disease.

The TP focality found so consistently in AD may provide us with topographical clues to the degeneration of the basal nucleus of Meynert (bnM) observed in AD. This basal forebrain region, the origin of most of the cholinergic innervation in the neocortex, has been found to be severely affected in AD. Mesulam and colleagues (1983) have recently reported that the posterior portion of the bnM (Ch4 posterior) projects mainly to the temporal lobe in the Rhesus monkey. The marked concentration of metabolic changes in the TP cortex may be a reflection of cell loss (or diminished neuronal firing) which is greatest in the posterior regions of the bnM.

Diminished FDG uptake in AD could be a reflection of a transport abnormality, particularly as there is much evidence to suggest that the blood-brain barrier (BBB) may be impaired in AD (for a review, see Friedland et al. 1984d). However, our initial studies of rubidium 82 and gallium 68 ethylene diaminetetraacetic acid (EDTA) uptake in brains of Alzheimer patients have not shown abnormal permeability of the brain to these two radionuclides (Friedland et al. 1983a; 1985b). In addition, our preliminary dynamic studies of the rate constants for FDG transport (k_1^*, k_2^*) have not shown differences between AD patients and healthy, aged subjects (Friedland et al. 1983c). However, because methodological aspects of this paradigm limit the accuracy of k_1^* and k_2^* determination (Budinger et al. 1985), this issue needs to be addressed further.

It is of interest to observe that in AD patients, impaired FDG uptake in the TP region is often asymmetrical (see Figs. 1, 2). Studies of lateral hemispheric percentage differences of FDG uptake have not found either hemisphere to be predominantly affected in a group of 18 AD subjects studied in our laboratory (Friedland et al. 1985b; Koss et al. 1985). However, approximately half the AD subjects have more metabolic asymmetry in the TP cortex than do healthy, age-matched controls. That is, group means show each hemisphere to be equally affected in the AD group, but more side-to-side differences were found in the AD group than in healthy, aged subjects. When this asymmetry is studied in absolute (nondirectional) units, we have found a mean of 13.9% (SD, 9.35%; $n=9$) asymmetry in the entire cortex (midventricular level) in AD patients, with a mean of 3.0% in healthy, aged subjects (SD, 3.75%; $n=6$; $P<0.005$) (Friedland et al.

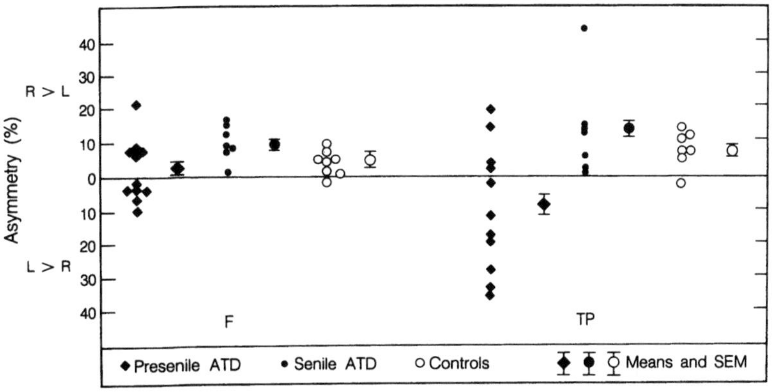

Fig. 4. Lateral asymmetries of glucose use in F and TP cortex. Percentage differences calculated as R-L/mean of R+L × 100 (activity densities, midventricular level). (*R*, right hemisphere; *L*, left hemisphere)

1985 b; Koss et al. 1985). Moreover, these asymmetries are related to the behavioral features of the illness. Most importantly, there was a negative correlation between memory abilities and absolute asymmetry in all regions ($P<0.05$) (Friedland et al. 1985 b).

These glucose utilization asymmetries are age-related and correspond to specific features of compromised performance. Figure 4 presents directional asymmetry values (percentage differences) for presenile AD ($n=11$; mean age, 59.2 years; SD, 3.2 years) and senile AD patients ($n=7$; mean age, 71.4 years; SD, 2.3 years) and healthy, aged controls ($n=7$; mean age, 63.0 years; SD 3.0 years). The presenile and senile AD groups did not differ in terms of duration of disease, performance IQ or verbal IQ (Koss et al. 1984). While the mean asymmetry of the senile subjects for the F and TP cortex did not differ from that of the controls, seven of the 11 presenile subjects displayed hypometabolism in the right TP cortex relative to the left TP cortex. This pattern was not observed in any of the senile AD patients or healthy, aged subjects. This asymmetry was related to cognitive performance: presenile subjects with greater right TP impairment performed much more poorly on the spatial tasks of the Wechsler Adult Intelligence Scale than either presenile subjects with relatively greater left hemisphere impairment ($P<0.001$) or senile subjects ($P<0.002$). Cognitive decline, as measured by the Mattis dementia rating scale, was also greater in presenile subjects with right hemisphere hypometabolism than in presenile patients with the reverse asymmetry ($P<0.02$).

Asymmetries in the disease processes of AD have not been recognized until recently. This is because anatomical and chemical studies of AD patients are usually performed on a single hemisphere, and asymmetries in previous rCBF and $rCMRO_2$ studies may have been masked by their overall nondirectionality. This lack of symmetry may be either a reflection of a patchy infectious or vascular process or a result of the degeneration of neurotransmitter systems which were asymmetrical prior to illness (Koss et al. 1985). In any event, these asymmetries provide us with more evidence linking AD to amyotrophic lateral sclerosis and Parkinson's disease, two other CNS degenerative disorders that are also known to have asymmetrical pathologic manifestations. The presence of a unique subset of presenile patients with right-sided hypometabolism corroborates the clinical impression of the presence of age-related subgroups of AD. Furthermore, depending on the hemispheric locus of greatest cerebral involvement, these findings provide a useful framework for understanding the marked behavioral heterogeneity of AD.

Conclusion

PET provides a valuable approach to the in vivo quantitation of aspects of brain physiology which cannot be studied with other methods, either pre- or postmortem. Our PET-FDG studies have demonstrated asymmetrical temporal-parietal hypometabolism in AD, findings related both to the behavioral features of the illness and to the age of the patient. These observations have important implications for differential diagnostic approaches to dementia and may suggest asymmetrical degeneration in the posterior region of the bnM. PET studies of cerebrovascular physiology and metabolism using new high-resolution instruments (Budinger et al. 1984) show great promise for further defining the metabolic function of the CNS in the dementias.

Note Added in Proof. Asymmetrical degeneration of the bnM in AD has recently been reported (Arent T et al. 1985, Neuroscience 14:1–14).

References

Benson DF, Kuhl DE, Hawkins RA, Phelps ME, Cummings JL, Tsai SY (1983) The fluorodeoxyglucose ^{18}F scan in Alzheimer's disease and multi-infarct dementia. Arch Neurol 40:711–714

Brun A (1984) An overview of light and electron microscopic changes. In: Alzheimer's disease: the standard reference. Free Press, New York, pp 37–47

Brun A, Englund E (1981) Regional pattern of degeneration in Alzheimer's disease: neuronal loss and histopathological grading. Histopathology 5:549–564

Budinger TF, Derenzo SE, Huesman RH (1984) Instrumentation for positron emission tomography. Ann Neurol [Suppl] 15:35–43

Budinger TF, Huesman RH, Knittel B, Friedland RP, Derenzo SE (1985) Physiological modeling of dynamic measurements of metabolism using positron emission tomography. In: Greitz T et al. (ed) The metabolism of the human brain: studies with positron emission tomography. Raven, New York, pp 165–183

Chase TN, Foster NL, Fedio P, Brooks R, Mansi L, DiChiro G (1984) Regional cortical dysfunction in Alzheimer's disease as determined by positron emission tomography. Ann Neurol [Suppl] 15:170–174

Cohen MB, Graham LS, Lake R, Metter EJ, Kulkami MK, Kling AS, Yamada JL, Fitten J (1984) SPECT imaging of 1–123 IMP in dementia. Clin Nucl Med 9:30

Frackowiak RSJ, Pozzilli C, Legg NJ, DuBoulay GH, Marshall J, Lenzi GL, Jones T (1981) Regional cerebral oxygen supply and utilization in dementia: a clinical and physiological study with oxygen-15 and positron tomography. Brain 104:753–778

Friedland RP, Yano Y, Budinger TF, Ganz E, Huesman RH, Derenzo SE, Knittel B (1983a) Quantitative evaluation of blood brain barrier integrity in Alzheimer-type dementia: positron emission tomographic studies with rubidium-82. Eur Neurol 22 [Suppl 2]:19–20

Friedland RP, Budinger TF, Ganz E, Yano Y, Mathis CA, Koss B, Ober BA, Huesman R, Derenzo SE (1983 b) Regional cerebral metabolic alterations in dementia of the Alzheimer-type: positron emission tomography with 18-fluorodeoxyglucose. J Comput Assist Tomogr 7:590–598

Friedland RP, Budinger TF, Yano Y, Huesman RH, Knittel B, Derenzo SE, Koss B, Ober BA (1983 c) Regional cerebral metabolic alterations in Alzheimer-type dementia: kinetic studies with 18-fluorodeoxyglucose. J Cereb Blood Flow Metabol 3 [Suppl 1]:510–511

Friedland RP, Budinger TF, Brant-Zawadzki M, Jagust WJ (1984 a) The diagnosis of Alzheimer-type dementia: a preliminary comparison of positron emission tomography and proton magnetic resonance. JAMA 252:2750–2752

Friedland RP, Prusiner SB, Jagust WJ, Budinger TF, Davis RL (1984 b) Bitemporal hypometabolism in Creutzfeldt-Jakob disease measured by positron emission tomography with [^{18}F]2-fluoro-deoxyglucose. J Comput Assist Tomogr 8:978–981

Friedland RP, Budinger TF, Jagust WJ, Yano Y, Huesman RH, Knittel B (1985 a) Positron emission tomography and the blood brain barrier in Alzheimer's disease. In: Lassen N, Cahn J (eds) Acute cerebrovascular diseases pathopharmacology: new brain imaging in cerebrovascular diseases. Libbey, Paris

Friedland RP, Budinger TF, Koss E, Ober BA (1985 b) Alzheimer's disease: anterior-posterior and lateral hemispheric alterations in cortical glucose utilization. Neurosci Lett 53:235–240

Friedland RP, Brun A, Budinger TF (1985 c) Pathological and positron emission tomographic correlations in Alzheimer's disease. Lancet I:228

Hill TC (1984) Clinical applications of single photon emission computed tomography. Society of Nuclear Medicine, Los Angeles

Jagust WJ, Friedland RP, Budinger TF (to be published) Positron emission tomography with [^{18}F] fluorodeoxyglucose differentiates normal pressure hydrocephalus from Alzheimer-type dementia. J Neurol Neurosurg Psychiatry (to be published)

Koss E, Friedland RP, Ober BA, Jagust WJ (1985) Lateral hemispheric asymmetries of glucose utilization are different in early and late onset Alzheimer-type dementia. Am J Psychiatry 142:638–640

Kuhl DE, Metter EJ, Riege WH, Phelps ME (1982) Effects of human aging on patterns of local cerebral glucose utilization determined by the [^{18}F]fluorodeoxyglucose method. J Cereb Blood Flow Metab 2:163–171

Kuhl DE, Metter EJ, Riege WH, Hawkins RA (1983) Determinations of cerebral glucose utilization in dementia using positron emission tomography. Proceedings of the International Conference on Alzheimer's Disease, 1983. WHO, Copenhagen, Danish medical Bulletin 32[1]:51–55

McKhann G, Drachman D, Folstein M, Katzman R, Price D, Stadlan EM (1984) Clinical diagnoses of Alzheimer's disease: report of the NINCDS-ADRDA work group under the auspices of department of health and human services task force on Alzheimer's disease. Neurology 34:939–944

Mesulam M-M, Mufson EJ, Levey AI, Wainer BH (1983) Cholinergic innervation of cortex by the basal forebrain: cytochemistry and cortical connections of the septal area, diagonal band nuclei, nucleus basalis (substantia innominata), and hypothalamus in the Rhesus monkey. J Comp Neurol 214:170–197

Phelps ME, Huang S-C, Hoffman EJ, Selin C, Sokoloff L, Kuhl DE (1979) Tomographic measurement of local cerebral glucose metabolic rate in humans with (F-18) 2-fluoro-2-deoxy-D-glucose: validation of method. Ann Neurol 6:371–388

Reivich M (1985) PET, NMR and XCT in brain diseases. In: Lassen N, Cahn J (eds) Acute cerebrovscular diseases pathopharmacology: new brain imaging technics in cerebrovascular diseases, Libbey, Paris

Reivich M, Kuhl D, Wolf A, Greenbeerg J, Phelps M, Ido T, Casella V, Fowler J, Hoffman E, Alavi A, Som P, Sokoloff L (1979) The (^{18}F)-fluorodeoxyglucose method for the measurement of local cerebral glucose utilization in man. Circ Res 44:127–137

Sokoloff L, Reivich M, Kennedy C, DesRosiers MH, Patlak CS, Pettigrew KD, Sakurada O, Shinohara M (1977) The [^{14}C]deoxyglucose method for the measurement of local cerebral glucose utilization: theory, practice and normal values in the conscious and anesthetized albino rat. J Neurochem 28:897–916

Investigation of Regional Cerebral Blood Flow and Metabolism in Dementia

W.-D. Heiss, G. Pawlik, K. Herholz, B. Szelies, C. Beil, and K. Wienhard [1]

Age-related disorders of the brain like the dementias may be caused by primary disturbances of cerebral blood flow (CBF) or of metabolism. Due to the coupling of functional activity and metabolism, impairment of higher brain function, on the other hand, may lead to a secondary decrease in physiologic variables. Therefore, investigation of CBF and metabolism of various substrates is useful for the detection of such brain disorders and may additionally yield quantifiable data on the severity of the disease. Such quantitative results can be used for a variety of purposes: to monitor the course of the disease in the patient, to formulate prognoses, and to constitute a basis for the objective comparison of various therapeutic protocols. During the last 40 years, various methods for the measurement of CBF and metabolism have been developed.

Determination of Flow and Metabolic Substrates in the Whole Brain

By determining the arteriovenous (AV) difference of metabolic substrate, e.g., of oxygen and glucose, age-dependent or pathologic changes of these metabolites in the brain can be quantified. Additionally, by measuring the AV difference of inhaled nitrous oxide, the flow of the whole brain can be calculated (Kety and Schmidt 1945). A large number of studies of age-related changes were performed with this method (summarized in Kety 1956) demonstrating high flow and oxygen consumption in childhood and a stable flow throughout adult life as long as no signs of vascular disease are present. Whether slight decreases of flow, oxygen consumption, and glucose metabolism occur with normal aging remains a controversial issue in the investigations using these methods (Lassen et al. 1960; Gottstein 1969; Gottstein and Held 1979; Sokoloff 1966). On the other hand, measurements of AV differences have clearly demonstrated that, in dementias, flow, oxygen consumption, and glucose uptake of the whole brain are sharply reduced (Lassen et al. 1960; Hoyer et al. 1975, 1977).

Regional Measurement of Cerebral Blood Flow

The first method permitting regional flow determinations with intact skull was introduced by Lassen and Ingvar (1963) and utilized the washout of ^{133}Xe from the

1 Max-Planck-Institut für neurologische Forschung, Ostmerheimer Str. 200, 5000 Köln 91 (Merheim), FRG

Senile Dementia of the Alzheimer Type
Ed. by J. Traber and W. H. Gispen

Table 1. Cerebral blood flow in multi-infarct dementia and primary degenerative dementia

Authors		Controls	Multi-infarct dementia	Primary degenerative dementia
Ingvar and Gustafson (1970)	F_B	49.8± 5.4		37.1± 7.8
	F_G	79.7±10.7		55.5± 9.2
	W_g	49.2± 3.9		42.0± 7.8
Obrist et al. (1970)	F_B	49.8± 5.4		36.2± 7.4
	F_G	79.7±10.7		57.5± 5.6
	W_g	49.2± 3.9		40.7± 9.4
Hachinski et al. (1975)	F_B	56	35.4± 9.1	47.7±20.7
	F_G	91	59.5±17.0	83.9±38.7
	W_g	49	42.7± 6.4	41.5± 5.5
Perez et al. (1977)	F_B		32.0± 5.5	34.1± 5.9
	F_G		56.3±16.8	69.3±32.9
	W_g		38.5± 8.9	48.6± 9.9
Lavy et al. (1978)	F_B	49.8		38.3
Harrison et al. (1979)	F_B	53.0±13.4	34.1±12.2	39.6±18.5
	F_G	85.2±20.5	56.9±20.5	67.2±34.2
	W_g	50.1± 4.5	42.9± 7.2	41.9± 4.9
Yamaguchi et al. (1980)	F_G	73.8± 6.3	70.7± 7.9	67.2± 9.0

F_B, mean weighted flow of cerebral hemisphere in ml/100 g/min (mean value ± standard deviation); F_G, flow of fast compartment (gray matter) in ml/100 g/min (mean value ± standard deviation); W_g, relative weight (%) of fast compartment (gray matter)

brain after invasive or noninvasive administration. Most studies performed with this technique demonstrated slight age-dependent decreases of CBF (e.g., Naritomi et al. 1979; Melamed et al. 1980). In patients with dementia, a marked decrease of CBF was found (Table 1). Hachinski et al. (1975), differentiating between degenerative dementias of the Alzheimer type and multi-infarct dementias, were the first to indicate that flow is initially more depressed in cases with multi-infarct syndrome than in others. These findings were also supported by Hoyer et al. (1975), who observed that metabolism is primarily affected in degenerative dementias, whereas flow decrease is the principal alteration produced in multi-infarct syndromes. These findings were not, however, reproduced in all investigations. Several authors found the severity and duration of organic brain syndrome to be the factors determining the extent of both flow and metabolic disturbances (Yamaguchi et al. 1980). Regional studies revealed the pattern of flow disturbances to vary, resulting in focal ischemic lesion in the cases of multi-infarct syndrome (Fig. 1) and a more diffuse, sometimes parietally pronounced flow decrease in degenerative forms (Fig. 2).

Three-Dimensional Quantification of Flow and Metabolism

The xenon clearance method performed with conventional technical equipment, suffers from a few limitations, the most serious being the overprojection of tissue volumes of low and high flow ("look through effect," Donley et al. 1975). Three-

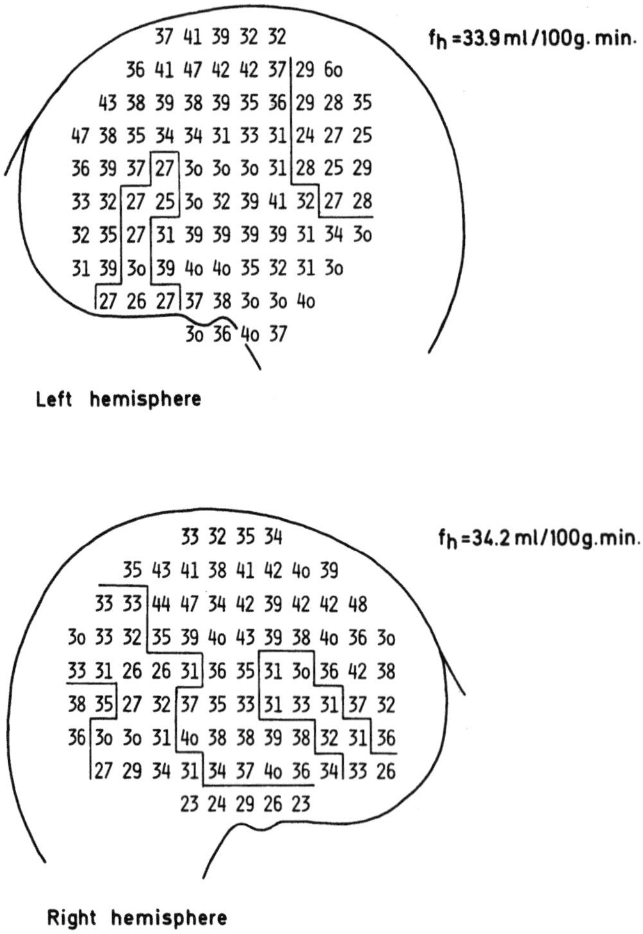

Fig. 1. Regional cerebral blood flow of both hemispheres, as measured with the two-dimensional Xe clearance techniqe, in a patient with multi-infarct dementia. Note several regions with markedly decreased flow values. Weighted mean flow values are given in ml/100 g/min; f_h, flow of the hemisphere

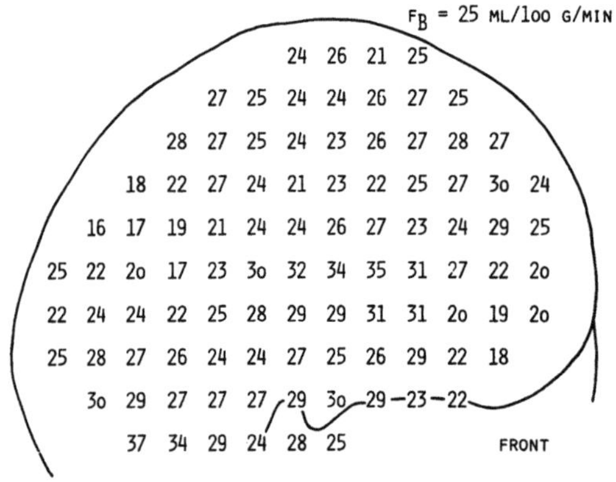

Fig. 2. Regional cerebral blood flow of the right hemisphere in a patient with dementia of the Alzheimer type. Note diffuse decrease in rCBF, pronounced decrease in the parietal lobe. F_B, flow of the whole hemisphere

dimensional methods can overcome this limitation. Such techniques can distinguish between gray and white matter and add important information by imaging anatomical details in the depths of the brain. Quantification of flow in small volumes is still limited by various technical problem arising from the implementation of computed tomography (CT) with stable xenon (Drayer et al. 1978), single-photon emission tomography with ^{133}Xe (Lassen 1981) or ^{123}I-isopropylamphetamine (Kuhl et al. 1982a), and magnetic resonance imaging. However, flow and metabolism of various substrates can be reliably measured by positron emission tomography (PET) (Ter-Pogossian et al. 1975; Phelps et al. 1982; Heiss and Phelps 1983).

Principles of Positron Emission Tomography

When positron-emitting radionuclides decay, a positively charged particle with the mass of an electron is released. Over a distance of 1–5 mm, this particle is decelerated to such a degree that it must combine with an electron. When these positively and negatively charged particles collide, their mass is annihilated, and two gamma quanta, each with an energy of 511 keV, are emitted traveling in opposite directions (180° angle). Without further collimation, the two photons can then be registered by electronically connected coincidence detectors that assign the decay event to the straight line between the two detectors. This electronic collimation permits construction of highly efficient detector systems, in which detectors arranged in circles or polygons are connected with each other in a fan-like fashion via coincidence counters. Cross-sections of the activity distribution in the examined structure are reconstructed from the many individual events that have been recorded in various directions, employing algorithms that resemble those used in X-ray computerized tomography. The tomographic images produced in this fashion represent an object thickness of about 10–15 mm at an in-plane resolution of 7–10 mm. The necessary attenuation and scatter corrections can be made with great accuracy because of the uniform and high energy of the gamma quanta. State-of-the-art machines containing numerous detector rings permit simultaneous scanning of up to nine brain slices during a single examination. A number of tracer compounds which make possible the examination of different physiologic processes can be labeled with the cyclotron-produced, short-lived, positron-emitting radionuclides ^{15}O, ^{11}C, or ^{18}F (reviews in Phelps et al. 1982; Heiss and Phelps 1983). As ^{18}F-labeled fluorodeoxyglucose (^{18}FDG, half-life of ^{18}F = 110 min) determinations of local glucose metabolism and ^{15}O (half-life = 2 min) measurements of oxygen consumption and blood flow are widely used both in functional studies on normal volunteers and in clinical examinations of various cerebral disorders, a description of these methods follows.

Determination of Local Glucose Metabolism with PET

The measurement of local glucose metabolism with ^{18}F-labeled 2-fluoro-2-deoxy-D-glucose (^{18}FDG) (Reivich et al. 1979) is derived from the ^{14}C-labeled deoxyglucose autoradiographic technique devised by Sokoloff et al. (1977). The technique developed by Sokoloff can be applied directly, as ^{18}FDG labeled in position 2 behaves like deoxyglucose. ^{18}FDG is transported into the cells by the same carrier system as glucose. Inside the cell, it is phosphorylated by hexokinase to ^{18}F-deoxyglucose-6-phosphate. Deoxyglucose-6-phosphate, however, cannot be metabolized to fructose-6-phosphate; rather, it accumulates in the cell because the phosphatase reaction that yields deoxyglucose again takes place much more slowly, and deoxyglucose-6-phosphate can penetrate the cell membrane in small amounts only. The kinetics of the accumulation of deoxyglucose-6-phosphate can be described in terms of the transport and enzyme constants of a three-compartment model. The local cerebral metabolic rate for glucose (LCMRGl) is then calculated employing the corresponding model equation which, in its original form, is rather complex, but which can be simplified for measurement purposes as follows:

$$\mathrm{LCMRGl} = \frac{(\mathrm{Gl})}{LC} \times \frac{C(^{18}\mathrm{F}) - C(^{18}\mathrm{FDG})}{A_b}$$

$C(^{18}F)$ corresponds to the entire radioactivity in the tissue and is determined directly by PET. $C(^{18}FDG)$ represents the concentration of free ^{18}FDG in the tissue, estimated on the basis of the plasma concentration at a given time T. The difference between the two values indicates the local tissue concentration of FDG-6-phosphate. A_b stands for the total amount of ^{18}FDG taken up by the tissue; it can be computed on the basis of the area under the ^{18}FDG concentration curve from time 0 to time T, taking into account the measured ^{18}FDG values in plasma and the appropriate model constants. The second ratio on the right side of the equation represents the phosphorylation rate of ^{18}FDG. Multiplication with plasma glucose concentration (Gl) would yield the rate of glucose phosphorylation if the behavior of glucose and ^{18}FDG were the same. However, as the AV extraction rate of glucose does not equal that of ^{18}FDG, the value has to be corrected by an experimentally determined constant (LC=lumped constant). In measuring cerebral glucose utilization after intravenous injection of 3–6 mCi ^{18}FDG, the plasma concentration curve of ^{18}FDG must be determined from the time of injection to the point of measurement. Likewise, the glucose concentration in plasma and the local ^{18}F activity in the brain must be determined after an equilibrium of ^{18}FDG between blood and tissue has been reached.

Determination of Regional Cerebral Blood Flow (rCBF) and Cerebral Oxygen Metabolism (rCMRO) by ^{15}O-PET

Water labeled with ^{15}O is a freely diffusible tracer which can be used for measurements of regional cerebral blood flow. It is administered continously by inhalation of ^{15}O-labeled carbon dioxide, which is converted to ^{15}O-labeled H_2O by carbonic anhydrase in the lung, using a steady-state model (Jones et al. 1976; Frackowiak et al. 1980). During inhalation of ^{15}O-labeled O_2 in a second run, the local brain activity as measured by PET mainly represents ^{15}O-labeled H_2O produced by aerobic metabolism in the tissue, which is also freely diffusible. Since the distribution of water between tissue and blood is known from the first run, the production rate of ^{15}O-labeled H_2O and hence the rCMRO may be calculated. Correction for the amount of unmetabolized oxygen bound to hemoglobin is possible by measurement of local cerebral blood volume using ^{11}C-labeled CO or ^{15}O-labeled CO as a hemoglobin marker (Lammertsma and Jones 1983). The relation between rCMRO and rCBF gives the regional oxygen extraction rate (rOER).

Studies in Normal Human Subjects

In normal volunteers, the average rate of cerebral glucose utilization is 29–32 μmol/100 g/min (Mazziotta et al. 1981; Heiss et al. 1984), as determined by means of ^{18}FDG and PET. Under control conditions (darkened laboratory and low noise background during examination), the anatomy of the brain is reflected in the metabolic activity of the transaxial cross sections. Individual metabolic rates can be estimated by direct comparison with the shades of gray or with the corresponding colors on the reference scale: The highest values are found in the visual cortex (45–50 μmol/100 g/min) and in the striatum (42–46 μmol/100 g/min). Values in other areas of the cortex, in the thalamus (35–42 μmol/100 g/min), and in the gray matter structures of the posterior fossa (25–30 μmol/100 g/min), are much lower. The lowest LCMRGl is found in white matter (15–22 μmol/100 g/min).

Studies of oxygen consumption and regional blood flow have also demonstrated comparable differences between gray and white matter: The mean value of CMRO was determined to be 5.9 ml/100 g/min for gray and 1.8 ml/100 g/min for white matter, while the mean rCBF values were 65.3 and 21.4 ml/100 g/min respectively (Frackowiak et al. 1980). The rOER was 0.48–0.49 for both tissues. Differences among various gray structures, as described for CMRGl, were not observed with the ^{15}O method, but this might be due to its low spatial resolution.

Age-related decreases of glucose metabolism and oxygen consumption observed in preliminary studies (Frackowiak et al. 1980; Kuhl et al. 1982c) were not confirmed in recent investigations on larger groups of volunteers: In 40 selected healthy men, neither the CMRGl of the whole hemispheres nor that of individual brain regions correlated with age (Rapoport et al. 1983). Similar results were reported by Metter et al. (1983) and Leon et al. (1983), but interregional correlations of older volunteers differed from those observed in younger men (Metter et al. 1983). The previously observed age-dependent changes in oxygen consumption were not confirmed in a recent study by Frackowiak et al. (1981).

Functional Activation During Sensory Stimulation

A number of studies (Greenberg et al. 1981; Phelps et al. 1982) have demonstrated that local glucose metabolism increases during functional activation of the corresponding brain structures. With visual stimulations, glucose metabolic rates rise in the primary visual cortex; moreover, this increase is dependent on stimulus intensity. For example, when the test person is given a complex scene to look at, the increase is about 50% and spreads to the visual association cortex. With auditory stimulation, different patterns are observed, depending on the modality of stimulation.

Eliminating sensory stimuli either by blindfolding the eyes or stopping the ears decreases the cerebral metabolic rate for glucose. The lowest metabolic rates are observed with complete sensory deprivation, which is, moreover asymmetric, revealing higher levels of activity in the left hemisphere. By blocking sensory input from the outside and reducing brain activity in sleep, a decrease in metabolic rates of between 10% and 20% compared with rates for wakefulness is found in all cortical and basal gray matter structures (Fig. 3), although during dreaming, brain metabolism is generally activated (Heiss et al. 1985).

Metabolic Disturbances in Dementia

Over the past few years, PET has contributed much to the understanding of neurologic disorders (for reviews, see Phelps et al. 1982; Heiss and Phelps 1983). Especially in cases of focal lesions, metabolic disturbances have been shown to extend far beyond the site of the primary lesions, and to include morphologically intact brain structures far away from the anatomical lesion. Decreased metabolism is particularly striking in patients with small infarctions which, although often undetectable by CT, are associated with extensive decreases in metabolic rate (Fig. 4). These remote metabolic effects may explain impairments which cannot be directly ascribed to the focal lesion. They underlie the psycho-organic syndrome in stroke patients and influence the outcome of rehabilitation after a stroke.

In disease such as dementia, where global impairment of brain function is often combined with unspecific CT findings, the decrease in metabolic rate is also generally diffuse and varies according to the severity of the psycho-organic syndrome. However, these metabolic disturbances are usually characteristic of each disease and its typical pattern of spread. In degenerative dementia of the Alzheimer type, cerebral glucose consumption is severely impaired (Fig. 5), even in the early stages before cerebral atrophy can be documented by CT. Corresponding metabolic changes are particularly pronounced in the parietotemporal cortex (Foster et al. 1983; Kuhl et al. 1983). In senile dementia, impaired glucose metabolism is evident in the frontal cortex (Alavi et al. 1982). In Pick's disease, the metabolic disturbance also afflicts the frontal lobe (Fig. 6). With multi-infarct dementias, glucose uptake is reduced more or less in proportion to the severity of clinical symptoms and in accordance with the multifocal destruction of cortical

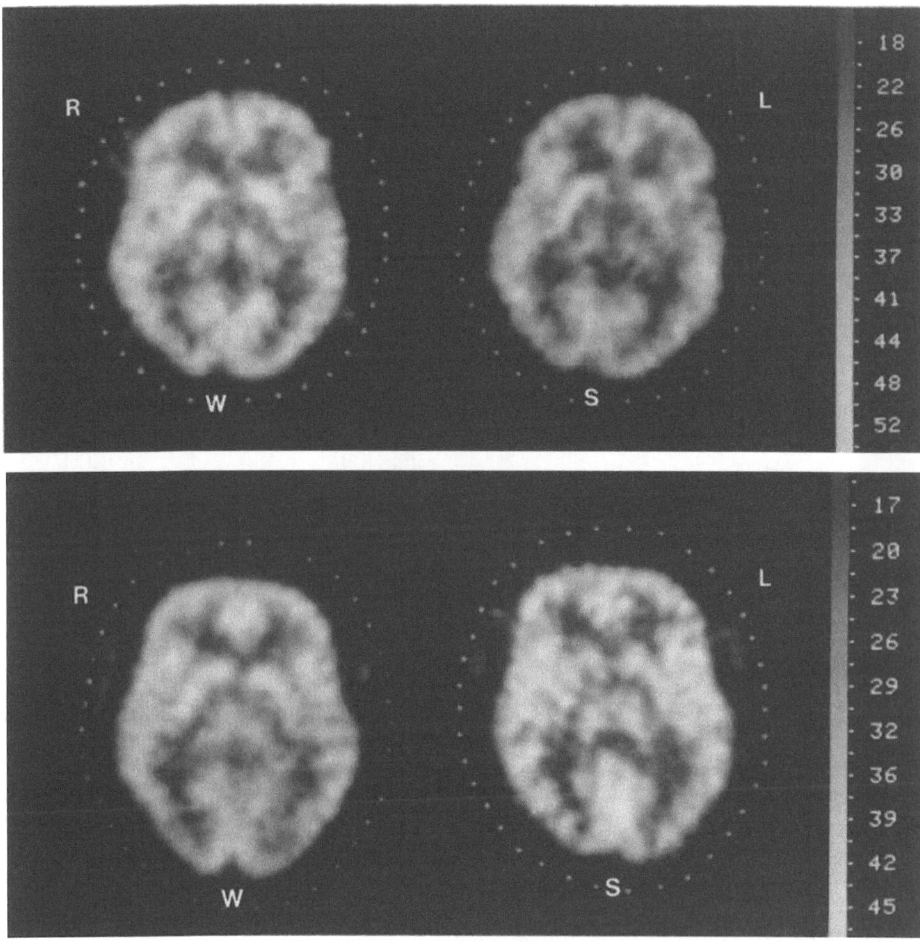

Fig. 3. a Corresponding images of the local cerebral metabolic rate for glucose determined by ^{18}FDG-PET in slices across the basal ganglia of a healthy 37-year-old male, showing a nonselective decrease in glucose utilization during sleep (*S*) as compared with wakefulness (*W*). **b** Metabolic maps of 29-year-old normal volunteer's brain slice showing generalized activation, most marked in the insular region, visual cortex, and hippocampal formations during sleep with dreaming (*S*) as compared with wakefulness (*W*) (from Heiss et al. 1985). Values on *reference gray scale* are in μmol/100 g/min

tissue, as demonstrated by CT; energy metabolism is affected mainly in small, old infarcts (Fig. 7).

In most patients suffering from dementia, CBF is decreased, but it has not yet been possible to discern typical patterns for the various types of dementia. The primary disturbance of flow in multi-infarct dementia and the primary impairment of metabolism in degenerative dementias postulated by Hoyer et al. (1975) has not been confirmed in PET studies (Frackowiak et al. 1981). In nine patients with multi-infarct dementia and in 13 Alzheimer patients, regional flow and oxygen consumption were similarly affected, and as a consequence, the rOER was

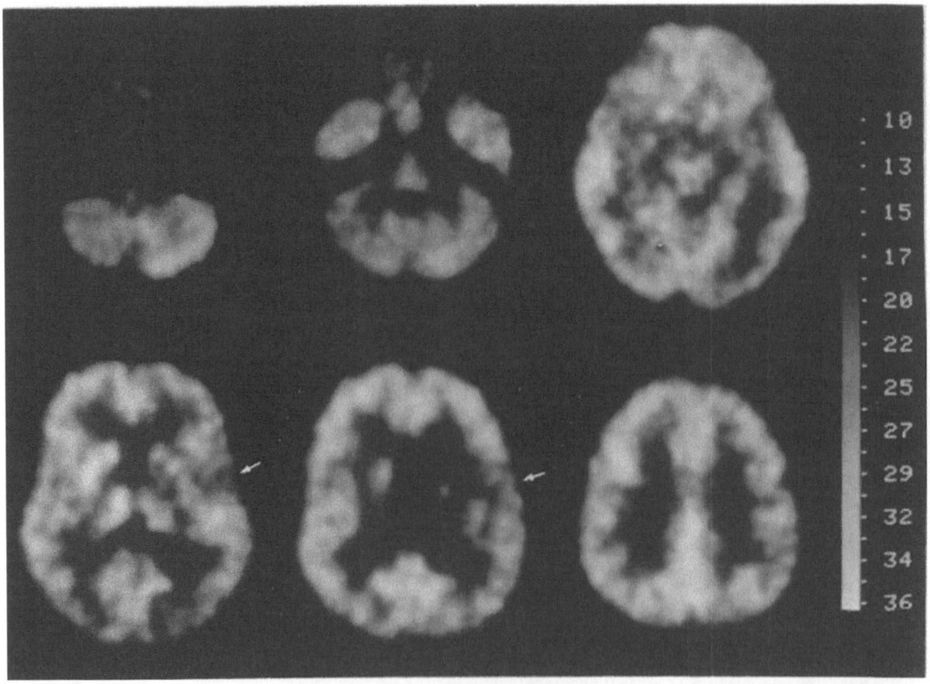

Fig. 4. Images of local cerebral metabolic rate for glucose at various levels above canthomeatal line in a patient with small ischemic infarct in the left temporal lobe. Marked reduction of glucose metabolism in the ischemic focus, but glucose metabolism is also decreased in morphologically intact brain structures, e.g., homolateral cortex, thalamus, and contralateral cerebellum. Scale as in Fig. 3

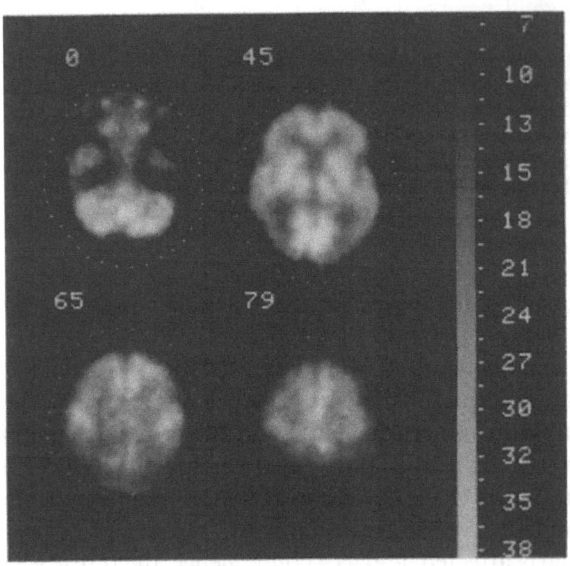

Fig. 5. Images of local cerebral metabolic rate for glucose at various levels above canthomeatal line (indicated in mm) in a patient with primary degenerative dementia of the Alzheimer type. Note marked reduction of glucose metabolism in parietal and temporal lobe. Scale as in Fig. 3

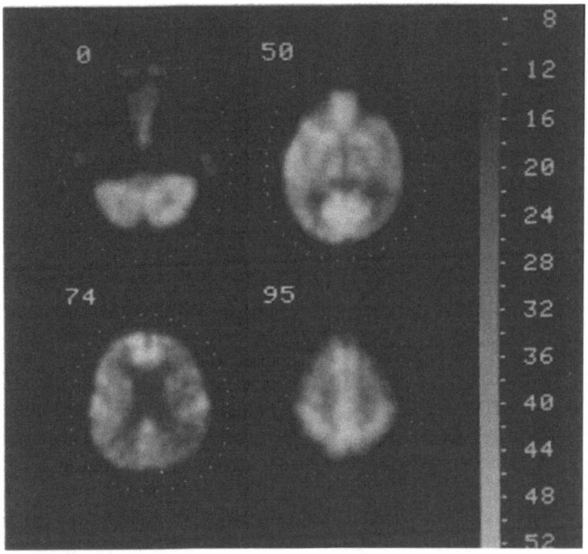

Fig. 6. Images of local cerebral metabolic rate for glucose at various levels above canthomeatal line (indicated in mm) in a patient with probable diagnosis of primary degenerative dementia of Pick's disease. In addition to marked decreases of glucose metabolism in parietotemporal regions, there is also a pronounced metabolic disturbance in the frontal lobe. Scale as in Fig. 3

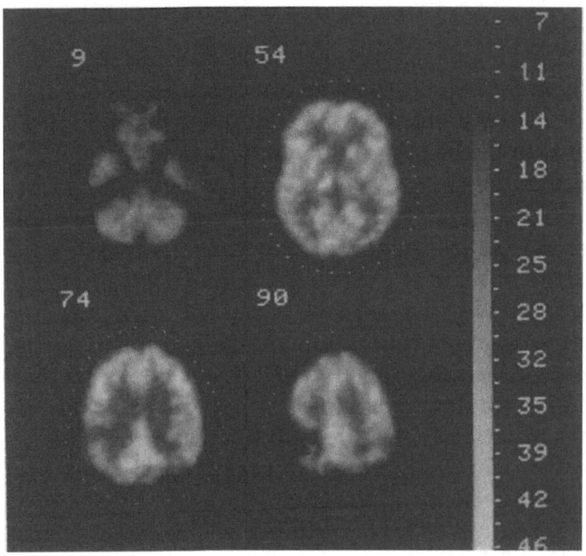

Fig. 7. Images of local cerebral metabolic rate for glucose at various levels above canthomeatal line (indicated in mm) in a patient with multi-infarct dementia. Glucose metabolism is focally decreased in several circumscript ischemic lesions. Scale as in Fig. 3

not changed. Decreases in flow and metabolism were related only to the duration and the severity of the mental impairment, but not to the type of dementia. An increase in the rOER was never observed, and therefore, a "chronic ischemic syndrome" could be ruled out. Regional differences of oxygen consumption were observed in both groups. In the vascular groups, disturbances were most prominent in the parietal lobe, but the pattern was highly influenced by focal ischemic lesions. In cases of moderate degenerative dementia, focal abnormalities were most frequent in the parietal and temporal lobe; in severe cases, disturbances were found primarily in frontal regions, while the occipital lobe was least affected.

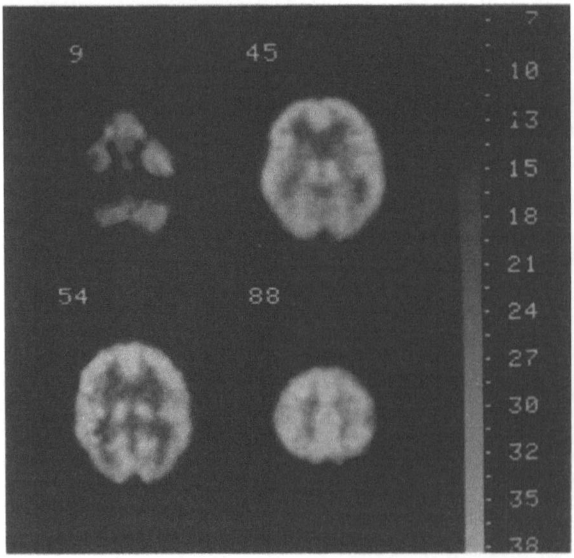

Fig. 8. Images of local cerebral metabolic rate for glucose at various levels above canthomeatal line (indicated in mm) in a patient with Huntington's chorea. Glucose metabolism is selectively impaired in the caudate and the lentiform nuclei. Scale as in Fig. 3

In Huntington's chorea, the most conspicuous metabolic changes are found in the basal ganglia, particularly in the caudate nucleus and putamen (Kuhl et al. 1982b) and reflect the severity of the clinical manifestations; even mild cases showing no characteristic atrophy of the head of the caudate nucleus through CT exhibit definite metabolic abnormalities (Fig. 8). The typical reduction of glucose uptake in the striatum of Huntington patients' family members may even allow detection of the disorder before any clinical symptoms become apparent.

Metabolic disturbances in dementia are related to the impairment of mental function: They may be the cause, but also the consequence of the brain's altered functional activity. In contrast to oxygen consumption and glucose metabolism, the synthesis of proteins, which can be determined with ^{11}C-labeled C-methyl-methionine (Bustany et al. 1983), is not directly coupled to nervous system functions. Decreases in protein synthesis of up to 40% for moderate and 62% for severe cases of Alzheimer dementia again predominate in parietal and frontal regions and could therefore be of pathogenetic importance.

These few examples of the application of PET to studies of local cerebral metabolism only serve to give an idea of the vast potential of the method. Many organic compounds can be labeled with positron emitters, e.g., ^{11}C, ^{13}N, and ^{18}F, to allow quantitative imaging of such processes as the metabolism of various substrates, protein synthesis, the function and distribution of receptors, tumor growth, and the distribution of drugs. With ^{15}O, produced directly in a cyclotron, local oxygen utilization can be measured. Simple compounds containing either ^{15}O or other radionuclides (^{11}C, ^{18}F), allow regional blood flow and blood volume to be determined quantitatively and three-dimensionally. All these applications of PET as a complex and yet noninvasive method grant insights into the functional anatomy, physiology, and pathology of the human brain unmatched by any other currently known technology.

References

Alavi A, Reivich M, Ferris S, Christman D, Fowler J, MacGregor R, Farkas T, Greenberg J, Dann R, Wolf A (1982) Regional cerebral glucose metabolism in aging and senile dementia as determined by 18F-deoxyglucose and positron emission tomography. In: Hoyer S (ed) The aging brain. Springer, Berlin Heidelberg New York, pp 187–195

Bustany P, Henry JF, Sargent T, Zarifian E, Cabanis E, Collard P, Comar D (1983) Local brain protein metabolism in dementia and schizophrenia: in vivo studies with ^{11}C-L-methionine and positron emission tomography. In: Heiss WD, Phelps ME (eds) Positron emission tomography of the brain. Springer, Berlin Heidelberg New York, pp 208–211

Donley RF, Sundt TM, Anderson RE, Sharbrough FW (1975) Blood flow measurement and the "look through" artifact in focal cerebral ischemia. Stroke 6:121–131

Drayer BP, Wolfson SK, Reinmuth OM, Dujovny M, Boenke M, Cook EE (1978) Xenon-enhanced CT for analysis of cerebral integrity, perfusion, and blood flow. Stroke 9:123–130

Foster NL, Chase TN, Fedio P, Patronas NJ, Brooks RA, DiChiro G (1983) Alzheimer's disease: focal cortical changes shown by positron emission tomography. Neurology 33:961–965

Frackowiak RSJ, Lenzi GL, Jones T, Heather JD (1980) Quantitative measurement of regional cerebral blood flow and oxygen metabolism in man using ^{15}O and positron emission tomography: Theory, procedure, and normal values. J Comput Assist Tomogr 4:727–736

Frackowiak RSJ, Pozzilli C, Legg NJ, DuBoulay GH, Marshall J, Lenzi GL, Jones T (1981) Regional cerebral oxygen supply and utilization in dementia. A clinical and physiological study with oxygen-15 and positron tomography. Brain 104:753–778

Gottstein U (1969) Interne Therapie der Altersprozesse des Gehirns und seiner Gefäße. Wien Klin Wochenschr 41:943

Gottstein U, Held K (1979) Effects of aging on cerebral circulation and metabolism in man. In: Gotoh F, Nagai H, Tazaki Y (eds) Cerebral blood flow and metabolism. Munksgaard, Copenhagen, pp 54–55

Greenberg JH, Reivich M, Alavi A, Hand P, Rosenquist A, Rintelmann W, Stein A, Tusa R, Dann R, Christman D, Fowler J, MacGregor B, Wolf A (1981) Metabolic mapping of functional activity in human subjects with the (^{18}F)fluorodeoxyglucose technique. Science 212:670–680

Hachinski VC, Iliff LD, Zilkha E, DuBoulay GH, McAllister VL, Marshall J, Ross Russell RW, Symon L (1975) Cerebral blood flow in dementia. Arch Neurol 32:632–637

Harrison MJG, Thomas DJ, DuBoulay GH, Marshall J (1979) Multi-infarct dementia. J Neurol Sci 40:97–103

Heiss WD, Phelps ME (1983) Positron emission tomography of the brain. Springer, Berlin Heidelberg New York

Heiss WD, Pawlik G, Herholz K, Wagner R, Göldner H, Wienhard K (1984) Regional kinetic constants and cerebral metabolic rate for glucose in normal human volunteers determined by dynamic positron emission tomography of (^{18}F)-2-fluoro-2-deoxy-D-glucose. J Cereb Blood Flow Metab 4:212–223

Heiss WD, Pawlik G, Herholz K, Wagner R, Wienhard K (1985) Regional cerebral glucose metabolism in man during wakefulness, sleep and dreaming. Brain Res 327:362–366

Hoyer S, Oesterreich K, Weinhardt F, Krüger G (1975) Veränderungen von Durchblutung und oxydativem Stoffwechsel des Gehirns bei Patienten mit einer Demenz. J Neurol 210:227–237

Hoyer S, Krüger G, Oesterreich K, Weinhardt F (1977) Effects of drugs on cerebral blood flow and oxidative metabolism in patients with dementia. In: Meyer JS, Lechner H, Reivich M (eds) Cerebral vascular disease. Excerpta Medica, Amsterdam, pp 25–28

Ingvar DH, Gustafson L (1970) Regional cerebral blood flow in organic dementia with early onset. Acta Neur Scand [Suppl] 43:42–73

Jones T, Chesler DA, Ter-Pogossian MM (1976) The continuous inhalation of oxygen-15 for assessing regional oxygen extraction in the brain of man. Br J Radiol 49:339–343

Kety SS (1956) Human cerebral blood flow and O_2 consumption related to aging. Ass Res Neur Ment Dis Proc 35:31–45 [NIH special issue]

Kety SS, Schmidt CF (1945) The determination of cerebral blood flow in man by the use of nitrous oxide in low concentration. Am J Physiol 143:53–66

Kuhl DE, Barrio JR, Huang SC, Selin C, Ackerman RF, Lear JL, Wu JL, Lin TH, Phelps ME (1982a) Quantifying local cerebral blood flow by *N*-isopropyl-*p*-(^{123}I)Iodoamphetamine (IMP) tomography. J Nucl Med 23:196–203

Kuhl DE, Phelps ME, Markham CH, Metter EJ, Riege WH, Winter J (1982b) Cerebral metabolism and atrophy in Huntington's disease determined by ^{18}FDG and computed tomographic scan. Ann Neurol 12:425–434

Kuhl DE, Metter EJ, Riege WH, Phelps ME (1982c) Effects of human aging on patterns of local cerebral glucose utilization determined by the (^{18}F)fluorodeoxyglucose method. J Cereb Blood Flow Metab 2:161–171

Kuhl DE, Metter EJ, Riege WH, Hawkins RA, Mazziotta JC, Phelps E, Kling AS (1983) Local cerebral glucose utilization in elderly patients with depression, multiple infarct dementia, and Alzheimer's disease. J Cereb Blood Flow Metab [Suppl 1] 3:S494–S495

Lammertsma AA, Jones T (1983) Correction for the presence of intravascular oxygen-15 in the steady-state technique for measuring regional oxygen extraction ratio in the brain: 1. Description of the method. J Cereb Blood Flow Metab 3:416–424

Lassen NA (1981) Regional activation of brain cortex in man revealed by ^{133}Xe inhalation flow tomography. Eur Neurol 20:291–293

Lassen NA, Ingvar DH (1963) Regional cerebral blood flow measurement in man. Arch Neurol (Chic) 9:615–622

Lassen NA, Feinberg I, Lane MH (1960) Bilateral studies of cerebral oxygen uptake in young and aged normal subjects and in patients with organic dementia. J Clin Invest 39:491–500

Leon MJ de, Ferris SH, George AE, Reisberg B, Christman DR, Kricheff II, Wolf AP (1983) Computed tomography and positron emission transaxial tomography evaluations of normal aging and Alzheimer's disease. J Cereb Blood Flow Metab 3:391–394

Lavy S, Melamed E, Bentin S, Cooper G, Rinot Y (1978) Bihemispheric decreases of regional cerebral blood flow in dementia: correlation with age-matched normal controls. Ann Neurol 4:445–450

Mazziotta JC, Phelps ME, Miller J, Kuhl DE (1981) Tomographic mapping of human cerebral metabolism: normal unstimulated state. Neurology 31:503–516

Melamed E, Lavy S, Bentin S, Cooper G, Rinot Y (1980) Reduction in regional cerebral blood flow during normal aging in man. Stroke 11:31–35

Metter EJ, Riege WH, Kuhl DE, Phelps ME (1983) Differences in regional glucose metabolic intercorrelations with aging. J Cereb Blood Flow Metab [Suppl 1] 3:S482–S483

Naritomi H, Meyer JS, Sakai F, Yamaguchi F, Shaw T (1979) Effects of advancing age on regional cerebral blood flow. Studies in normal subjects and subjects with risk factors for atherothrombotic stroke. Arch Neurol 36:410–416

Obrist WD, Chivian E, Cronqvist S, Ingvar DH (1970) Regional cerebral blood flow in senile and presenile dementia. Neurology 20:315–322

Perez FI, Mathew NT, Stump DA, Meyer JS (1977) Regional cerebral blood flow statistical patterns and psychological performance in multi-infarct dementia and Alzheimer's disease. Can J Neurol Sci 4:53–62

Phelps ME, Mazziotta JC, Huang SC (1982) Study of cerebral function with positron computed tomography. J Cereb Blood Flow Metab 2:113–162

Rapoport SI, Duara R, Horwitz B, Kessler RM, Sokoloff L, Ingvar DH, Gray C, Cutler N (1983) Brain aging in 40 healthy men: rCMRglc and correlated functional activity in various brain regions in the resting state. J Cereb Blood Flow Metab [Suppl 1] 3:484–485

Reivich M, Kuhl D, Wolf A, Greenberg J, Phelps M, Ido T, Casella V, Fowler J, Hoffman E, Alavi A, Som P, Sokoloff L (1979) The (^{18}F)fluorodeoxyglucose method for the measurement of local cerebral glucose utilization in man. Circ Res 44:127–137

Sokoloff L (1966) Cerebral circulatory and metabolic changes associated with aging. Res Publ Assoc Res Nerv Ment Dis 41:237–254

Sokoloff L, Reivich M, Kennedy D, DesRosiers MH, Patlak CS, Pettigrew KD, Sakurada O, Shinohara M (1977) The ^{14}C-deoxyglucose method for the measurement of local cerebral glucose utilization: theory, procedure, and normal values in the conscious and anesthetized albino rat. J Neurochem 28:897–916

Ter-Pogossian MM, Phelps ME, Hoffman EJ, Raichle ME (1975) A positron emission transverse tomograph (PETT) for the three-dimensional and non-invasive measure of cerebral hemodynamics and metabolism. In: Harper AM, Jennett WB, Miller JD, Rowan JO (eds) Blood flow and metabolism in the brain. Churchill Livingstone, Edinburgh, p 7.20–7.24

Yamaguchi F, Meyer JS, Yamamoto M, Sakai F, Shaw T (1980) Noninvasive regional cerebral blood flow measurements in dementia. Arch Neurol 37:410–418

Novel Developments in the Neuropathology of Senile Dementia of the Alzheimer Type

Are Neurons of the Human Cerebral Cortex Really Lost During Aging? A Morphometric Examination*

H. Haug[1]

Introduction

This description of the aging human brain centers on the biological or physiological aspects of the aging process. All pathologic changes, including presenile dementia, are omitted from the discussion.

Even today, some scientists are still of the opinion that increasing numbers of neurons are lost during life. This belief is based on research published about 30 years ago, the basis of which was the work of Brody (1955). Brody himself expressed this theory of neuron loss in vague terms because his statistical basis was too small to make definite statements. However, subsequent interpretations of his work by other scientists and in the press have created the conviction that neurons are lost throughout life.

Morphometry is the name given to modern and improving procedures of measuring histologic sections. The data obtained in this manner can be transformed into three-dimensional values with the help of stereological techniques which were unknown 30 years ago (Haug 1979; Weibel 1979). These and other new procedures now make possible more efficient methods of examining the question of neuron loss and will also enable other important aspects of brain aging to be described. The following observations concerning brain morphology can be made:

1. Secular acceleration in body size leads to concomitant increases in brain volume for successive generations.
2. Modern procedures allow estimates not only of whole brain weight but also of the volume fraction of gray and white matter for various parts of the brain. With the help of stereology, it is possible to determine whether various parts of the brain undergo changes in size at the same rate.
3. The effect of preparative techniques on morphometric results can be accurately determined in order to correct the morphometric data evaluated and achieve precise results for neuron density and size.
4. Because changes in the ultrastructure of the human brain are difficult to describe, they should be examined by means of electron microscopy. With this method, tissue should be fixed as early as possible after death. However, this is impossible with human brain material because dissection can be performed only after a period of several hours after death.

* This investigation was kindly supported by the *Deutsche Forschungsgemeinschaft* (Ha 239, 13–18)

1 Medical University Lübeck, Department of Anatomy, Ratzeburger Allee 160, D-2400 Lübeck 1, FRG

Senile Dementia of the Alzheimer Type
Ed. by J. Traber and W. H. Gispen

Future developments in the preparation of specimens and techniques of measurement can also be expected to lead to good ultrastructural results. Other investigations of aging have been performed by physiologists and behaviorists. Further results gained through animal research can, with caution, be extrapolated to human aging. Some psychological investigations have also opened up new vistas on human brain aging.

All these efforts to increase our knowledge of aging processes require highly sensitive techniques and large quantities of material. This means that future investigations of aging in the human brain will be accompanied by increasing expense. Both the extreme variability of human external and internal structures as well as tissue changes affects results of aging behavior, a fact which also necessitates investigating a large amount of material in order to reach statistical significance. This high variability has made it necessary to revise older measurements which had been based on less material.

Material and Methods

Our investigations of the aging human brain require different types of material. For details concerning the material used in this study to analyze the effect of secular acceleration and aging on brain size, see Haug (1984b). This investigation was based on the analysis of 24,000 brains.

Changes brought about by aging in various parts of the human brain are evaluated for 12 human brains up to 90 years in age. This relatively small base is attributable to the high expense of this type of investigation (Eggers et al. 1984).

To examine alterations of neuron density and size, we used a large amount of material. A total of five cortical areas were measured:

1. Area 6 in the frontal lobe, which has an extrapyramidal function and has recently been designated the "supplementary motor area" by some investigators
2. Area 11 in the orbital part of the frontal lobe, which is linked to psychosocial functions
3. Area 7 in the convexity of the parietal lobe, which is related to sensory and, especially, speech analysis
4. The projection area 17, or visual cortex, in the occipital lobe
5. Area 20 at the basis of the temporal lobe, which probably plays a role in higher integrative activities. Sharp localization of functions in this area is impossible

Morphometric analyses of neurons were performed on over 120 human brains. A total of 230 single evaluations of brain areas have been made. Each single evaluation resulted in measurements of 1,500–2,000 neurons for all layers. Since details of how these analyses were carried out can be found in Haug (1979, 1982), it is sufficient here to note that each cell was measured over the drawing mirror of a microscope with a computerized digitizer (KONTRON, MOP). This investigation was performed over about 8–9 years.

Effects of Techniques of Tissue Preparation on Morphometric Results

As the procedures used can greatly affect the results obtained, a brief description of methodology is necessary. In this way, the considerable discrepancies in the literature concerning morphological aspects of the aging process might be explained.

Since remarkable change in volume can be observed during the preparation (fixation, dehydration, embedding in paraffin wax, sectioning, and staining) of tissue, we have systematically measured this alteration. Figure 1 shows that the magnitude of these changes during methyl benzoate embedding depends on age. The embedding shrinkage of brain tissue belonging to a young person is more pronounced than for tissue from an older individual, probably because of the different water content.

The increased shrinkage of young tissue tends to compress the neurons on the stained slide, resulting in higher cell density in the microscopic image. On the other hand, the less pronounced shrinkage of tissue from aged individuals produces a lower neuron density. However, the cell density of both kinds of tissue is distinctly higher than for fresh tissue. The difference in embedding shrinkage between tissue specimens taken from individuals 20 and 75 years old amounts to about 15%. Consequently, we observe a 15% lower neuron density in microscopic images of tissue of the aged, making it necessary to estimate the degree of shrinkage in order to be able to correct the primary results.

That embedding shrinkage is age-dependent was unknown to early investigators, who probably correctly counted the number of neurons, but erroneously postulated neuron losses which were in fact caused by differences in the shrinkage of brain tissue (Haug 1980; Sass 1982).

This fact shows that, as in other scientific disciplines, many findings are influenced by the complex reaction of the tissue as a whole. Therefore, results may be falsified if all aspects of the problem are not taken into account. Since it is possible that investigators might not at present be aware of certain factors, erroneous find-

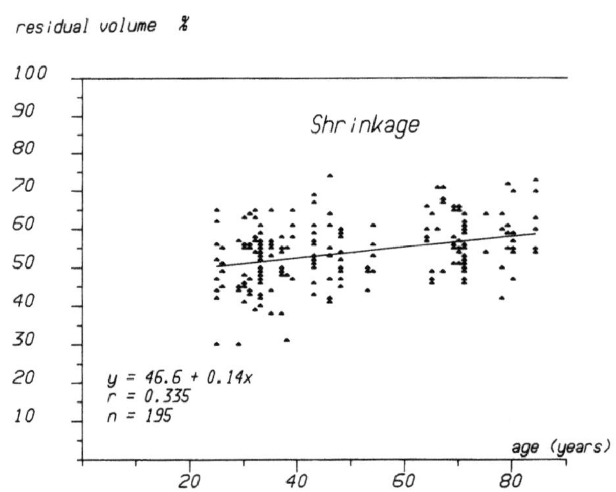

Fig. 1. Brain tissue shrinkage during embedding (expressed residual volume, *ordinate*) as compared with age. 100% residual volume corresponds to unfixed fresh tissue. The degree of shrinkage is the difference between 100% and the volume of the stained slide. $P = 0.001$

ings may result despite the most conscientious efforts. It goes without saying, of course, that we have made an effort to avoid all possible falsifying influences.

Influence of Secular Acceleration on Brain Weight and Aging

Secular acceleration is the increase in human body size from generation to generation. *Developmental acceleration* refers to the accelerated development of a single individual, leading to earlier maturity. The latter process is probably caused by increased standards of living. Because secular acceleration is virtually independent of the living standards, it can be observed in many parts of the world (Haug 1984 b).

The increase in height due to secular acceleration amounts to about 1 mm/year, meaning that mean body height is presently 10 cm greater than 100 years ago. However, it must be noted that the average secular acceleration during the last century represents only half that rate. Human body size remained constant between the birth of Christ and about 1750 A. D.

The larger the body, the larger the brain. Brain weight increases by an average of 0.6 g/year. This means that taking secular acceleration into account, the brain weight of one generation is proportionately higher than that of the preceding generation as measured in youth. Brain weights during one investigation are normally determined within a short time span (transverse examination). Consequently, older generations reveal lower brain weights than subsequent ones, but this lower weight is not actually caused by brain shrinkage.

We have tried to calculate the fraction of the generational difference in brain weights due to secular acceleration, with the aim of estimating the age at which the weight of the human brain actually begins to diminish. Figure 2 shows that the mean human brain weight is constant up to 60 years of age. After the 65 years of age, we can observe a real loss in human brain volume. After the age of eighty,

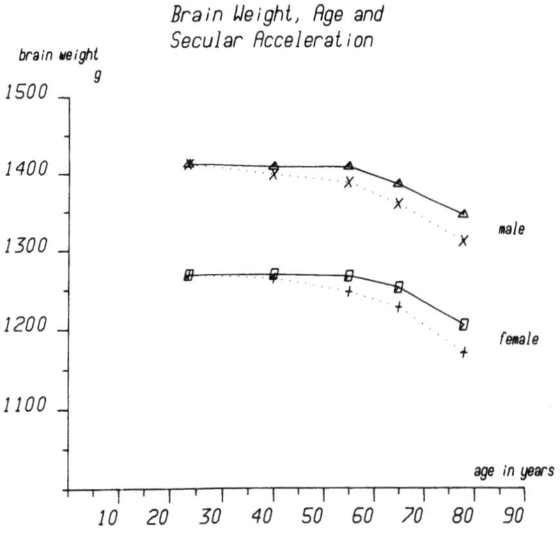

Fig. 2. Mean human brain weight (*ordinate*) as related to age in years (*abscissa*). The *broken line* reflects the average weights for a total or 24,000 brains. The *solid line* takes secular acceleration into consideration and illustrates the change in brain weight occurring during the life span of a hypothetical individual

Table 1. Age-related change in volume of whole human brain and of brainregions expressed in % of the main brain size of a 25-year-old and a 75-year-old person

	Age groups		Brain volume of a 75-year-old as compared with that of a 25-year-old	Change of volume in a 75-year-old relative to a 25-year-old
	30–60 years	61–90 years		
Entire brain	100	100	94	− 6
Entire cortex	48.4	49.3	46.6	− 4
Frontal cortex	15.6	14.5	13.6	−13
Parietal cortex	16.8	17.8	16.7	± 0
Substantia alba	31.0	30.8	28.9	− 7
Basal ganglia	3.75	3.31	3.11	−17

this loss amounts to about 8%–10% and is statistically significant (Haug 1984b).

At the same time, our results demonstrate that the onset of brain volume loss is highly divergent. For instance, one can find extremely high brain weights in very old individuals. This means that the onset and rate of aging events in the human brain differ widely from individual to individual.

Aging of Various Brain Regions

With the help of new morphometric procedures, we (Eggers et al. 1984) have measured the gray and white matter in different regions of the brain. Our results are expressed in percentages on account of the large discrepancies in brain size. Calculations of whole brain size were based on our estimates of the effects of secular acceleration.

Table 1 summarizes the most important results. The entire brain of a 75-year-old is, on the average, about 6% lighter than that of the average 25-year-old. However, the 15% decrease in the weight of the frontal cortex (in front of the motor area) is not proportional. On the other hand, the regions involving sensory and speech functions in the parietal and occipital lobes do not change in size. A larger loss of volume during aging can be found in the central ganglia (thalamus and corpus striatum). White matter also decreases in size.

To summarize, the various regions of the brain undergo different macroscopic alterations during aging. This also applies to the cerebral cortex, where the frontal cortex undergoes marked shrinkage during aging, whereas the parieto-occipital cortex does not change in size.

Effects of Aging on the Neurons of the Cerebral Cortex

Morphometric assessments of the number and size of neurons in the aging cortex must take into account the variability within a population. Figures 3 and 4 show the variability in neuron density and size. Our estimates are based on measure-

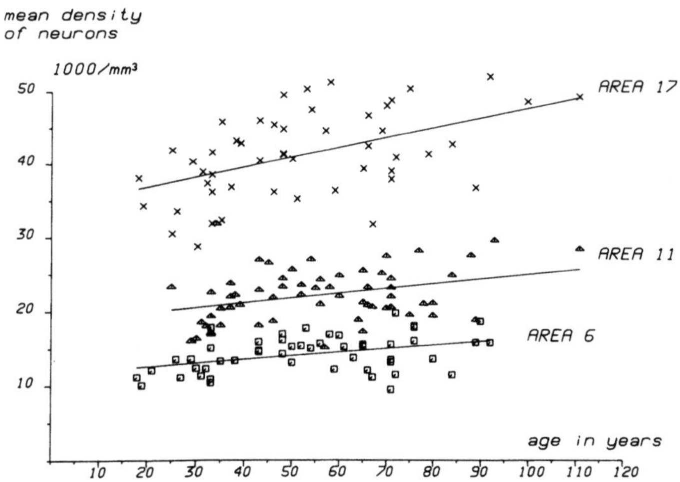

Fig. 3. Mean neuron density in areas 6, 11, and 17, expressed in 1,000/mm^3 (*ordinate*). In spite of marked individuall variability, the significance of the age-related increase in density for area 17 (visual cortex) is high ($P = 0.001$). In areas 6 and 11, the significance of this increase is $P = 0.01$, while in areas 7 and 20, the variability is insignificant

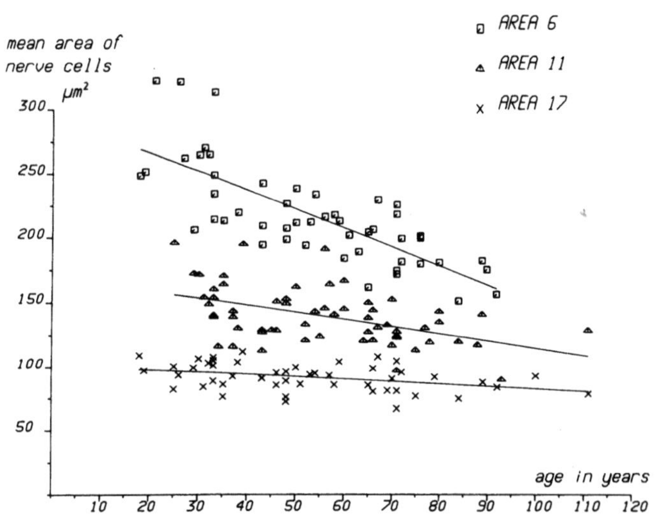

Fig. 4. Mean size of perikarya in brain areas 6, 11, and 17, expressed as the projection area in µm^2 (*ordinate*). The decrease in size is highly significant, ($P = 0.001$) for areas 6 and 11, significant ($P = 0.05$) for area 17, barely significant ($P = 0.1$) for area 20, and insignificant for area 7

ments of at least 50 brains in each area, except for area 20 of the temporal cortex, for which measurements of only 20 brains are provided.

All cases with pathologic or psychologic alterations were eliminated from our study in order to focus on biological aspects of aging. A surprising observation was that neuron density does not diminish during aging, after allowing for embedding shrinkage (Fig. 1). All the results of the microscopic morphometry discussed here are based on fresh or unfixed human brain. Therefore, the neuron densities represent the actual number of neurons in living brain tissue for the brain areas examined (Haug 1984a; Haug et al. 1983; Haug et al. 1984).

It is striking that, with age, some areas show an increase in neuron density per mm^3. This is primarily true of area 6 (extrapyramidal cortex). On the other hand, we found that macroscopically speaking, this area decreases in size. The increase in density is probably connected with this decrease in volume. This question is discussed further.

Figure 3 compares the neuron density of three of the five evaluated areas. Areas 7 and 20, which are not shown here, show the same tendencies as area 11. An increase in neuron density with age can be observed in all areas except areas 7 and 20.

Perikaryon size shows different tendencies. Figure 4 demonstrates the changes in neuron size for three brain areas. Area 6 exhibits a striking degree of diminution of neuron size with age. Area 17 shows a lower, though still statistically significant reduction in size, while area 7 shows little diminution of neuron size.

A first glance at area 11 (psychosocial functions) reveals similarities to area 6. However, the decrease in neuron size does not occur continuously. Figure 5 demonstrates this by illustrating the reduction in cell size occurring with age. Cell area remains constant up to age with a slight increase possible around age 50. After 60 years of age, mean size shrinks noticeably. We feel that our results are valid, in view of the fact that 70,000 neurons were examined.

As far as neuron density and size are concerned, area 20 shows a pattern similar to that of area 11, despite the fact that only 20 brains were studied. It is probable that the neurons in this area also diminish in size after 60 years of age.

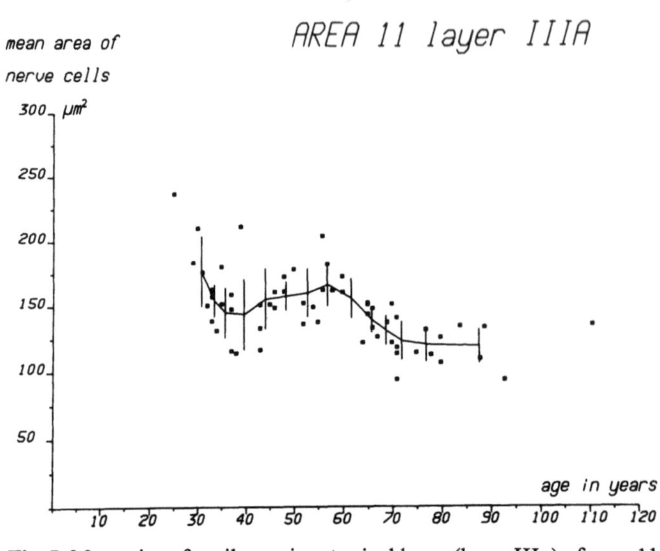

Fig. 5. Mean size of perikarya in a typical layer (layer IIIa) of area 11, as expressed by an empirical regression (Peil and Schmerling). The graph demonstrates that neuronal shrinkage can be clearly observed only after 60 years of age. The tendency toward an increase in area from age 50–60 is not significant

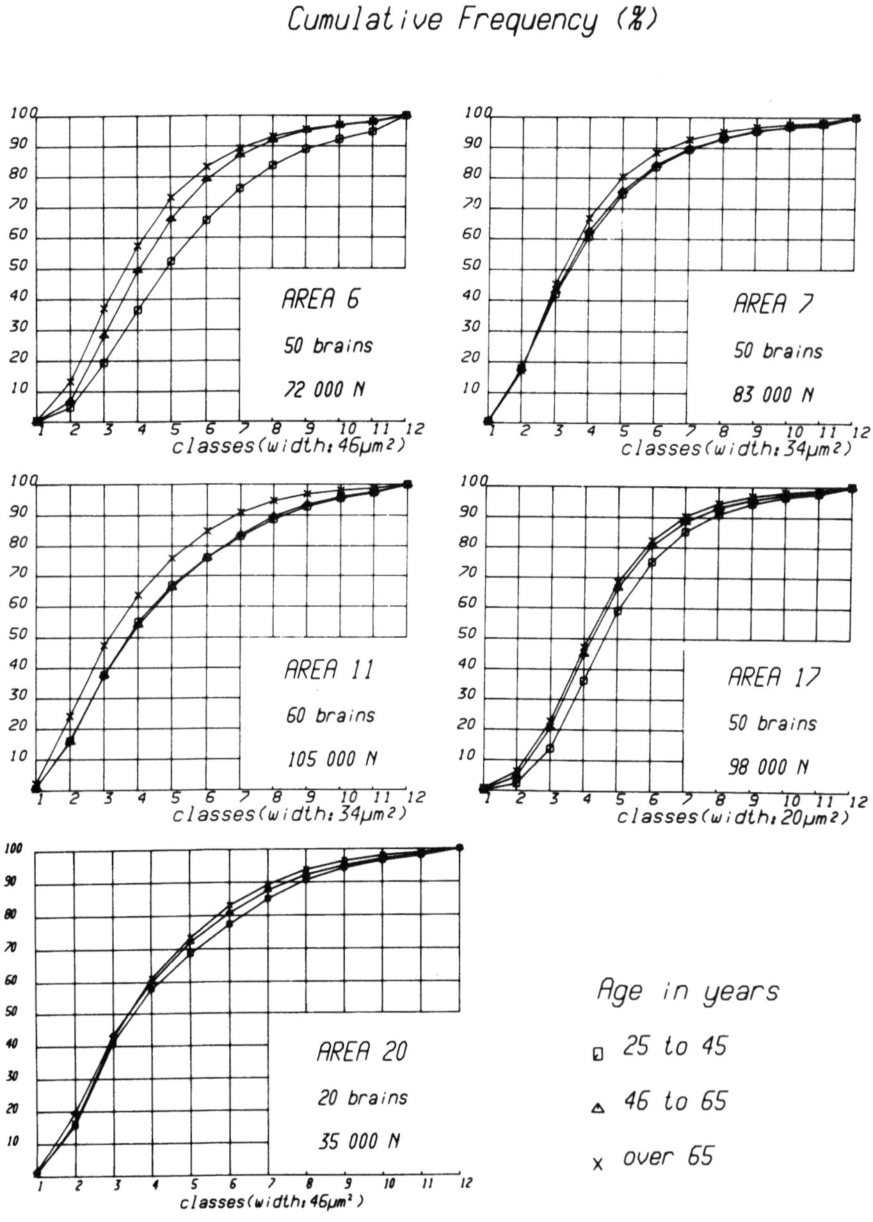

Fig. 6. Size distribution of cortical neurons in five human cortical areas shown for three age groups. Curves represent cumulative frequencies beginning with the smallest cell class. The cell classes differ according to the size of the neurons in each brain area. Curves at the *left* represent small neuron distributions and, at the *right*, larger size distributions

The higher parietal cortex (area 7) and the visual cortex (area 17) reveal decreases in nerve cell size that remain relatively small until old age, with a shrinkage amounting to about 10% in volume. Area 6 undergoes a mean volume decrease of 30%–35%, while areas 11 and 20 are diminished by between 10% and 30%.

Figures 4 and 5 do not demonstrate how the different neuron sizes contribute toward the overall reduction in mean projection area. This is illustrated with the size distribution graphs in Fig. 6. The five graphs show the overall neuronal size distribution for 12 size classes expressed in curves of sum frequencies. Such curves can answer further questions concerning the degree and rate of age changes for different sizes of neurons. The total number of cells analyzed for each curve corresponds to 100%.

The scales of the cortical areas studied vary as to the arrangement of size distribution according to differences in mean neuronal size. Steep sections of the curves indicate that the corresponding size classes contain many cells, while flat sections describe classes with few cells. The curves in one graph depict three age groups. The curves lying more to the right are based on larger cell size distributions and, vice versa, the curves at the left are based on smaller ones. The distance between the curves expresses the difference in size between the projection area of neuronal sizes for the various age groups.

The large distance separating the age curves for area 6 means that cell size diminishes continuously for all size classes in the three age groups. The curves for area 7 show that only a very small decrease in cell size takes place during the aging process. Area 11 exemplifies yet another pattern. Cell size remains nearly unchanged up to age 65, after which a distinct decrease in size can be observed. This accords with the distribution of mean sizes shown in Fig. 5. The visual cortex, with its relatively small cells, shows a slight, but continuous decrease in cell size with age.

The graphs in Fig. 6 demonstrate that the decreases in size undergone by cells in one area of the brain during aging are similar. After evaluating 20 brains, we believe that area 20 of the temporal cortex shows aging patterns similar to those seen in area 11 (Nass 1985).

Similar observations regarding neuron size have been made by Uemura and Hartmann (1978). Our own examinations involve the various layers of the cerebral cortex. Though some smaller discrepancies can be observed, they have no implications for our view of the aging process.

Total Number of Neurons in the Human Cerebral Cortex

The neuron density and cortical volume of which it was possible to calculate from individual brain weights allow an estimation of the total number of neurons in the whole cortex. Cortical volume, in turn, amounts to about 47.5% of the total brain (Schlenska 1969; Haug 1970; Eggers et al. 1984).

Figure 7 shows that the number of neurons varies considerably. It should be noted here that Fig. 7 records only those brains for which values based on two or more areas were available. The mean number of neurons in the human cerebral cortex totals 13.9×10^9 (billions), with a range of between 10 and 20×10^9

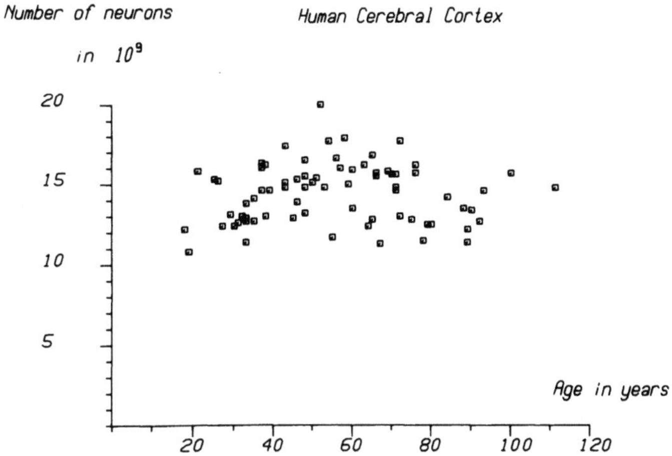

Fig. 7. Total number (in billions) of neurons in the entire human cerebral cortex (*ordinate*). Each mean value contains values for at least two areas. The values are calculated according to normalized mean density; the weight of cerebral cortex represents 47.5% of the average whole brain. Total number of neurons does not appear to change with age

neurons. We cannot discern any tendency for the number of neurons to diminish with age, but it must be noted that the decrease in brain size is counterbalanced by an increase in neuron density (Fig. 3).

In summary, the following statement is possible: the total number of neurons in the human cerebral cortex does not change during the aging process, if all pathologic material is excluded from consideration. However, this result is not representative of brain regions other than the cortex. Furthermore, it is probable that pathologic material reveals degeneration, as for example, in Alzheimer's desease (Terry 1983).

Aging of Cortical Ultrastructures

The analysis of the ultrastructure covers the entire neuron, including the perikaryon, dendrites, neurites, synapses, and glia with processes and vessels, and implements high-power images, usually produced by electron microscopy. Methodologically the morphometry of these structures has not yet been satisfactorily resolved. Two procedures are important. However, because of the effort involved, they have not been used very frequently:

1. The neurons and their processes can be stained by Golgi staining with silver. In conjunction with light microscopy, this stain reveals that the larger dendrites have spines representing a kind of synaptic contact from neuron to neuron. It is possible to count this type of synapse. Marin-Padilla and Marin-Padilla (1982), Scheibel and Scheibel (1978), Schierhorn (1978), and Schönheit and Schulz (1978) have shown that the number of spines decreases with age, bringing about a concomitant decrease in the numbers of synaptic contacts.

Some investigations suggest that the reduction in synaptic contacts is accompanied by a decrease in functional ability (see below). However, it should be mentioned that at present little research on this issue has been done.

2. Contrary to the autolysis of other ultrastructural components, it is possible to stain the synapses in the human brain for electron microscopy with a phosphotungstic procedure. Huttenlocher (1979) has found out that the density of synapses decreases slightly with age. With this procedure, it is possible to examine more types of synapses than with light microscopy, which reveals only spine synapses.

Such examinations should be increasingly used in the future, on the grounds that the slight aging changes discovered by light microscopy force us to look more closely for age changes at the ultrastructural level, especially those involving synapses, neuronal processes, and vessel walls.

Uemura and Hartmann (1978) and Higatsberger et al. (1982) report a loss of DNA and other neurochemical substances in the nerve cell bodies of human brain. Carlsson (1981) found a slight decrease in neurotransmitter levels, which are sometimes diminished at an increasing rate after 60 years of age.

Aging and the Human Brain: New Insights

These and other developments have led to new insights in our understanding of morphological and functional changes taking place in the human brain during the aging process:

1. Morphometric results of macroscopy and light microscopy show that, up to 60–65 years of age, no or only small changes occurring as a result of aging can be observed in the human cerebral cortex with the exception of area 6, see point 2. It should be pointed out that this is a statement of statistical probability, meaning that, on an average, the onset of morphological age changes in the human cortex may be expected to occur around age 60–65. However, on an individual basis, the age at which such alterations may occur varies. The time of onset and speed of aging probably depend on a genetic program.
2. Aging differs in time, extent, and rate for the gray matter of different regions. Aging changes in area 6 of the human cortex begin very early (Between the ages of 25 and 40 years). Those taking place in the visual cortex (area 17) and the parietal lobe (area 7), which play a role in sensory processes, begin late in life, as revealed by macroscopic and microscopic morphometric examinations.

   Psychosocial functions regulated by the orbital part of the frontal lobe (area 11) exhibit special traits. Neuron measurements do not show changes until retirement age. After the age of 65, pericaryon size diminishes noticeably.
3. At present, the effects of aging changes in the ultrastructure of the human cortex are too slight to have been convincingly demonstrated. However, preliminary examinations suggest that the density of synapses decreases with advancing age, though details of how this occurs remain unknown (see point 4). It is

to be hoped that more studies using ultrastructural techniques will broaden our knowledge in this field.

4. Experiments with aged rats have shown that environment exerts a strong influence on the aging process (Connor et al. 1981, 1982; Diamond and Connor 1982). Rats identical in age were housed in a narrow cage comparable to the restrictive environment of a home for the elderly. After a certain amount of time had elapsed, they showed a considerable loss of spine synapses in the cerebral cortex. On the other hand, rats of similar age and breeding which are put into large cages with an enriched environment together with rats of other ages reveal no loss of spine synapses after the same period of observation. This finding suggests the following conclusion: the use of cortical neuronal connections permits conservation of these structures and their functions. This is not a new statement, as it is well-established, for example, that muscles which are not used undergo atrophy.
5. It is well-known in human psychology that work and activity help to conserve mental ability, while an impoverished environment (like certain inferior homes for the elderly), by imposing a life of relative inactivity, leads to atrophy of brain structures.
6. Our own results demonstrate that the extrapyramidal human cortex (area 6) begins to age relatively early, as a result of a decrease in motor activity. On the other hand, the sense organs continue to be used, even in old age or in an environment of poor quality, which permits long maintenance of structure and function. With such findings in mind, we can more easily grasp the observations regarding area 11 in the basal frontal cortex, which are related to psychosocial functions. Cortical structures are preserved until retirement age. After retirement, the need for preservation diminishes and, consequently, one can begin to observe changes in the cortical structure.
7. The genetically determined timetable of age changes occurring in various parts of the cerebral cortex is slowed or accelerated, depending on the degree to which brain functions are put to use. With this in mind, we can understand why individuals who work beyond the normal retirement age retain their mental faculties into old age. Political leaders in a number of countries are examples of this.
8. Some studies have shown that metabolic changes also occur during aging (Ulfert et al. 1982; Sarkander et al. 1982).

The current discussion in the Federal Republic of Germany regarding the appropriate age for retirement shows little concern for the aged. However, the individual's own experience and the observations of science make us realize that the normal working life should be extended. In the USA, some changes have been brought about as a consequence of this viewpoint. The enormous changes taking place in the workplace compel us to find new solutions concerning the length of our working life. I think retirement age should be very flexible, so that it can be adapted to the capabilities of the individual. Furthermore, it should not be forgotten, that, in a few years, the age groups beginning their working life will be very small, according to demographers. This will probably lead to the extension of the normal working life, because the problem of financing retirement pensions will provide additional incentives for a longer working life.

Acknowledgements. I would like to thank Dr. Spann, Institute for Forensic Medicine, Munich, for his collaboration and for the samples he provided. I also want to express my thanks to my co-workers U. Barmwater, R. Eggers, D. Fischer, S. Kühl, E. Naß, N.-L. Sass, K. Wasner, G. Knebel, E. Mecke, P. Oesterle, C. Örün, and W. Schließer.

References

Brody H (1955) Organization of the cerebral cortex. III. A study of aging in the human cerebral cortex. J Comp Neurol 102:511–556

Carlsson A (1981) Aging and brain neurotransmitters. In: Platt D (ed) Funktionsstörungen des Gehirns im Alter. 7. Rothenburger Gespräch, 6. und 7. November 1980. Schattauer, Stuttgart, pp 66–81

Connor JR, Melone JH, Yuen AR, Diamond MC (1981) Dendritic length in aged rats' occipital cortex: An environmentally induced response. Exp Neurol 73:827–830

Connor JR, Beban SE, Hopper PA, Hansen B, Diamond MC (1982) A golgi study of the superficial pyramidal cells in the somatosensory cortex of socially reared old adult rats. Exp Neurol 76:35–45

Diamond MC, Connor JR (1982) Plasticity of the aging cerebral cortex. Exp Brain Res [Suppl] 5:36–44

Eggers R, Haug H, Fischer D (1984) Preliminary report on macroscopic age changes in the human prosencephalon. A sterologic investigation. J Hirnforsch 25:129–139

Haug H (1970) Der makroskopische Aufbau des Großhirns. Qualitative und quantitative Untersuchungen an den Gehirnen des Menschen, der Delphinoideae und des Elefanten. Ergebn Anat Entwicklungsgesch 43:4

Haug H (1979) The evaluation of cell-densities and of nerve-cell-size distribution by stereological procedures in a layered tissue (cortex cerebri). Microsc Acta 82:147–161

Haug H (1980) Die Abhängigkeit der Einbettungsschrumpfung des Gehirngewebes vom Lebensalter. Verh Anat Ges 74:699–700

Haug H (1982) The location and size distribution of neurons in the layered cortex. Acta Stereol 1:259–267

Haug H (1984 a) Alterungsprozesse im Gehirn. Morphometrische Methoden ermöglichen neue Einblicke. Umschau 84:455–458

Haug H (1984 b) Der Einfluß der säkularen Akzeleration auf das Hirngewicht des Menschen und dessen Änderung während der Alterung. Gegenbaurs Morphol Jahrb 130:481–500

Haug H, Barmwater U, Eggers R, Fischer D, Kühl S, Sass N-L (1983) Anatomical changes in aging brain: morphometric analysis of the human prosencephalon. Aging 21:1–12

Haug H, Kühl S, Mecke E, Sass N-L, Wasner K (1984) The significance of morphometric procedures in the investigation of age changes in cytoarchitectonic structures of human brain. J Hirnforsch 25:353–374

Higatsberger MR, Budka H, Bernheimer H (1982) Neurochemical investigations of aged human brain cortex. Exp Brain Res Suppl 5:112–117

Huttenlocher PR (1979) Synaptic density in human frontal cortex – developmental changes and effects of aging. Brain Res 163:195–205

Lehr V (1984) Vorruhestand – ist das human? Umschau 84:300

Marin-Padilla M, Marin-Padilla TM (1982) Origin, prenatal development and structural organization of layer I of the human cerebral (motor) cortex. Anat Embryol 164:161–206

Naß E (1985) Altersabhängige Veränderungen im Lobus temporalis (Area 20 nach Brodmann) des Menschen. Eine lichtmikroskopische Untersuchung mit morphometrischer Bestimmung von Zelldichte und Zellgröße, verbunden mit einer Betrachtung von Geschlechtsunterschieden. Inauguraldissertation Med. Hochschule Lübeck

Peil J, Schmerling S (1982) Empirical regression for trend elimination and smoothing of time series. Gegenbaurs Morphol Jahrb 128:324–332

Sarkander H-I, Lux R, Cervos-Navarro J (1982) Histone-DNA-interactions in neuronal chromatin during aging. Exp Brain Res [Suppl] 5:45–50

Sass N-L (1982) The age-dependent variation of the embedding-shrinkage of neurohistological sections. Mikroskopie 39:278–281
Scheibel ME, Scheibel AB (1978) The dendritic structure of the human Betz cell. In: Brazier MAB, Petsche H (eds) Architectonics of the cerebral cortex. Raven, New York, pp 43–57
Schierhorn H (1978) Die postnatale Entwicklung der Lamina V-Pyramidenzellen im sensomotorischen Cortex der Albinoratte. Gegenbaurs Morphol Jahrb 124:1–23, 24–42, 230–255
Schlenska G (1969) Messungen der Oberfläche und der Volumenanteile des Gehirnes menschlicher Erwachsener mit neuen Methoden. Z Anat Entwicklungsgesch 128:47–59
Schönheit B, Schulz E (1978) Der Einfluß sensorischer Deprivation auf die Lamina-V-Pyramidenneurone des Gyrus cinguli der Ratte. Z Mikrosk Anat Forsch 92:374–384
Tery RD (1983) Cortical morphometry in the Alzheimer's disease. Banbury Report 15:95–103
Uemura E, Hartmann HA (1978) Prefrontal cortex in aging normal and demented patients. Neuropathol Exp Neurol 37:487–496
Ulfert G, Schmidt U, Hoyer S (1982) Glucose and energy metabolism of rat cerebral cortex during aging. Exp Brain Res [Suppl] 5:102–111
Weibel ER (1979) Stereological Methods, vol 1. Practical methods for biological morphometry. Academic, London

Senile Dementia of the Alzheimer Type: Morphological and Immunocytochemical Studies*

J. P. Brion[1], P. van den Bosch de Aguilar[2], and J. Flament-Durand[1]

Introduction

Although recent progress in the isolation of neurofibrillary tangles (NFT) has been made (Ihara et al. 1983; Iqbal et al. 1984), little information is available on the biochemical nature of NFT, their precise relationship with neuron organelles and their etiopathogenesis. Difficulties in carrying out the biochemical analysis of NFT until now have been attributed to their unusual insolubility (Selkoe et al. 1982), although this property also seems a matter of debate (Iqbal et al. 1984). Ultrastructural studies have also clearly pointed out their unique morphological features (Terry 1963; Kidd 1963). Immunohistochemistry offers an interesting approach, since well-defined antibodies reacting with NFT in tissue sections (Anderton et al. 1982; Gambetti et al. 1983) have recently been described.

We have employed light and electron microscopy to undertake immunocytochemical studies of NFT, using antibodies raised against cytoskeletal proteins and an antibody raised against isolated NFT, as described by Ihara et al. (1983). We have tried to correlate, on morphological grounds, lesions such as senile plaques (SP) and NFT with the described impairment of the cholinergic system in senile dementia of the Alzheimer type (SDAT) (Davies and Maloney 1976). We are also investigating the consequences of implantations in animals of SDAT brain tissue, in the hopes of finding a valid animal model of SDAT.

Material and Methods

Ultrastructural Studies

Brain biopsies from the frontal lobe of patients with SDAT were observed by transmission electron microscopy (TEM). Fractions enriched in NFT were prepared from brain taken postmortem from patients with SDAT, according to a modified Selkoe's procedure (1982). They were studied by TEM after negative staining before and after treatment with sodium dodecyl sulfate (SDS) as well as after rotatory shadowing with platinum iridium.

* Supported by grants from the *Fonds de la Recherche Fondamentale Collective* (No. 2.4517.82)
1 Université Libre de Bruxelles/Laboratoire d'Anatomie pathologique, Route de Lennik, 808, B-1070 Bruxelles, Belgique
2 Université Catholique de Louvain

Senile Dementia of the Alzheimer Type
Ed. by J. Traber and W. H. Gispen

Implantation Studies

Small tissue blocks containing NFT taken from the cortex of a SDAT patient were transplanted into the occipital cortex of 7-week-old rats according to the method of Das et al. (1979). Fragments of normal brain from an elderly patient were used as a control. After 8 weeks, the brain was removed and processed by routine methods for light and TEM studies.

Antigen and Antibody Preparations

NFT were prepared by the procedure of Ihara et al. (1983) and injected in rabbits. Microtubule proteins from rat and human brain were prepared by the assembly-disassembly method (Shelanski et al. 1973) and microtubule-associated proteins (MAP) by the method of Fellous et al. (1977). After electrophoreses on SDS-polyacrylamide gel, gel slices corresponding to high molecular weight MAP 2 and tau protein were homogenized and injected into rabbits. The sera were checked by immunocytochemistry and immunoblotting. Human brain filament fractions, mainly containing the three components of neurofilaments (NF) and the glial fibrillary acidic protein (GFAP), were prepared according to Chiu and Norton (1982). The anti-GFAP was kindly supplied by Lowenthal (UIA) and the anti-tubulin by De Mey (Janssen Pharmaceutica).

Immunohistochemistry

Hippocampal and cortical tissue blocks from SDAT and normal patients were fixed in 10% formalin and embedded in paraffin. Other blocks were fixed in 4% paraformaldehyde, and thick sections were obtained using a vibratome. The peroxidase–anti-peroxidase method of Sternberg (1979) was used for immunohistochemistry. For immunoelectron microscopy, postmortem material, fixed in 4% paraformaldehyde and 0.5% glutaraldehyde, was embedded in Epon and processed by the immunogold staining method (De Mey et al. 1981). Isolated NFT were labeled by the same method. In addition to the usual immunohistochemical and antibody controls, absorption studies were conducted as follows: overnight preincubation at 4 °C of the antibody with the antigenic preparation under investigation, centrifugation at 100,000 g for 60 min, and use of the final supernatant as "primary" antiserum.

Histochemistry

Tissue blocks (hippocampus and cortex) were fixed as suggested by Rossor et al. (1982) and cryostat sections stained for acetylcholinesterase (ACE) according to the protocol of Tsuji (1974). (The sulfide deposits were intensified by the use of silver nitrate.) Ethopropazine was included in the incubation medium to inhibit nonspecific cholesterase.

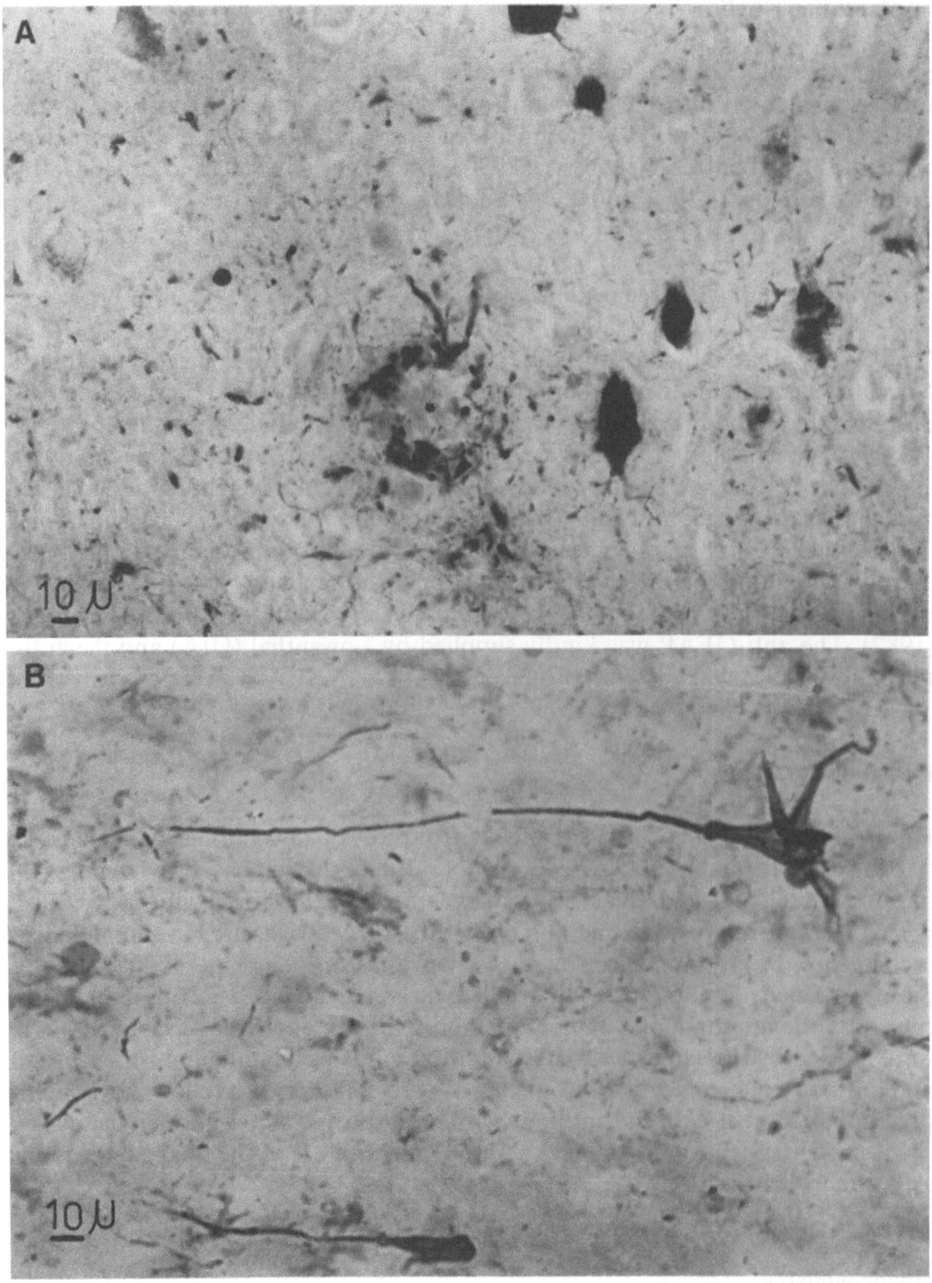

Fig. 1 A, B. Anti NFT labeling (PAP method). **A** Paraffin-embedded temporal lobe of SDAT, counterstained with Congo red. The antibody selectively labels the tangles and the abnormal neurites surrounding the central core of the plaque. Note that this amyloid (*) is not labeled. **B** Section (50 μm thick) obtained with a vibratome: labeling of the tangles in the pericaryon and in the cell processes

Results

Our TEM observations of brain biopsies have confirmed the well-known lesions of SDAT. The NFT were observed at both pre- and postsynaptic sites and, occasionally, in myelinated fibers. NFT-containing neurites are practically devoid of normal neurotubules and demonstrate a pronounced accumulation of dense, osmiophilic bodies, lysosomes, and altered mitochondria (Flament-Durand and Couck 1978). Spongiform alterations similar to those observed in Jakob-Creutzfeld disease have also been observed.

The preparation of NFT-enriched fractions has allowed better visualization of the ultrastructure of paired helical filaments (PHF) by negative staining and shadowing. This has revealed a protofilamentous substructure (at least six protofilaments, each of them 2 nm wide) in PHF exhibiting a right-handed helix every 80 nm (Brion et al. 1984).

The graft of SDAT brain tissue induces some modifications in the rat cortex, including an intense, fibrous, astrocytic reaction; occasionally, twisted filaments were found in the bundle of normal filaments of these glial processes (van den Bosch et al. 1984). An activation of fibrillary astrocytes around the SP and in the vicinity of NFT is also clearly shown in human tissue by anti-GFAP labeling (Flament-Durand et al. 1983).

The serum obtained from rabbits immunized with isolated tangles (anti-NFT) labeled NFT only on paraffin sections. Numerous fine neurites were also detected in affected areas. The immunohistochemical labeling seemed to detect NFT at

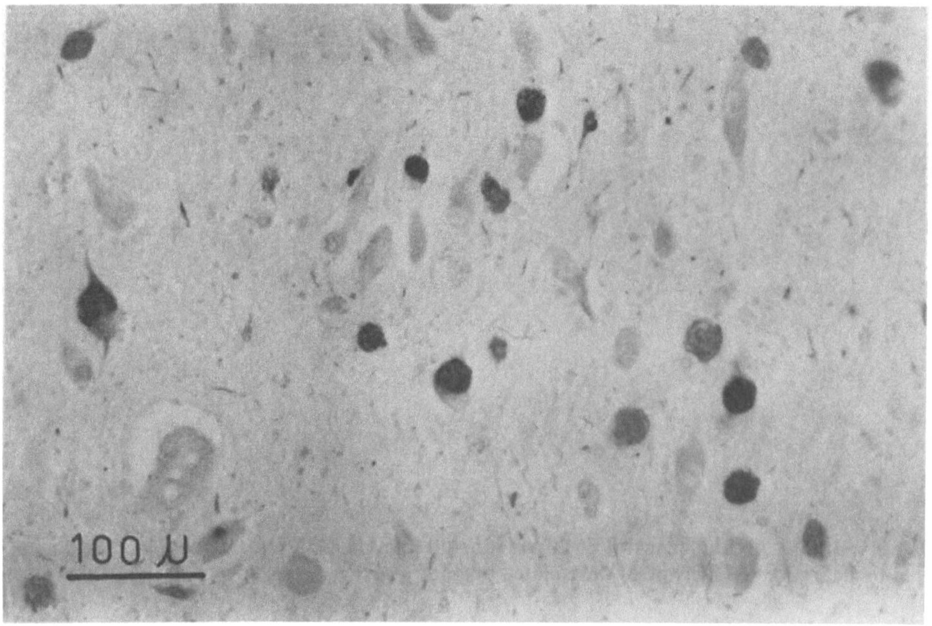

Fig. 2. Anti-NFT labeling of some neurons of the nucleus of Meynert (paraffin-embedded tissue)

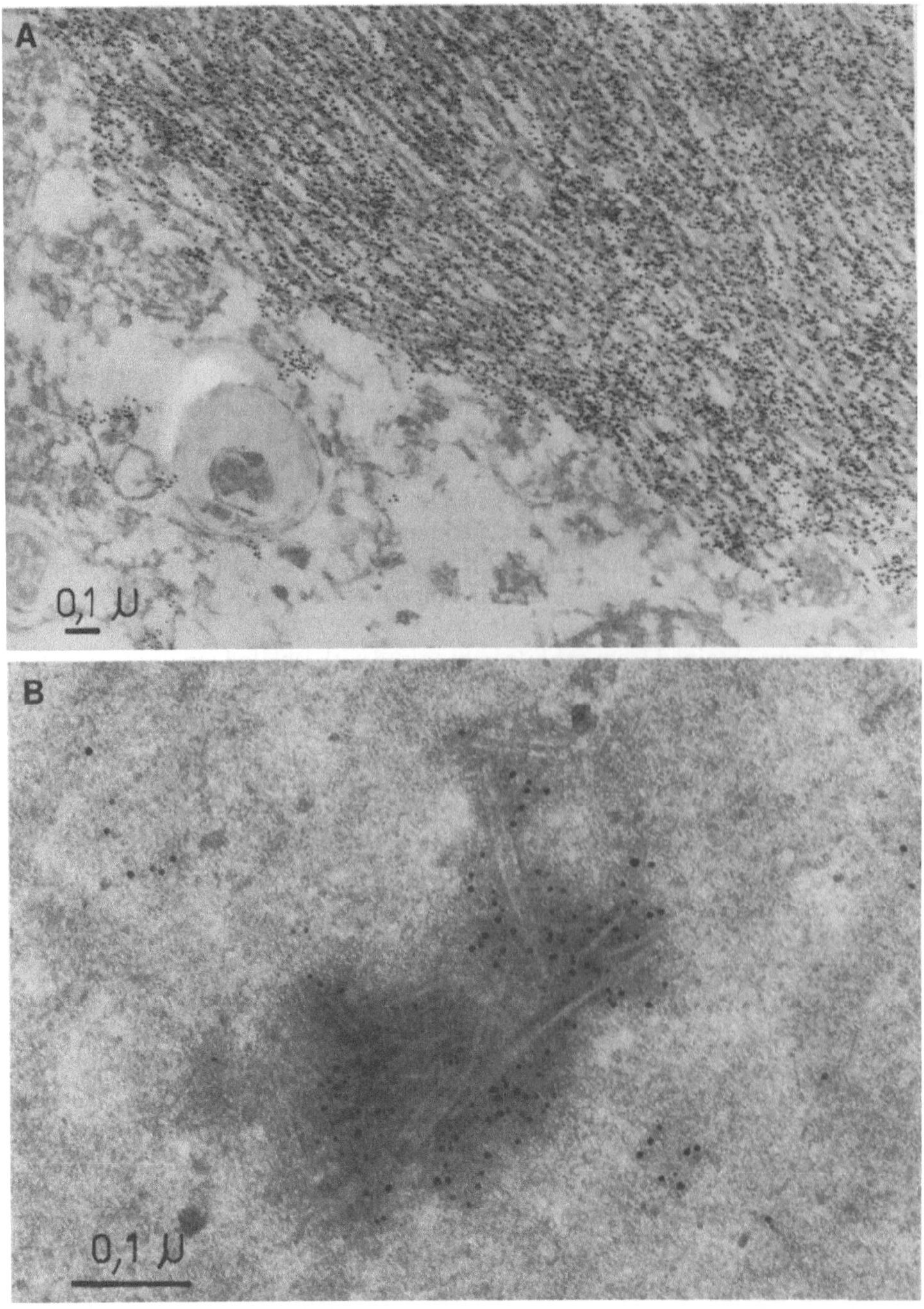

Fig. 3 A, B. Anti-NFT labeling in TEM (immunogold stainind method). **A** Labeling of the tangles in a tissue section. **B** Labeling of the isolated tangles

least as efficiently as Congo red or silver staining performed on adjacent sections. Many plaques were also detected by the labeling of their periphery, while their central amyloid core, which remained unlabeled, was demonstratable by Congo red counterstaining (Fig. 1 a). The same observations were made on thick human vibratome sections, which allowed a more stereological view of the affected neurons (Fig. 1 b). NFT were detected not only in the Ammon's horn and the temporal and frontal cortex, but also in the nucleus basalis and septal nuclei (Fig. 2). With TEM, the tangles were the only structure recognized by anti-NFT on tissue sections (Fig. 3 a) (Brion et al. 1985). PHF isolated in SDS were labeled by anti-NFT (Fig. 3 b). No consistent labeling of NFT was obtained with the antisera against either MAP 2 or tubulin, although normal neurons adjacent to NFT were labeled.

Interestingly, we observed labeling of NFT with anti-tau antiserum in tissue sections: the pictures obtained with this antibody are very similar to those obtained with anti-NFT (Fig. 4). Labeling of NFT was also observed on tissue sections with TEM. However, the anti-tau antiserum was not capable of labeling the PHF isolated in denaturing conditions at the TEM level. Results of the absorption experiments of anti-NFT are summarized in Table 1. No absorption was obtained with human brain filaments or liver homogenate for the range of protein concentrations tested. Anti-NFT was absorbed with isolated tangles or brain homogenates taken from SDAT patients. It was only moderately absorbed with brain homogenates taken from young patients without neurologic lesions. A complete absorption was however observed with high protein concentrations of

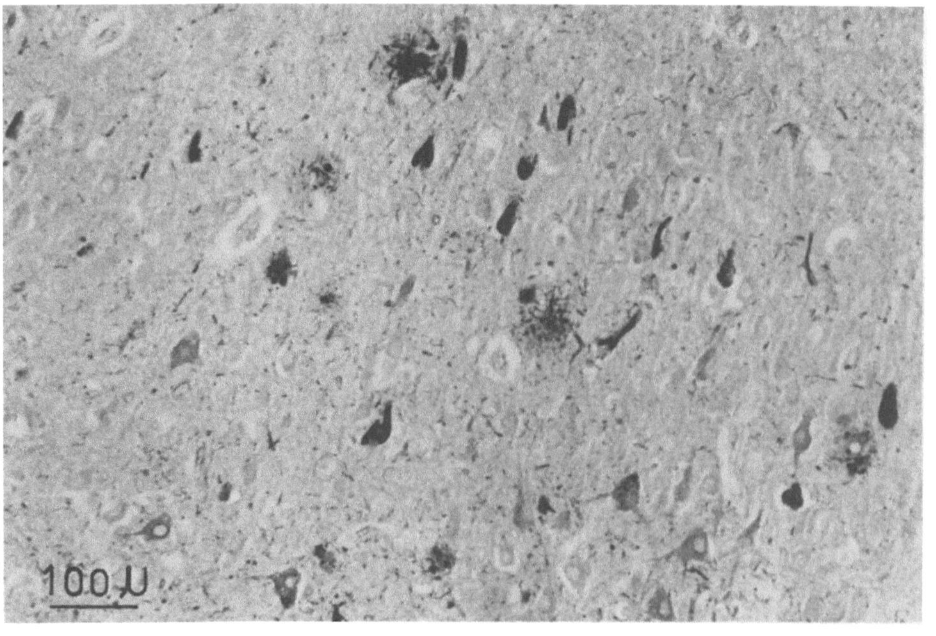

Fig. 4. Anti-tau labeling of NFT in some neurons of the temporal cortex (paraffin-embedded material)

Table 1. Absorption studies of anti-NFT

	Sex	Age (years)	Proteins used in absorption/ ml antibody[a]	Tangles in tissue blocks[b]	Decrease in immuno-labeling[c]
SDAT brain tissue (temporal cortex)	F	86	5 mg (1)	++	++++
Down syndrome brain tissue (temporal cortex)	M	50	5 mg (2)	+++	++++
Control cases (temporal cortex)	F	31	8.5 mg (1)	/−/	+
			21.5 mg (2)	/−/	+
	F	38	22 mg (1)	/−/	+
	M	50	25 mg (1)	/−/	++
	F	86	10 mg (1)	/−/	++
			25 mg (1)	/−/	++++
	F	84	4 mg (1)	/−/	0
			25 mg (1)	/−/	+++
	F	81	7.5 mg (1)	/−/	+
	F	83	25 mg (1)	/−/	+++
	M	88	25 mg (2)	rare	++++
	F	86	25 mg (1)	(+)	++++
	M	82	25 mg (1)	/−/	++++
Rar brain		6 months	12 mg (1)	/	0
Rat liver		6 months	83 mg (1)	/	0
Isolated NFT	F	83	47 μg (2)	++	++++
Human brain filaments	M	81	250 μg (1)	/−/	0
Human microtubule	F	38	2.3 mg (1)	/−/	++++
Rat MAPs		3 months	200 μg (1)	/	+++

[a] Number of experiments are listed in parentheses
[b] /−/, absent; +, few; ++, numerous; +++, very numerous
[c] 0, null; +, moderate; ++, partial; +++, pronounced; ++++, total

brain homogenates from aged normal brain. Congo red staining of sections adjacent to the tissue blocks used for absorption did not reveal NFT. Absorption was also observed with the preparations of rat MAP and human total microtubule proteins. The histochemical detection of ACE in the human hippocampus was drastically reduced in some cases of SDAT (Fig. 5). This was paralleled by marked decrease in ACE-positive fibers in the fimbria. Some SP were detected owing to their ACE-positive staining. These positive SP, which sometimes contained an amyloid core, were especially frequent in the molecular layer of the gyrus dentatus. In other sectors, e.g., the subiculum areas, which occasionally contained many plaques both with and without amyloid, as judged from silver impregnations on adjacent sections, the SP were not ACE-positive.

Discussion

TEM observations of brain biopsies makes possible the enhancement of unusual data such as the presence of NFT in postsynaptic sites and in myelinated fibers.

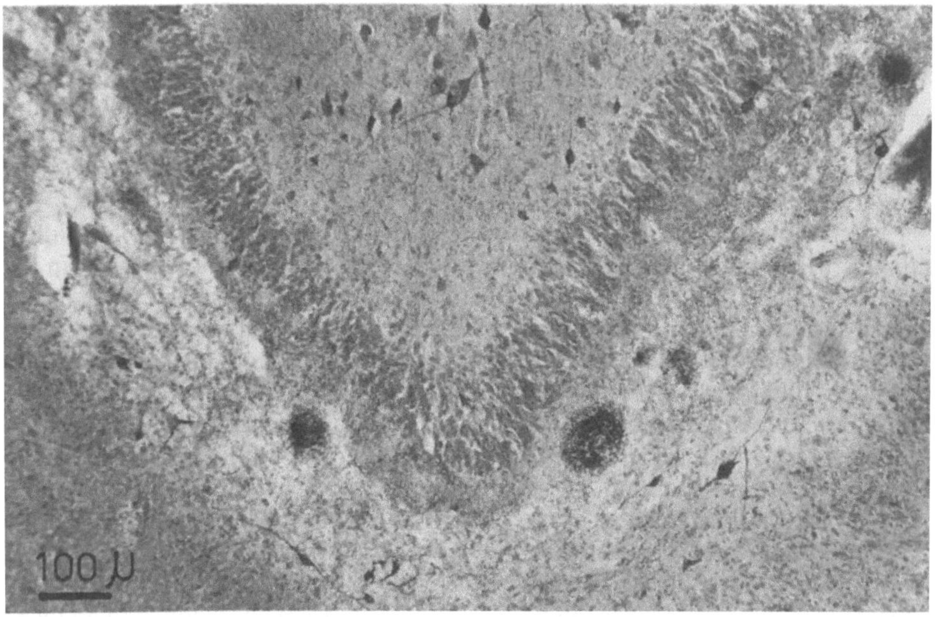

Fig. 5. Cryostat section of SDAT brain stained for ACE. Detection of ACE in some of the plaques close to the gyrus dentatus

The axoplasmic flow appears to be impaired, as demonstrated on morphological grounds, by the loss of microtubules and the accumulation of altered organelles in NFT-containing neurites (Dustin and Flament-Durand 1982). These alterations of the axoplasmic flow, either primary or secondary to the presence of NFT, certainly contribute to the impairment of neuronal function. The presence of spongiform alterations (Flament-Durand and Couck 1979) similar to those observed in Jakob-Creutzfeld disease might support the hypothesis of the possible role of a transmissible agent in the genesis of SDAT (Gibbs and Gajduzek 1978). A case can also be made for the role of a transmissible agent or neurotoxic factor on the basis of the glial cytoskeletal anomalies observed after implantation of SDAT cortex in rat cortex (van den Bosch et al. 1984).

The ultrastructural features of PHF differentiate them from normal constituents of the cytoskeleton (Brion et al. 1984). Similarly, immunohistochemical studies on human brain tissue with anti-NFT reveal the latter's lack of reactivity with tissue components other than NFT, a finding also shown by Ihara et al. (1983). Clearly, the amyloid central core of some SP differs from NFT on both immunologic and ultrastructural grounds, although they both exhibit birefringence after Congo red staining, a property that is possibly related to their beta-pleated configuration. These observations were extended at the TEM level in tissue sections of postmortem material. The PHF are the only structures recognized by anti-NFT. We were still able to obtain labeling in TEM of PHF isolated after denaturing treatment (i.e., under conditions in which it is hoped that all normal fibrous proteins are removed), confirming that this antibody recognizes at least selectively some antigens characteristic of PHF.

The labeling of NFT with anti-tau was confirmed at the TEM level on tissue sections, but not on PHF isolated in denaturing conditions. Rasool et al. (1983) and Ihara et al. (1983) also have shown that antibodies against NF proteins which labeled NFT in tissue sections failed to react with them after SDS treatment, suggesting that these antibodies are able to detect antigens not inherent to PHF but possibly, belonging either to normal fibers trapped in NFT or to a moderately soluble, abnormal fibrous structure.

The notion that our anti-tau can recognize antigens on microtubules intermingled with PHF can be discarded, since TEM revealed no microtubules in the labeled tangles. PHF and tau proteins thus might well share antigenic determinants, although the former possess inherent antigens (demonstrated by anti-NFT). Normal microtubules contain tau proteins, and the latter remain associated with tubulin and other MAP in a constant ratio through several cycles of assembly and disassembly (Cleveland et al. 1977). In rat, tau proteins are composed of four types with an apparent molecular weight of between 52 and 69 kd. Interestingly, Grundke-Iqbal et al. (1979) and Yen et al. (1981) have obtained labeling of NFT with antisera raised against microtubule proteins. Polyacrylamide gel electrophoresis of PHF preparations (Iqbal et al. 1984) have shown protein bands in the range of 45–62 kd. Antibodies prepared with these isolated NFT (Grundke-Iqbal et al. 1984) labeled NFT in tissue sections and were absorbed with an identically prepared fraction from a normal brain, suggesting that a PHF-like antigen occurs in normal brain.

Our absorption studies suggest the existence of a PHF-like antigen in normal aged brain, possibly present in the MAP fraction. The significance of the labeling with anti-tau is a puzzling question. Qualitative and quantitative variations in tau proteins related to the maturation of the microtubule system are known to occur in rat during brain development (Mareck et al. 1980). The possibility that such variations might occur in aging human brain deserves attention and might account for our immunohistochemical results. In any case, these immunohistochemical results emphasize the relation of NFT to the neuronal cytoskeleton.

It has recently been proposed that all the degenerating neurites constituting SP are cholinergic axons of the nucleus basalis of Meynert and the septum (Struble et al. 1982). This would be reflected by the positive histochemical detection of ACE in "primitive" SP, whereas "end-stage" SP with an amyloid core fail to be detected by this method. ACE staining of some SP in the hippocampus has also been described previously by Perry et al. (1980). At the level of the hippocampus, we have confirmed that some SP are detected by the histochemical reaction, although predominantly in certain areas such as the molecular layer of the gyrus dentatus. In other areas (subiculum), SP without an amyloid core were not often detected by ACE staining. This might suggest that the neuritic constituents of SP do not all originate exclusively in basal brain areas. Using the Golgi method, Probst et al. (1983) have observed that local neurons of the hippocampus might participate in the formation of SP.

In conclusion, our results indicate that the abnormal filaments wich constitute the most distinctive lesion in SDAT exhibit unique morphological features which differentiate them from normal constituents of the cytoskeleton. To understand better their biochemical nature and etiopatholoy, more studies are needed.

Acknowledgement. We are grateful to A. M. Couck for expert technical assistance, J. L. Conreur for photographic work, and J. De Ligne for typing the manuscript.

References

Anderton BH, Breinburg D, Downes MJ, Green PJ, Tomlinson BE, Ulrich J, Wood JN, Kahn J (1982) Monoclonal antibodies show that neurofibrillary tangles and neurofilaments share antigenic determinants. Nature 298:84–86

Brion JP, Couck AM, Flament-Durand J (1984) Ultrastructural study of enriched fractions of "tangles" from human patients with senile dementia of the Alzheimer type. Acta Neuropathol 64:148–152

Brion JP, Couck AM, Passeirero E, Flament-Durand J (1985) Neurofibrillary tangles in Alzheimer's disease: an immunohistochemical study. J Submicrosc Cytol 17:89–96

Chiu FC, Norton WT (1982) Bulk preparation of CNS cytoskeleton and the separation of individual neurofilament protein by gel filtration: dye-binding characteristics and amino acid compositions. J Neurochem 39:1252–1260

Cleveland DW, Hwo SH, Kirschner MW (1977) Purification of tau, a microtubule-associated protein that induces assembly of microtubules from purified tubulin. J Mol Biol 116:207–225

Das GD, Hallas BH, Das KG (1979) Transplantation of neural tissues in the brains of laboratory mammals: technical details and comments. Experientia 35:143–153

Davies P, Maloney AJ (1976) Selective loss of central cholinergic neurons in Alzheimer's disease. Lancet II:1403

De Mey J, Moeremans M, Geuens G, Nuydens R, De Brabander M (1981) High-resolution light and electron-microscopic localization of tubulin with the IGS (immunogold staining) method. Cell Biol Int Rep 5:889–899

Dustin P, Flament-Durand J (1982) Disturbances of axoplasmic transport in Alzheimer's disease. In: Weis DG, Gorio A (eds) Axoplasmic transport in physiology and pathology. Springer, Berlin Heidelberg New York, pp 131–136

Fellous A, Francon J, Lennon AM, Nunez J (1977) Microtubule assembly in vitro. Purification of assembly-promoting factors. Eur J Biochem 78:167–174

Flament-Durand J, Couck AM (1978) Ultrastructural observations in brain biopsies of Alzheimer's dementia. VIIIth International congress of neuropathology, Washington. J Neuropathol Exp Neurol 37:613

Flament-Durand J, Couck AM (1979) Spongiform alterations in brain biopsies of presenile dementia. Acta Neuropathol 46:159–162

Flament-Durand J, Couck AM, Brion JP (1983) New morphological data observed in human brains with senile dementia of the Alzheimer type (SDAT). In: Knook DL, Calder G, Amaducci L (eds) Aging of the brain and senile dementia: the inventory of EEC potentialities. Eurage Meeting, San Miniato, pp 65–70

Gambetti P, Autilio-Gambetti L, Perry G, Shecket G, Crane RC (1983) Antibodies to neurofibrillary tangles of Alzheimer's disease raised from human and animal neurofilament fractions. Lab Invest 49:430–435

Gibbs CJ, Gajduzek DC (1978) Subacute spongiform virus encephalopathies: the transmissible virus dementia. In: Katzman R, Terry RD, Prick KL (eds) Alzheimer's disease dementia and related disorders. Raven, New York, pp 559–577

Grundke-Iqbal I, Johnson AB, Wisniewski HM, Terry RD, Iqbal K (1979) Evidence that Alzheimer neurofibrillary tangles originate from neurotubules. Lancet I:578–580

Grundke-Iqbal I, Iqbal K, Tung YC, Wisniewski HM (1984) Alzheimer paired helical filaments: immunochemical identification of polypeptides. Acta Neuropathol 62:167–177

Ihara Y, Abraham C, Selkoe DJ (1983) Antibodies to paired helical filaments in Alzheimer's disease do not recognise normal brain proteins. Nature 304:727–730

Iqbal K, Zaidi T, Thompson CH, Merz PA, Wisniewski HM (1984) Alzheimer paired helical filaments: bulk isolation, solubility, and protein composition. Acta Neuropathol (62):167–177

Kidd M (1963) Paired helical filaments in electron microscopy of Alzheimer's disease. Nature (Lond) 197:192–193

Mareck A, Fellous A, Francon J, Nunez J (1980) Changes in composition and activity of microtubule-associated proteins during brain development. Nature 284:353–355

Perry RH, Blessed G, Perry EK, Tomlinson BE (1980) Histochemical observations on cholinesterase activities in the brains of elderly normal and demented (Alzheimer-type) patients. Age Ageing 9:9–16

Probst A, Basler V, Bron B, Ulrich J (1983) Neuritic plaques in senile dementia of Alzheimer type: a Golgi study in the hippocampal region. Brain Res 268:249–254

Rasool C, Anderton B, Kahn J, Ihara Y, Selkoe D (1983) Differential reaction of Alzheimer neurofibrillary tangles with antineurofilament and anti-PHF antibodies. J Neuropathol Exp Neurol 42:335

Rossor MN, Svendsen C, Hunt SP, Mountjoy CQ, Roth M, Iversen LL (1982) The substantia innominata in Alzheimer's disease: an histochemical and biochemical study of cholinergic marker enzymes. Neurosci Lett 28:217–222

Selkoe DJ, Ihara Y, Salazar FJ (1982) Alzheimer's disease: insolubility of partially purified paired helical filaments in sodium dodecyl sulfate and urea. Science 215:1243–1245

Shelanski ML, Gaskin F, Cantor CR (1973) Microtubule assembly in the absence of added nucleotides. Proc Natl Acad Sci USA 70:765–768

Sternberger LA (1979) Immunocytochemistry. Wiley, New York

Struble RG, Cork RC, Whitehouse PJ, Price DL (1982) Cholinergic innervation in neuritic plaques. Science 216:413–415

Terry RD (1963) The fine structure of neurofibrillary tangles in Alzheimer's disease. J Neuropathol Exp Neurol 22:629–642

Tsuji S (1974) On the chemical basis of thiocholine methods for demonstration of acetylcholinesterase activities. Histochemistry 42:99–110

van den Bosch de Aguilar P, Langhendries-Weverberg C, Goemare-Vanneste J, Flament-Durand J, Brion JP, Couck AM (1984) Transplantation of human cortex with Alzheimer's disease into rat occipital cortex: a model for the study of Alzheimer's disease. Experientia 40:402–403

Yen SH, Gaskin F, Terry RD (1981) Immunocytochemical studies of neurofibrillary tangles. Am J Pathol 104:77–89

Neurotransmitter Receptor Alterations in Alzheimer's Disease*

P. J. WHITEHOUSE[1] and K.-S. AU[2]

Introduction

Alzheimer's disease (AD) is a neurodegenerative disorder characterized neuropathologically by senile plaques and neurofibrillary tangles occurring in association with dysfunction and eventual death of several specific neuronal populations. In brainstem and diencephalon, the neurotransmitter specificity of some affected populations of neurons is known. For example, the medial septum, nucleus of the diagonal band of Broca, and nucleus basalis of Meynert are components of the basal forebrain cholinergic system (Hedreen et al. 1984; Mesulam et al. 1984). In AD, dysfunction in this system (Whitehouse et al. 1981, 1982; Price et al. 1983) is the probable substrate for the loss of presynaptic cholinergic markers in the telencephalon (Bowen et al. 1976; Davies and Maloney 1976b). This cholinergic deficit has been linked to the severity of clinically apparent dementia and to the magnitude of neuropathologic changes (Blessed et al. 1968). In the brainstem, neuronal dysfunction occurs in the noradrenergic locus ceruleus and serotonergic raphe nuclei (Forno 1978; Bondareff et al. 1982; Curcio and Kemper 1984). Loss of neurons also occurs in the amygdala, hippocampus, and neocortex, although the neurotransmitter specificity of these affected populations of neurons is less clear (Colon 1973; Terry et al. 1981; Ball 1977; Herzog and Kemper 1980; Hooper and Vogel 1976). Reductions in cortical somatostatin and gamma-aminobutyric acid (GABA) levels can probably be linked to dysfunction in populations of interneurons (Perry et al. 1977a; Davies et al. 1980; Rossor et al. 1980).

A component of the neurotransmitter circuit which has not been extensively studied in AD is the neurotransmitter receptor. Since receptors are markers for specific neuronal populations, i.e., only certain neurons maintain certain receptors, dysfunction in specific neural systems should lead to specific receptor changes. The maintenance of receptors on membranes may be disrupted early in the disease (prior to the actual death of neurons), and, thus, may serve as a sign of initial pathophysiologic events. In addition, neurotransmitter receptors are a specific kind of neural marker in that they indicate synaptic connectivity. That is, receptors found on the surface of neurons reflect the neurotransmitter specificity of the input to that cell. In some disorders, the receptor itself appears to be

* This work was supported by grants from the U.S. Public Health Service (NIH AG 03359, NS 20471, and AG 05146) as well as Fellowships from the McKnight Foundations, the Commonwealth Fund, and the Sloan Foundation

1 Neuropathology Laboratory, Departments of Neurology and Neuroscience
2 Division of Geriatrics, Department of Medicine, The Johns Hopkins University School of Medicine Baltimore, Maryland, USA

Senile Dementia of the Alzheimer Type
Ed. by J. Traber and W. H. Gispen

the target of the disease process. In myasthenia gravis, for example, an autoimmune attack on the nicotinic cholinergic receptor can be linked to muscle weakness (Drachman 1983). Finally, many neuroactive drugs act by modifying receptors; a better understanding of receptor changes in disease may lead to improvements in therapy.

In this paper, we review alterations in neurotransmitter and related receptors reported for AD, focusing on cholinergic, noradrenergic, serotonergic, and GABAergic systems. We will conclude by discussing several new approaches to studying receptors which may be helpful in elucidating the role of receptors in the pathophysiology of AD.

Alterations in Neurotransmitter and Related Receptors

Cholinergic Receptors

In contrast to the general agreement that presynaptic cholinergic markers, such as the activity of choline acetyltransferase (ChAT), are markedly reduced in the amygdala, hippocampus and neocortex of patients with AD (Bowen et al. 1976; Davies and Maloney 1976a), the pattern of changes in cholinergic receptors is unclear. Using the drug ligands [^{3}H]quinuclidinyl benzilate (QNB) (Davies and Verth 1978), [^{3}H]*N*-methyl scopolamine (Perry et al. 1977b), and [^{3}H]atropine (White et al. 1977), early studies showed no significant alterations in muscarinic receptor density in the frontal, parietal, and temporal cortices, hippocampus, dentate nucleus, caudate nucleus, putamen, and substantia nigra of AD patients when compared with controls. Recently, however, Rinne et al. (1984), using [^{3}H]QNB, showed a significant reduction of muscarinic receptors in the amygdala, nucleus accumbens, and hippocampus in brains of patients with AD. Scatchard's analysis of hippocampal samples revealed that the decrease in [^{3}H]QNB binding is due to a decrease in the number of receptors rather than to a change in affinity of the receptor for the drug ligand. Reduction in hippocampal [^{3}H]QNB binding was also found by Reisine et al. (1978).

Mash and Potter (1983) have recently claimed that densities of muscarinic receptors are decreased in the cortices of patients with AD. They report, however, that loss is limited to the M-2 receptor, a subtype of the muscarinic receptor characterized by high affinity for muscarinic agonists (such as carbachol) and low affinity for certain antagonists (notably pirenzepine) (Hammer et al. 1980). In animals, the same authors showed that lesions of basal forebrain cholinergic neurons produce a similar decrease in cortical M-2 receptor density and concluded that the M-2 receptor represents a presynaptic receptor (Mash and Potter 1983). However, the finding of altered M-2 receptors in AD was not confirmed in a study by Caulfield et al. (1982).

In some neurodegenerative disorders, neuronal loss is associated with an upregulation of neurotransmitter receptors on postsynaptic sites due to a compensatory denervation supersensitivity (Whitehouse et al., to be published a). In AD, London and Waller (to be published) have reported finding increased QNB binding in several regions of the cortex. In addition, a negative correlation between ChAT activity and muscarinic receptor densities has been taken as evidence for receptor upregulation in the face of presynaptic dysfunction (Nordberg et al. 1983).

Although muscarinic cholinergic receptors are the predominant cholinergic receptor type in the central nervous system, some central cholinergic receptors have nicotinic pharmacologic and physiologic characteristics (Morley et al. 1979). Davies and Feisullin (1981) demonstrated a reduced density of ^{125}I-labeled alpha-bungarotoxin binding sites in the temporal cortices of patients with AD, although this finding was not confirmed in another study (Lang and Henke 1983). It is not clear, however, whether ^{125}I-labeled alpha-bungarotoxin represents an appropriate ligand for nicotinic cholinergic receptor sites in the central nervous system (Morley et al. 1979).

Monoamine Receptors

Subtypes of both serotonin and noradrenergic receptors have been studied in the brains of patients with AD. Alterations in these receptors bear an unclear relationship to dysfunction of neurons in the raphe nucleus and locus ceruleus. Serotonin receptors in the central nervous system have been classified into several types: S-1 receptors have a high affinity for serotonin; S-2 receptors have a lower affinity for serotonin, but a higher affinity for the dopamine antagonist spiperone. Lysergic acid diethylamide (LSD) binds to both receptor types. Bowen et al. (1983 a) demonstrated a significant reduction in [^{3}H]LSD binding in temporal cortices and in [^{3}H]serotonin binding in the frontal cortices of patients with AD. Cross et al. (1984a), using [^{3}H]LSD binding displaced by serotonin and spiperone, found a marked reduction of both S-1 and S-2 receptors in the frontal and temporal cortices and hippocampus. In a more recent study using [^{3}H]serotonin and [^{3}H]ketanserin, Cross et al. (1984b) reported a reduction of S-1 receptors in the amygdala, hippocampus, and temporal cortex and a more extensive reduction of S-2 receptors in the frontal, temporal, and cingulate cortices and the amygdala. In this study, a greater reduction of [^{3}H]serotonin binding was found in AD patients with a younger age of onset, consistent with other studies which reported more extensive dysfunction in monoaminergic cell groups in younger patients (Bondareff et al. 1982).

To date, the few postmortem studies of noradrenergic receptor densities in brains of patients with AD have not shown any significant alterations as compared with controls. Bowen et al. (1983b), measuring [^{3}H]dihydroalprenol (DHA) binding, found no significant changes in beta-adrenergic receptors in frontal and temporal cortices. In another study, Cross et al. (1984a), measuring [^{3}H]WB4101, [^{3}H]Rauwolscine, and [^{3}H]DHA binding, found no changes in alpha$_1$-, alpha$_2$-, and beta-receptor densities respectively in the hippocampus and the occipital cortex.

GABA-Related Receptors

In some studies, presynaptic markers for GABAergic neurons, such as the activity of glutamic acid decarboxylase, have been found to be reduced in patients with AD (Bowen et al. 1974; Perry et al. 1977a). Using [^{3}H]GABA, Reisine et al. (1978) reported a marked reduction in GABA receptors in the caudate nucleus and frontal cortex, but no significant difference in the putamen and hippocampus in AD patients. In two other studies, however, [^{3}H]muscimol binding was found to be unaltered in the temporal and occipital cortices (Bowen et al. 1979, 1983b). Muscimol is a GABA agonist which binds to a subpopulation of high-affinity GABA receptors. Benzodiazepine binding sites have been linked to GABA receptors (Unnerstall et al. 1981). Recently, Owen et al. (1983) reported a small but significant reduction in [^{3}H]flunitrazepam binding in the temporal cortices of patients with AD.

Other Receptors

Dopaminergic receptor density measured by [^{3}H]spiroperidol was found to be reduced in the caudate nucleus in AD patients, but unaltered in the frontal cortex, hippocampus, and putamen (Reisine et al. 1978). Opiate receptor densities, using [^{3}H]naloxone, were also found to be unchanged in the temporal lobes of patients with AD (Bowen et al. 1979).

New Approaches to the Study of Receptors in Disease

Although studies of neurotransmitter receptors in brain homogenates have contributed to our understanding of the neurotransmitter-specific pathology of AD, certain problems in the interpretation of these studies need to be addressed. Several new approaches to the study of receptors in disease which may assist in resolving these difficulties are discussed here.

Although consistent alterations in serotonin receptors have been reported by several groups, the nature and extent of other receptor changes are less clear. Studies of cholinergic receptors, in which increases and decreases in density or a lack of density change for several subtypes have been reported, are particularly inconsistent. Differences in methods of tissue dissection and receptor assays may explain some of these discrepancies. Another source of variance in these studies may relate to the characteristics of the patients studied. Age at death, duration of disease, drug history, severity and pattern of cognitive impairment, agonal status, cause of death, and postmortem delay in processing tissues may all affect receptor assays (Whitehouse et al. 1984b). Recently, another potential reason for discrepancies between studies, the existence of subtypes of AD, has received attention. For example, presynaptic cholinergic and somatostatinergic deficits appear to be less severe in patients who experience the onset of the disease at a later age (so-called senile dementia of the Alzheimer type) than in those individuals with disease onset at an earlier age (so-called presenile AD). Moreover, subtypes of AD may be definable on neuropathologic as well as clinical grounds. For example, although alterations in cholinergic neurons appear to be a consistent feature of the disease, neuronal loss in the locus ceruleus and raphe may be more variable. Bondareff et al. (1982) suggested that two subtypes of AD may be defined based on the magnitude of neuronal loss in the locus ceruleus.

Current studies of receptor alterations in AD are also limited by our inability to interpret the functional significance of receptor alterations. Not all pharmacologically defined binding sites necessarily represent physiologically active receptor complexes. Thus, some binding site alterations in disease are not easily interpretable in terms of known cellular alterations in disease. In addition, until we can more accurately define the pharmacologic characteristics of pre- and postsynaptic receptors and differentiate them, our interpretations of the anatomy of receptor changes will be limited.

Most studies of receptor change in AD have used tissue homogenates, so that only limited correlations with neuropathologic features of the disease can be made. In vitro receptor autoradiography (ARG) allows mapping of neurotransmitters with a high degree of anatomic resolution (Kuhar 1985; Whitehouse, to be published). The pharmacologic principles of receptor ARG are identical to homogenate drug-binding assays, although ARG is applied to frozen tissue thaw-mounted to glass slides rather than tissue homogenates. ^{3}H- or ^{125}I-labeled drug ligands can then be incubated with these tissue sections, and the pattern of binding to the tissue can be determined. Preincubation, incubation and wash times, temperatures, and buffers are chosen to maximize specific binding and to minimize the effect of endogenous ligands. After incubation and washings, the tissue is dried as rapidly as possible to prevent diffusion of the ligand from the binding site. The autoradiogram is produced by juxtaposing this labeled tissue to a piece of [^{3}H]-sensitive film or emulsion-covered coverslip. Development of the emulsion results in an image of distribution of radioactivity in the tissue.

The higher anatomical resolution of ARG allowed one group of authors to claim that the distribution of muscarinic cholinergic receptors in the cortices of some patients with AD was altered (Lang and Henke 1983). Another ARG study failed to find these receptor changes in the hippocampus and, in addition, reported no changes in the frontal, cingulate, and temporal cortices (Palacios 1982). Furthermore, these two ARG studies provided evidence that senile plaques contain muscarinic cholinergic receptors.

We have used receptor ARG to map neurotransmitters in the nucleus basalis of Meynert (Whitehouse et al. 1984a). Homogenate studies of this region are difficult because of its small size and extensive distribution in the basal forebrain. We have found relatively high concentrations of cholinergic receptors, reflecting the cholinergic nature of these neurons, and of GABA-related receptors probably associated with an inhibitory GABAergic afferent pathway. In addition, we have used ARG to map muscarinic receptors in telencephalic distribution areas of the basal forebrain cholinergic system (Whitehouse et al., to be published b). For example, we mapped the distribution of subtypes of muscarinic cholinergic receptors in the amygdala and found that the greatest reduction in receptor density occurred in the basolateral nucleus, which receives a dense innervation from the basal forebrain cholinergic system. Moreover, the high-affinity agonist subtype of muscarinic receptor was preferentially affected. As mentioned previously, this high-affinity agonist subtype has been claimed by others to be the presynaptic cholinergic receptor (Mash and Potter 1983). One might expect that the presynaptic receptor would be preferentially lost in areas to which this system projects.

The interpretation of receptor alterations in human disease can also be facilitated by studying animal models. Lesion experiments can be used to examine whether receptor alterations, which accompany acute lesions, parallel those found in a disease process which affects the same population of neurons. However, receptor changes seen in acute lesions often follow a time course different from that produced by the gradual cell death which occurs in disease. Using natural animal models of human degenerative disorders, it is possible to follow the evolution of receptor changes in a slowly progressive disease, since animal tissue can be examined at different points in the disease process (Troncoso et al. 1984). Recently, it has become possible to measure neurotransmitter receptors in living human subjects using positron emission tomography (Wagner et al. 1983). This technique will allow serial studies of receptor alterations in human disease and will improve our ability to correlate receptor alterations with clinical features of the disorder.

In summary, several new approaches to measuring neurotransmitter receptors in human disease offer the hope that we can better define the anatomy of receptor alterations in AD and link these alterations more closely to the clinical and neuropathologic features of this disorder.

Acknowledgements. The authors thank M. J. Kuhar and D. L. Price for helpful discussions, C. Marine and C. Jordon for excellent secretarial assistance, and B. Jones and T. Kopajtic for technical assistance.

Note Added in Proof. Recently, reduction of density of several other neurotransmitter receptors has been reported in cortex in AD, including receptors for glutamate (Greenamyre et al. 1985) and somatostatin (Beal et al. 1985). In addition, we have used a new approach to measure nicotinic cholinergic receptors (using [^{3}H] acetylcholine and [^{3}H] nicotine) and found a consistent reduction in nicotinic receptors in four areas of cortex in AD (Whitehouse et al. 1985).

References

Ball MJ (1977) Neuronal loss, neurofibrillary tangles and granulovacuolar degeneration in the hippocampus with ageing and dementia. A qualitative study. Acta Neuropathol (Berl) 37:111–118

Beal MF, Mazurek MF, Tran VT, Chattha G, Bird ED, Martin JB (1985) Reduced numbers of somatostatin receptors in the cerebral cortex in Alzheimer's disease. Science 229:289–291

Blessed G, Tomlinson BE, Roth M (1968) The association between quantitative measures of dementia and of senile change in the cerebral grey matter of elderly subjects. Br J Psychiatry 114:797–811

Bondareff W, Mountjoy CQ, Roth M (1982) Loss of neurons or origin of the adrenergic projection to cerebral cortex (nucleus locus ceruleus) in senile dementia. Neurology (NY) 32:164–168

Bowen DM, Flack RHA, White P, Smith CB, Davison AN (1974) Brain decarboxylase activities as indices of pathological change in senile dementia. Lancet I:1247–1249

Bowen DM, Smith CB, White P, Davison AN (1976) Neurotransmitter-related enzymes and indices of hypoxia in senile dementia and other abiotrophies. Brain 99:459–496

Bowen DM, Spillane JA, Curzon G, Meier-Ruge W, White P, Goodhardt MJ, Iwangoff PO, Davison AN (1979) Accelerated ageing or selective neuronal loss as an important cause of dementia? Lancet I:11–14

Bowen DM, Allen SJ, Benton JS, Goodhardt MJ, Haan EA, Palmer AM, Sims NR, Smith CCT, Spillane JA, Esiri MM, Neary D, Snowdon JS, Wilcock GK, Davison AN (1983a) Biochemical assessment of serotonergic and cholinergic dysfunction and cerebral atrophy in Alzheimer's disease. J Neurochem 41:266–272

Bowen DM, Davison AN, Sims NR (1983b) The cholinergic system in the ageing brain and dementia. In: Samuel D, Algeri S, Gershon S, Grimm VE, Toffano G (eds) Aging of the brain. Raven, New York, pp 183–190 (Aging, vol 22)

Caulfield MP, Straughan DW, Cross AJ, Crow T, Birdsall NIM (1982) Cortical muscarinic receptor subtypes and Alzheimer's Disease. Lancet 2:1277

Colon EJ (1973) The cerebral cortex in presenil dementia. A quantitative analysis. Acta Neuropathol (Berl) 23:281–290

Cross AJ, Crow TJ, Johnson JA, Perry EK, Perry RH, Blessed G, Tomlinson BE (1984a) Studies on neurotransmitter receptor systems in neocortex and hippocampus in senile dementia of the Alzheimer-type. J Neurol Sci 64:109–117

Cross AJ, Crow TJ, Ferrier IN, Johnson JA, Bloom SR, Corsellis JAN (1984b) Serotonin receptor changes in dementia of the Alzheimer type. J Neurochem 43:1574–1581

Curcio CA, Kemper T (1984) Nucleus raphe dorsalis in dementia of the Alzheimer type: neurofibrillary changes and neuronal packing density. J Neuropathol Exp Neurol 43:359–368

Davies P, Feisullin S (1981) Postmortem stability of alpha-bungarotoxin binding sites in mouse and human brain. Brain Res 216:449–454

Davies P, Maloney AJF (1976a) Selective loss of central cholinergic neurons in Alzheimer's disease. Lancet 2:1403

Davies P, Maloney AJF (1976b) Selective loss of central cholinergic neurons in Alzheimer senile dementia. Nature 288:279–280

Davies P, Verth AH (1978) Regional distribution of muscarinic acetylcholine receptor in normal and Alzheimer's-type dementia brains. Brain Res 138:385–392

Davies P, Katzman R, Terry RD (1980) Reduced somatostatin-like immunoreactivity in cerebral cortex from cases of Alzheimer disease and Alzheimer senile dementia. Nature 288:279–280

Drachman DB (1983) Myasthenia gravis: immunobiology of a receptor disorder. Trends Neurosci 6:446–451

Forno LS (1978) The locus caeruleus in Alzheimer's disease. J Neuropathol Exp Neurol 37:614

Greenamyre JT, Penney JB, Young AB, D'Amato CJ, Hicks SP, Shoulson I (1985) Alterations in L-glutamate binding in Alzheimer's and Huntington's diseases. Science 227:1496–1499

Hammer R, Berrie CP, Birdsall NJM, Burgen ASV, Hulme EC (1980) Pirenzepine distinguishes between different subclasses of muscarinic receptors. Nature 283:90–92

Hedreen JC, Struble RG, Whitehouse PJ, Price DL (1984) Topography of the magnocellular basal forebrain system in human brain. J Neuropathol Exp Neurol 43:1–21

Herzog AG, Kemper TL (1980) Amygdaloid changes in aging and dementia. Arch Neurol 37:625–629

Hooper MW, Vogel FS (1976) The limbic system in Alzheimer's disease. A neuropathologic investigation. Am J Pathol 85:1–20

Kuhar MJ (1985) Receptor localization with the microscope. In: Yamamura HI, Enna SJ, Kuhar MJ (eds) Neurotransmitter receptor binding, 2nd edn. Raven, New York, pp 153–176

Lang W, Henke H (1983) Cholinergic receptor binding and autoradiography in brains of non-neurological and senile dementia of Alzheimer-type patients. Brain Res 267:271–280

London ED, Waller SB (to be published) Relations between choline acetyltransferase and muscarinic binding in aging and Alzheimer's disease. In: Hanin I (ed) Dynamics of cholinergic function. Plenum, New York

Mash DS, Potter LT (1983) Changes in M1 and M2 muscarine receptors in Alzheimer's disease and aging, and with lesions of cholinergic neurons in animals. Soc Neurosci Abstr 9:582

Mesulam M-M, Mufson EJ, Levey AI, Wainer BH (1984) Atlas of cholinergic neurons in the forebrain and upper brainstem of the macaque based on monoclonal choline acetyltransferase immunohistochemistry and acetylcholinesterase histochemistry. Neuroscience 12:669–686

Morley BJ, Kemp GE, Salvaterra P (1979) Alpha-bungarotoxin binding sites in the CNS. Life Sci 24:859–872

Nordberg A, Larsson C. Adolfsson R, Alafuzoff I, Winblad B (1983) Muscarinic receptor compensation in hippocampus of Alzheimer patients. J Neural Transm 56:13–19

Owen F, Poulter M, Waddington JL, Mashal RD, Crow TJ (1983) ^{3}H-RO5-4864 and ^{3}H-flunitrazepam binding in kainate-lesioned rat striatum and in temporal cortex of brains from patients with senile dementia of the Alzheimer type. Brain Res 278:373–375

Palacios JM (1982) Autoradiographic localization of muscarinic cholinergic reeptors in the hippocampus of patients with senile dementia. Brain Res 243:173–175

Perry EK, Gibson PH, Blessed G, Perry RH, Tomlinson BE (1977a) Neurotransmitter enzyme abnormalities in senile dementia. J Neurol Sci 34:247–265

Perry EK, Perry RH, Blessed G, Tomlinson BE (1977b) Necropsy evidence of central cholinergic deficits in senile dementia. Lancet 1:189

Price DL, Whitehouse PJ, Struble RG, Price DL Jr, Cork LC, Hedreen JC, Kitt CA (1983) Basal forebrain cholinergic neurons and neuritic plaques in primate brain. Biological aspects of Alzheimer's disease. Banbury Rep 15:65–77

Reisine TD, Yamamura HI, Bird ED, Spokes E, Enna SJ (1978) Pre- and postsynaptic neurochemical alterations in Alzheimer's disease. Brain Res 159:477–481

Rinne JO, Rinne JK, Laakso K, Paijarvi L, Rinne UK (1984) Reduction in muscarinic receptor binding in limbic areas of Alzheimer brain. J Neurol Neurosurg Psychiatry 47:651–653

Rossor MN, Emson PC, Mountjoy CQ, Roth M, Iversen LL (1980) Reduced amounts of immunoreactive somatostatin in the temporal cortex in senile dementia of Alzheimer type. Neurosci Lett 20:373–377

Terry RD, Peck A, DeTeresa R, Schechter R, Horoupian DS (1981) Some morphometric aspects of the brain in senile dementia of the Alzheimer type. Ann Neurol 10:184–192

Troncoso JC, Cork LC, Whitehouse PJ, Kuhar MJ, Price DL (1984) Canine inherited ataxia: neurotransmitter receptors in the cerebellum. Ann Neurol 16:135

Unnerstall JR, Kuhar MJ, Niehoff DL, Palacios JM (1981) Benzodiazepine receptors are coupled to a subpopulation of gamma-aminobutyric acid (GABA) receptors: evidence from a quantitative autoradiographic study. J Pharmacol Exp Ther 218:797–804

Wagner HN Jr, Burns HD, Dannals RF, Wong DF, Langstrom B, Duelfer T, Frost JJ, Ravert HT, Links JM, Rosenbloom SB, Lukas SE, Kramer AV, Kuhar MJ (1983) Imaging dopamine receptors in the human brain by positron tomography. Science 221:1264–1266

White P, Goodhardt MJ, Keet JP, Hiley CR, Carrasco LH, Williams IEI, Bowen DM (1977) Neocortical cholinergic neurons in elderly people. Lancet 1:668–670

Whitehouse PJ (to be published) Receptor autoradiography: applications in neuropathology. Trends Neurosci

Whitehouse PJ, Price DL, Clark AW, Coyle JT, DeLong MR (1981) Alzheimer disease: evidence for selective loss of cholinergic neurons in the nucleus basalis. Ann Neurol 10:122–126

Whitehouse PJ, Price DL, Struble RG, Clark AW, Coyle JT, DeLong MR (1982) Alzheimer's disease and senile dementia: loss of neurons in the basal forebrain. Science 215:1237–1239

Whitehouse PJ, Jones BE, Kopajtic TA, Price DL, Kuhar MJ (1984a) Receptors in the nucleus basalis of primates: an *in vitro* autoradiographic study. Ann Neurol 16:118

Whitehouse PJ, Lynch D, Kuhar MJ (1984b) Effects of postmortem delay and temperature on neurotransmitter receptor binding in a rat model of the human autopsy process. J Neurochem 43:553–559

Whitehouse PJ, Martino AM, Price DL, Kellar KJ (1985) Reductions in nicotinic but not muscarinic cholinergic receptors in Alzheimer's disease measured using [^{3}H]acetylcholine. Ann Neurol 18:145

Whitehouse PJ, Trifiletti RR, Jones BE, Folstein S, Price DL, Snyder SH, Kuhar MJ (to be published a) Neurotransmitter receptor alterations in Huntington's disease: autoradiographic and homogenate studies with special reference to benzodiazepine receptor complexes. Ann Neurol

Whitehouse PJ, Kopajtic T, Jones BE, Kuhar MJ, Price DL (to be published b) An *in vitro* receptor autoradiographic study of muscarinic cholinergic receptor subtypes in the amygdala and neocortex of patients with Alzheimer's disease. Meeting of the American Academy of Neurology, 1985

Co-Localization of Aluminium and Silicon in Senile Plaques: Implications for the Neurochemical Pathology of Alzheimer's Disease

J. M. CANDY[1], J. A. EDWARDSON[1], J. KLINOWSKI[3], A. E. OAKLEY[1], E. K. PERRY[2], and R. H. PERRY[1]

Introduction

The neuropsychiatric features of Alzheimer-type senile dementia (SDAT) are accompanied by a constellation of histopathological and biochemical abnormalities. At present, it is not known how the major structural changes associated with the disease such as senile plaques, neurofibrillary tangles (NFT) and granulovacuolar degeneration are related to the growing list of neurochemical deficits which have been reported in recent years. The latter include a reduction of neurotransmitters and related enzymes in the cholinergic, noradrenergic and serotoninergic pathways which project diffusely to the cortex from subcortical nuclei (for recent reviews, see Bowen et al. 1984; Bloxham et al. 1985; Hardy et al. 1985). Depletion of the cholinergic markers choline acetyltransferase (ChAT) and acetylcholinesterase (AChE) are amongst the earliest and most severe of the biochemical changes to occur, and loss of these enzymes correlates well with the degree of cognitive impairment (Perry and Perry 1980). In addition to abnormalities in extrinsic cortical systems, there is also evidence for biochemical changes in intrinsic neurones. Thus, the level of immunoreactive somatostatin is reduced, especially in the temporal cortex, (for review, see Rossor et al. 1984), and there is a significant loss of cortical serotonin receptors (Cross et al. 1984). In addition, an increase in ^{3}H-labelled glutamate binding in the caudate nucleus has been interpreted as the consequence of a loss of corticostriatal neurones which use this amino acid as a transmitter (see Davison et al., this volume).

This study reports high, focal concentrations of aluminium and silicon in the core of senile plaques isolated from SDAT and normal elderly brains. Co-localization of these elements in plaques provides a common feature with NFT-bearing neurones, where elevated intracellular concentrations of both aluminium and silicon have previously been reported. The possible relationships between these observations and the transmitter deficits found in SDAT are discussed.

1 MRC Neuroendocrinology Unit and
2 Department of Neuropathology, Newcastle General Hospital, Westgate Road, Newcastle upon Tyne NE4 6BE, UK
3 Department of Physical Chemistry, Lensfield Road, University of Cambridge, Cambridge CB2 1EP, UK

Senile Dementia of the Alzheimer Type
Ed. by J. Traber and W. H. Gispen

Composition of Core Material from Senile Plaques

Senile plaques and NFT comprise the two major histopathological features of SDAT. They are also present in the normal elderly brain, but at a much lower density (Tomlinson et al. 1968). Plaques are complex structures, consisting of abnormal neuronal processes and glial cells surrounding a central core of fibrillary material, which is generally assumed to consist of classic amyloid, i.e. polymeric protein fibrils in β-pleated sheet conformation (Glenner et al. 1974). Senile plaques are largely, although not entirely, restricted to the cortex (Tomlinson 1982), and their density has been shown to correlate with the degree of cognitive impairment in SDAT (Blessed et al. 1968). The chemical composition of the so-called amyloid core is of interest for several reasons. Histochemical staining for AChE suggests a contribution by cholinergic neurones to the neuritic processes which surround the core (Perry et al. 1980, 1983 a), although it is likely that other types of neurones are also involved. Amyloid in peripheral endocrine tissues is composed of polymeric aggregates of proteins which, in some cases, represent abnormal secretory products (Westermark et al. 1977). We have shown (Oakley et al. 1981; Perry et al. 1981) that a number of neuropeptides including substance P, cholecystokinin octapeptide (CCK-8) and somatostatin-14 are in vitro capable of forming polymeric aggregates which have ultrastructural dimensions and staining properties resembling amyloid (Fig. 1). Prusiner (1982, 1984) has suggested that some "amyloid" fibrils associated which plaques which occur in transmissible encephalopathies such as scrapie, Creutzfeldt-Jakob disease and kuru are composed of linear arrays of a protease-resistant, self-replicating protein, the so-called "prion." Whatever the true nature of plaque amyloid in SDAT, an outstanding feature of this material is its extreme resistance to extraction procedures which readily solubilize peripheral amyloid. We have recently (Candy et al. 1984, 1985) isolated core material from unfixed cortex of patients which SDAT using a procedure involving incubation of homogenates with a protease (subtilisin), overnight treatment witch 2% sodium dodecyl sulphate to solubilize proteins, further treatment with 4 *M* hydroxylamine to remove collagen and final purification on a sucrose gradient.

Core material isolated in this way has the staining reactions characteristic of plaque amyloid in situ, i.e. apple green birefringence with Congo red staining under polarized light, crystal violet metachromasia and silver staining with King's procedure. Individual cores appear under the scanning electron microscope as roughly spherical particles, some 8–20 μm in diameter (Fig. 2). After centrifugation onto an electron microscopic grid and negative staining, these cores show a fibrillary structure resembling that of plaque amyloid in situ with a subunit diameter of approximately 30 Å (Fig. 3). Isolated core material was found to have a remarkably low protein content (<5%), as measured by amino acid determination, fluorescamine assay and infrared analysis. Accordingly, elemental composition was studied using energy dispersive X-ray microanalysis (EDX) on intact isolated plaque cores and sections of Epon-embedded cores. EDX analysis showed aluminium and silicon to be co-localized within the centre of the core in amounts ranging from 4% to 19% and from 6% to 24% of the total core material respec-

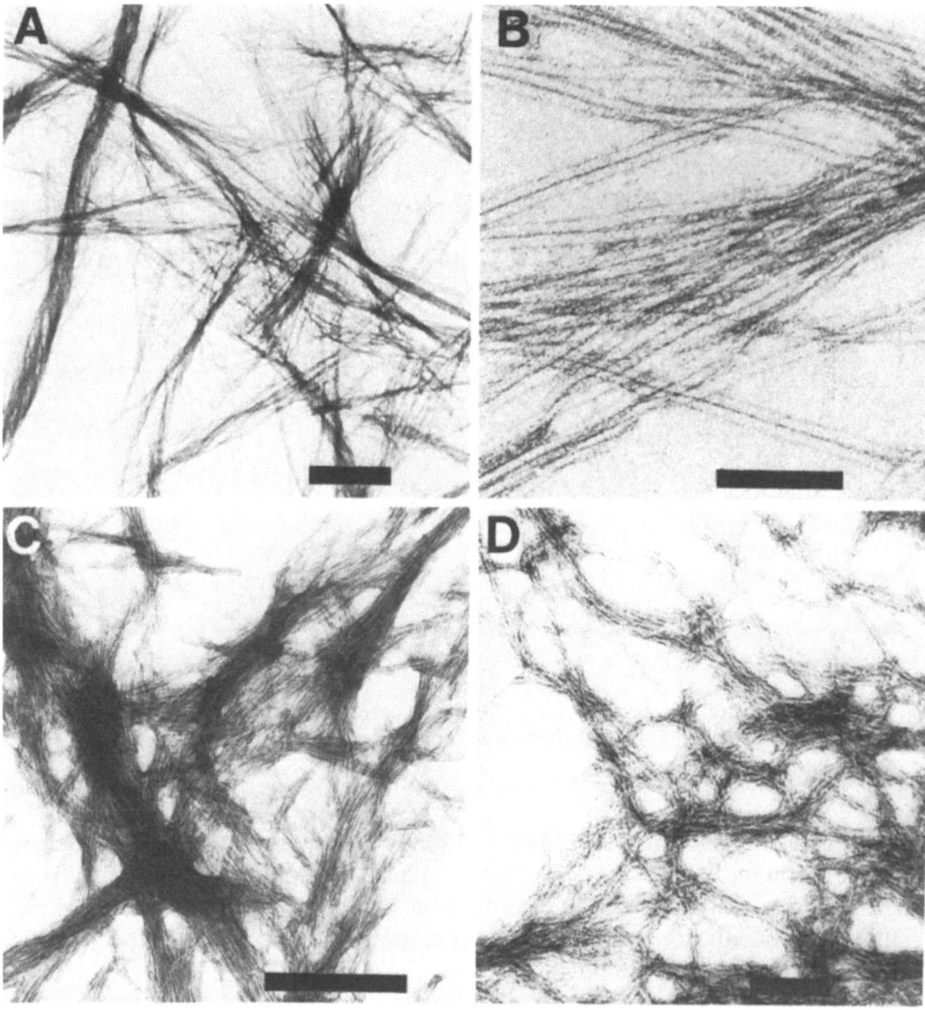

Fig. 1 A–D. Fibrillary polymeric forms of substance P, sulphated CCK-8 and the reduced form of somatostatin in 2% NaCl. For electron microscopic examination, 5 µl aliquots of the peptide solutions were centrifuged (160,000 g for 30 min) onto electron microscope grids coated with formvar and carbon, followed by negative staining with 1% uranyl acetate. **A** Low-power appearance of substance P fibrillary aggregates, *calibration bar* 1 µm. **B** High-magnification detail of **A** showing individual substance P fibrils, which have diameters ranging from 70–90 Å. The *calibration bar* represents 1,000 Å. **C** Fibrillary aggregates formed by sulphated CCK-8. The width of the CCK-8 fibrils is dependent on the number of laterally associated subunits (30–40 Å in diameter); *calibration bar* represents 0.5 µm. **D** Fibrillary polymeric aggregates produced by somatostatin after reduction of the disulphide bridge by dithiothreitol (10 m*M*, pH 8.0). The fibrils are 50–70 Å in diameter. The *calibration bar* is 1,000 Å

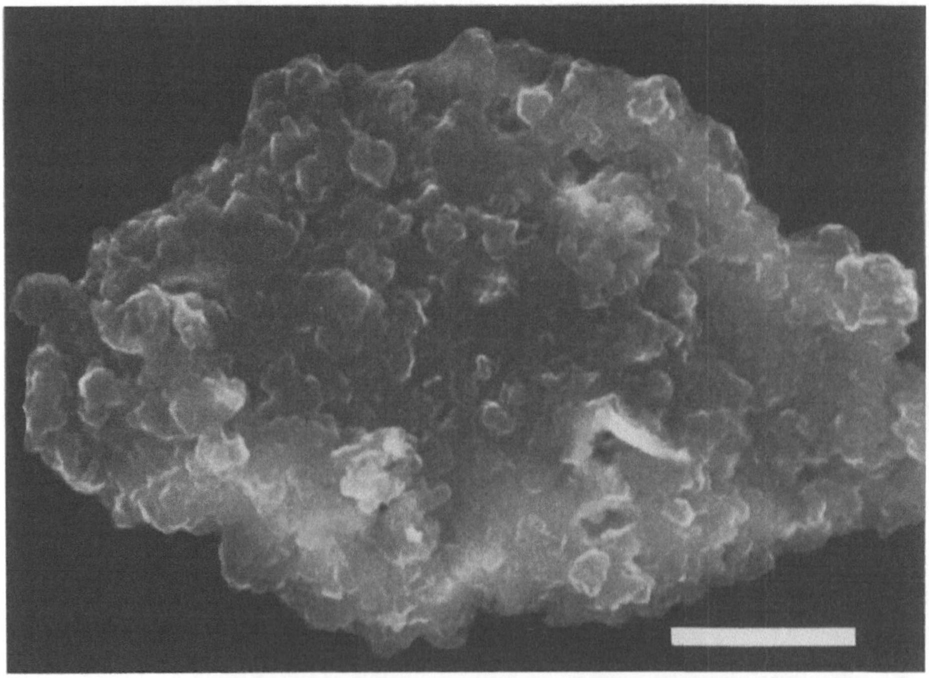

Fig. 2. Scanning electron micrograph of a senile plaque core isolated from the cerebral cortex of a patient with senile dementia of Alzheimer type. The *calibration bar* represents 5 μm

tively (Fig. 4). Further analysis of isolated plaque cores using solid-state nuclear magnetic resonance (NMR) of ^{27}Al with magic angle spinning gave a spectrum which indicates the presence of aluminium in two coordination states (tetrahedrally and octahedrally coordinated with respect to oxygen). The spectrum is typical of an amorphous aluminosilicate.

When cryostat sections of formalin-fixed frontal or temporal cortex from SDAT patients were stained using King's silver procedure, it was possible, using EDX analysis, to demonstrate co-localization of aluminium and silicon in situ in senile plaques that had prominent central cores. Material from five patients with senile dementia and two patients with presenile dementia which had been assessed clinically and pathologically were examined in this way. Over 75% of plaques with a central core showed a focal concentration of aluminium and silicion. It is likely that, in the remainder, either the core was located within the section, at a depth beyond X-ray penetration (about 10 μm) or that masking by the silver deposits produced in staining had occurred. Analyses were therefore carried out on unfixed, unstained frozen sections from two SDAT patients. Focal aluminium- and silicon-rich areas identical in size and distribution to plaque cores were observed (Fig. 5). Silver-stained sections from the frontal cortex of five intellectually normal, elderly cases were also analyzed by EDAX, and 25 out of 27 plaques with central cores were found to have high levels of aluminium and silicon co-localized in a manner identical to the cases of SDAT (Fig. 6).

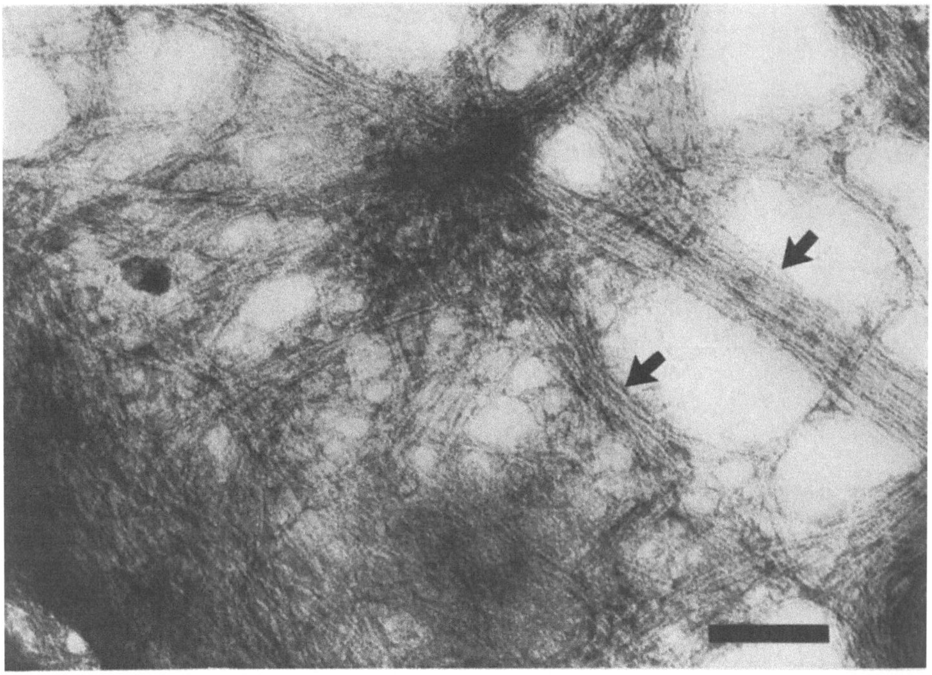

Fig. 3. Transmission electron micrograph of a senile plaque core isolated from the cerebral cortex in senile dementia of Alzheimer type. The isolated senile plaque cores were centrifuged (160,000 g for 30 min) onto an electron microscope grid coated with formvar and carbon, followed by negative staining with 1% uranyl acetate. Areas showing the fibrillary nature of the core at its periphery can be seen (↗); the fibrils had a subunit diameter of about 30 Å. The *calibration bar* represents 1,000 Å

The presence of aluminium in senile plaques was first claimed by Duckett and Galle (1976), but a later report by these workers (1980) implies that only a small proportion of plaques contain aluminium. Silicon has also previously been reported to be present in isolated core material and in the rims of senile plaques (Nikaido et al. 1972). Our finding of the co-localization of aluminium and silicon at the centre of the core and the presence of these elements as aluminosilicates has not previously been described.

The high content of aluminium and silicon and the relatively low protein content of plaque cores do not, at first, seem compatible with the fibrillary ultrastructure and staining properties observed with isolated plaque core material. Thus, it is of interest to note that some naturally occurring aluminosilicates exist in fibrillary form (Farmer et al. 1983). The aluminosilicate imogolite (Fig. 7) shows a structure resembling that of core material and exhibits apple green birefringence with Congo red staining under polarized light. Definitive identification of the exact species of aluminosilicate in plaques will require solid-state NMR of ^{29}Si on greater quantities of isolated core material. In addition, NMR of ^{13}C should yield information on the nature of other material present.

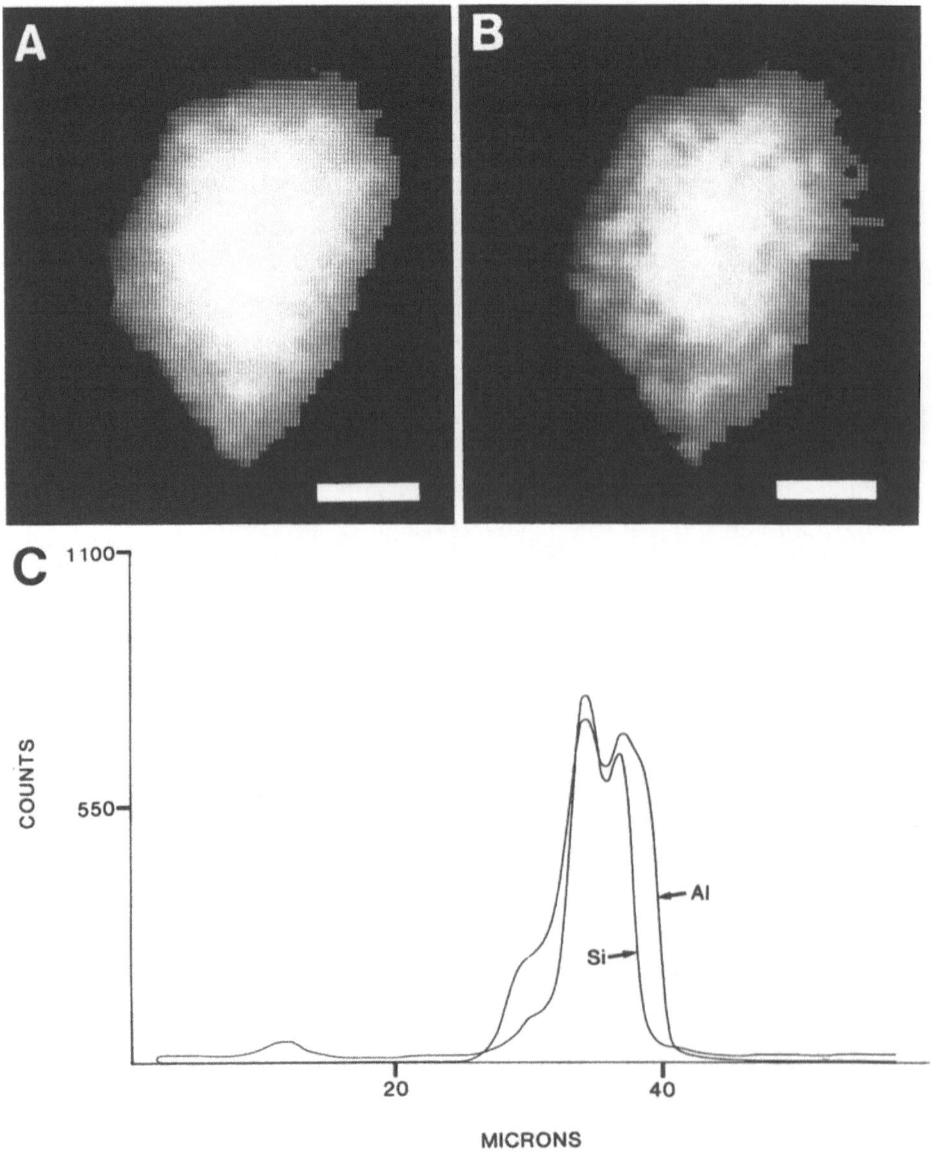

Fig. 4 A–C. Co-localization of silicon and aluminium in senile plaque cores isolated from the cerebral cortex of a case of senile dementia of the Alzheimer type and embedded in Epon. The distribution of **A** silicon and **B** aluminium in an Epon section (3–4 μm is shown). It can be seen that silicon and aluminium have a similar discrete localization in the central region of the plaque core. These maps of elemental distribution were produced using a scanning electron microscope and an energy-dispersive X-ray microanalytical system with digimap facilities. The maps represent the distribution of silicon and aluminium after background subtraction to eliminate the continuum effect (accelerating voltage was 25 keV with a dwell time per point of 50 ms. The *calibration bars* in **A** and **B** represent 2 μm. **C** Line scan (X-ray signal intensity plotted against distance) of the distribution of silicon and aluminium across an isolated senile plaque core. It can be seen that the distributions of silicon and aluminium in the plaque core are coincident (accelerating voltage 15 keV, dwell time per point 25 s

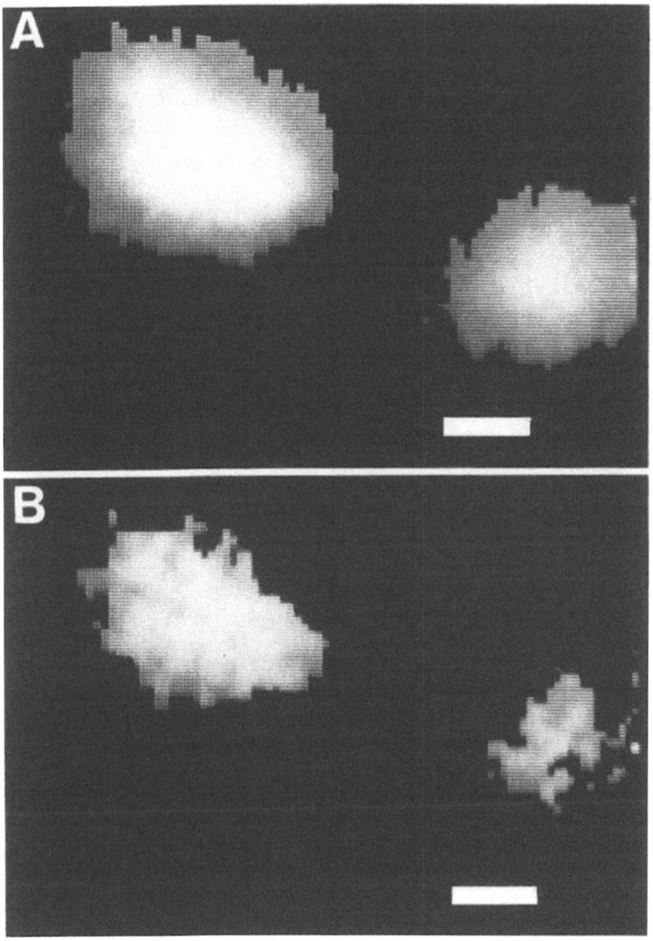

Fig. 5 A, B. Silicon and aluminium in presumed senile plaque cores in the cerebral cortex in senile dementia of Alzheimer type. Cryostat sections (20 μm) of unfixed frontal cortex were mounted on melinex (ICI) and carbon coated. Digimap distribution of **A** silicon and **B** aluminium in the same area of the section (accelerating voltage 25 keV, dwell time per point 150 ms). It can be seen that silicon and aluminium are co-localized in presumed senile plaque cores. The *calibration bars* represent 5 μm

Aluminium in the Brain in SDAT: Possible Aetiological Implications

Involvement of aluminium in the aetiology of senile dementia was first proposed following reports that the brain content of this element is significantly elevated in SDAT (Crapper et al. 1973, 1976). While these results have been disputed (McDermott et al. 1979), there is general agreement that brain levels of aluminium are increased in old age. Even if total amounts of brain aluminium do not increase in SDAT, it is clear that the pattern of distribution is altered and that aluminium is associated with prominent neuropathological features of this dis-

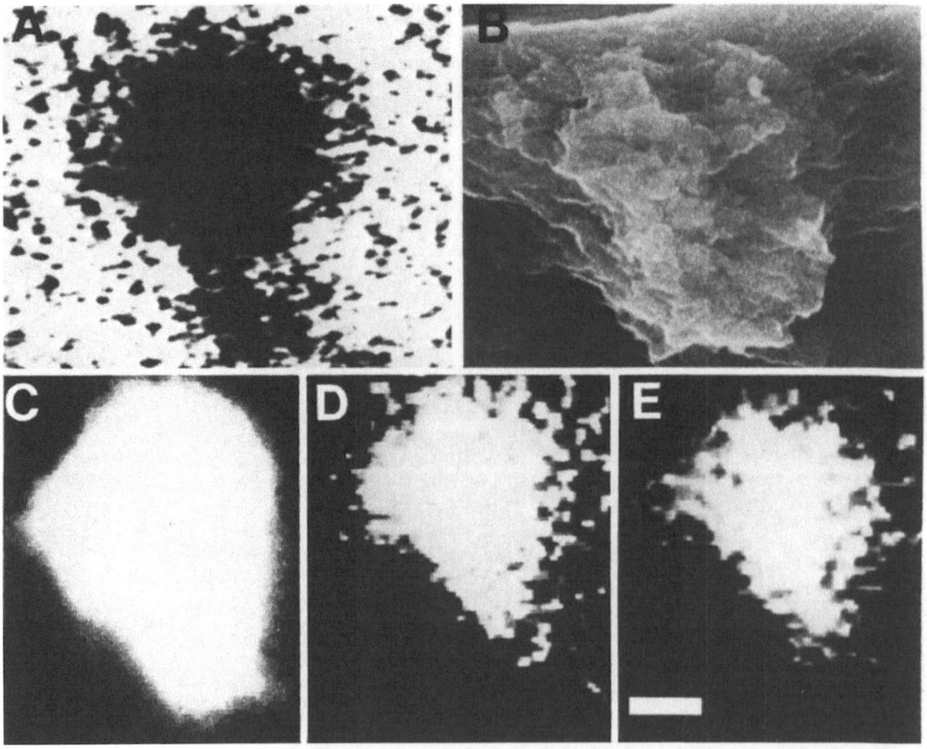

Fig. 6 A–E. Aluminium and silicon in senile plaques from the cerebral cortex of an elderly nondemented patient. Cryostat sections (20 μm) of formalin fixed were silver-stained and mounted on melinex (ICI). **A** Senile plaque with a silver-stained core visualized with light microscopy. **B** Scanning electron microscope appearance on the plaque core demonstrated in **A**. **C** Digimap distribution of silver in the area shown in **A** after background subtraction. The silver-stained core is readily visible. Digimap distribution of **D** silicon and **E** aluminium in the same area. It can be seen that silicon and aluminium are co-localized in the senile plaque core obtained from this elderly, nondemented patient. Micrographs are all at the same magnification; *calibration bar* represents 2 μm

order. Thus, the amount of aluminium localized in plaque cores and present intracellularly in NFT-bearing neurones (Perl and Brody 1980) is significantly increased, as a simple consequence of the greater density of these features in SDAT brain as compared with control brains.

The localization of aluminium and silicon at the very centre of the plaque core suggests a primary or early involvement of these substances in the mechanism of core formation. A secondary deposition would presumably be more likely to show a homogeneous or even peripheral pattern of distribution. The fact that some plaques may not contain a visible core at light microscopic level does not exclude the possibility of an initiating role for aluminium or silicon (or aluminosilicates), since the local profusion of abnormal neurites and glial processes in early plaques indicates some highly focalized change in the extracellular environment, thereby causing this disarray. A focal deposit of aluminosilicate without the

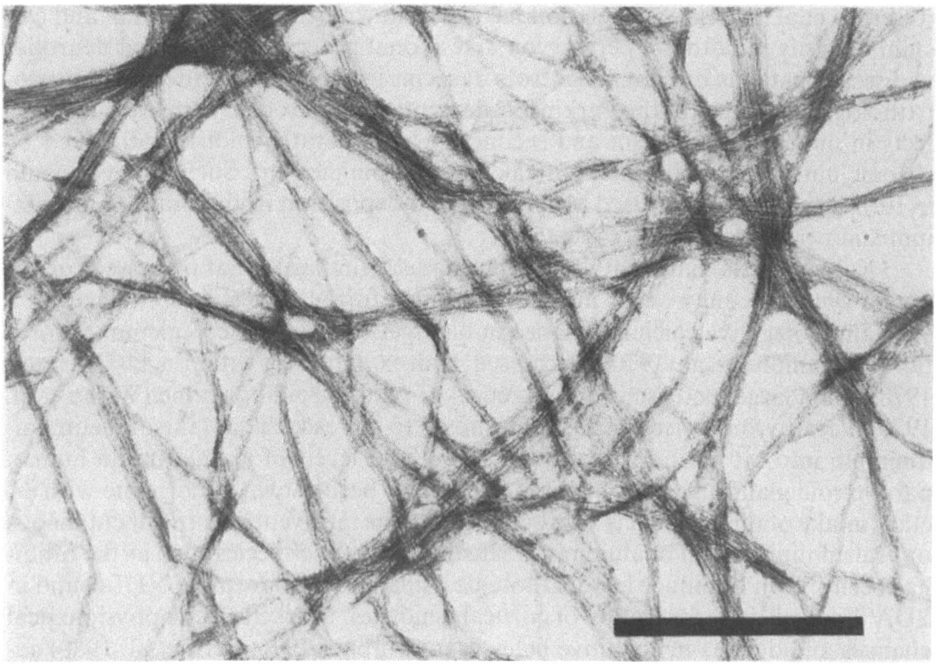

Fig. 7. Fibrillary appearance of the aluminosilicate imogolite. Synthetic imogolite was centrifuged onto an electron microscope grid coated with formvar and carbon, then negatively stained with 1% uranyl acetate. Note the apparent flexible nature of the fibrillary aggregates. The *calibration bar* represents 0.5 μm

outer layer of core material may be present at this stage. Indeed, the peripheral material may represent an attempt to isolate the aluminosilicate from the surrounding tissue.

The finding of aluminium and silicon in the plaque core provides a possible link with the other prominent neuropathological feature of SDAT, the NFT. Thus, studies using X-ray microprobe analysis have shown that the content of aluminium is higher in NFT-bearing neurones than in adjacent normal cells (Perl and Brody 1980). These workers also reported that intracellular levels of silicon were higher in SDAT patients than in normal controls, although in the former group both NFT-containing neurones and cells which appeared normal showed similar silicon levels. This is at variance with an earlier report (Nikaido et al. 1972) claiming that silicon levels in NFT-bearing cells were higher than those in adjacent normal cells. The presence of aluminium and silicon in neurones with NFT raises the possibility that both elements are involved in NFT formation. While the accumulation of aluminium and silicon in plaques and NFT-containing neurones may reflect secondary deposition following as yet unknown pathogenic changes, the hypothesis that these substances may have a primary involvement cannot be excluded.

Deposits of intracellular calcium and aluminium have been described in NFT-bearing neurones from cases of the Parkinsonian-dementia complex of Guam

(Garruto et al. 1984). A correlation has been shown between aluminium and calcium deposits in both the perikaryon and axonal processes of affected neurones in diseased patients but not in controls. It seems likely that the widespread neuropathological changes of the Parkinson-dementia complex of Guam are due to defects in mineral metabolism and secondary hyperparathyroidism, provoked by chronic nutritional deficiencies of calcium and magnesium. Such changes could in turn result in the increased absorption and deposition in the brain of aluminium and perhaps other toxic metals.

The hypothesis that a pathogenic mechanism similar to that proposed for the Guam syndrome may occur in SDAT requires further investigation. There is a substantial negative calcium balance in old age, with decreased calcium absorption (Bullamore et al. 1970), decreased hydroxylation of vitamin D (Rushton 1978) and a large increase in the secretion of parathyroid hormone (Wiske et al. 1979). Parathyroid hormone has been shown to increase the uptake of dietary aluminium into rat brain (Mayor et al. 1980), and levels of aluminium in human parathyroid glands measured post mortem have been shown to correlate with dietary intake of this element (Cann et al. 1979). The intraventricular, subcutaneous or oral administration of aluminium salts in susceptible species such as the rabbit has been shown to induce histopathological changes similar to the NFT found in SDAT, as well as degeneration of cortical dendrites. Marked electrophysiological changes and deficits in cognitive behaviour (Crapper 1976; Petit et al. 1980) accompany these neuropathological changes.

Dissociation between the density of plaques and tangles in individual cases of SDAT is well described (Tomlinson 1982), and even if aluminium or aluminosilicates are implicated in their pathogenesis, the mechanisms could be independent. Aluminium has a wide spectrum of neurotoxic effects on biochemical mechanisms in vitro (for a review, see Boegman and Bates 1984), many of which are attributable to interference with calcium-mediated processes. Aluminium binds with high affinity to a variety of macromolecules, including DNA (Karlik et al. 1980), transmitter-related enzymes such as AChE (Marquis and Black 1984) and the calcium-regulating protein calmodulin (Siegel and Haug 1983). Since calcium-activated proteinase has been implicated in the disaggregation of neurofilament protein (Malik et al. 1981), it is at least possible that aluminium could initiate tangle formation through the inhibition of such a mechanism.

The occurrence of the greatest densities of plaques and tangles in the cerebral cortex of SDAT patients would, on the basis of a hypothesis implicating aluminium or aluminosilicates in their pathogenesis, suggest that this region is the primary site of pathology and that the biochemical and histopathological abnormalities in subcortical nuclei are perhaps secondary. A substantial weight of evidence is consistent with this view.

The Cerebral Cortex as the Primary Site for Pathological Change in Alzheimer's Disease

Dementia is frequently associated with the late stages of Parkinson's disease, in which there is undoubtedly a primary degeneration of cells in the substantia nigra and other subcortical nuclei (see Lee, this volume). It has been claimed that the dementia of Parkinson's disease is traceable to the coexistence of Alzheimer's disease (Marsden 1982), but there is now evidence that both cognitive impairment and depletion of presynaptic cholinergic markers occur in cases lacking Alzheimer-type pathology in the cortex (Perry et al. 1983 b, 1985). In Parkinson's disease, as in SDAT, there are neuropathological changes in the Meynert nucleus, dorsal raphe nucleus and locus ceruleus (see Bloxham et al. 1985 for a review). However, the loss of cells in these nuclei is greater than that which occurs in SDAT, even though the dementia of Parkinson's disease is less severe. Loss of neurones from the nucleus basalis of Meynert in nondemented cases of Parkinson's disease exceeds that in elderly (70–90 years) SDAT patients (Perry et al. 1985), and it is the reduction of activity in the cortical cholinergic system which seems to correlate best with the severity of cognitive impairment. Thus, the cholinergic deficit is greater in demented cases of Parkinson's disease (Table 1) where it is as great as that seen in SDAT. in contrast with Parkinson's disease, the relatively modest loss of cells in the nucleus of Meynert in SDAT (33%) is accompanied by a much more severe loss of ChAT activity (90%) from this region (Perry et al. 1982). This discrepancy may indicate the down-regulation of cholinergic activity in neurones of the basal forebrain as a consequence of some change which occurs in their terminal regions in the cerebral cortex (Bloxham et al. 1985). Such retrograde degeneration might be related to the involvement of cholinergic processes in cortical plaques. It appears that, in SDAT, it is mainly subcortical neurones projecting to the cortex of intrinsic cortical neurones that have a high density of NFT or show signs of severe biochemical abnormality. This is in contrast to Parkinson's disease, where there is a significant loss of neurones or marked evidence of histopathological change in nuclei such as the substantia nigra or dorsal vagus nuclei, which do not project to the cortex. Thus, a comparison between Parkinson's disease and SDAT points to the primary involvement of the cortex in the latter.

The cortical hypothesis is supported by the work of Bigl et al. (1984), who have shown that degeneration in different subdivisions of the nucleus basalis of Meynert is not homogeneous, but rather that the pattern of cell loss correlates significantly with the density of senile plaques in the related cortical target areas. A high degree of individual variation occurs between different regions of the nucleus basalis and even between the same region in both hemispheres. The correlation of subcortical cell loss with plaque density in the specific area of projection points strongly to a primary cortical involvement. Similarly, Mann and Marcyniuk (1984, personal communication) have described a greater loss of locus ceruleus neurones from areas thought to project topographically to the plaque-rich frontal and temporal cortex than from regions which project to occipital cortex where the density of plaques is normally low.

Table 1. Presynaptic cholinergic markers in the cerebral cortex[a]

Cortical lobe	Normal		Parkinson's disease without dementia		Parkinson's disease with dementia		Alzheimer-type senile dementia	
	ChAT	AChE	ChAT	AChE	ChAT	AChE	ChAT	AChE
Occipital	3.50 (1.27)	0.56 (0.20)	1.44 (0.39)[b]	0.38 (0.11)	0.91 (0.31)[b]	0.39 (0.18)	1.42 (0.60)[b]	0.46 (0.14)
Parietal	6.09 (1.37)	0.95 (0.41)	2.98 (0.30)[b]	0.48 (0.14)[c]	1.31 (0.89)[b]	0.45 (0.09)[c]	1.08 (0.85)[b]	0.46 (0.15)[c]
Temporal	4.64 (1.93)	0.68 (0.15)	3.22 (1.52)	0.58 (0.13)	1.21 (1.13)[b]	0.41 (0.17)[c]	1.10 (0.67)[b]	0.40 (0.12)[c]
Frontal	8.61 (2.65)	0.86 (0.17)	5.43 (1.00)	0.70 (0.08)	2.70 (1.12)[b]	0.44 (0.10)[b]	3.50 (1.03)[b]	0.52 (0.18)[b]

[a] Choline acetyltransferase (ChAT) activity expressed as nmol/h/mg protein and acetylcholinesterase (AChE) activity expressed as µmol/h/mg protein; values expressed are means and, in parentheses, standard deviations of mean

[b] $p < 0.001$ (as determined by Student's *t*-test)

[c] $p < 0.01$ (as determined by Student's *t*-test)

Alzheimer-type pathological and neurochemical changes also occur in older subjects with Down's syndrome, and it has been shown that, in this disorder, plaques appear earlier and in greater densities than NFT-bearing neurones (Burger and Vogel 1973). Although plaques do occur in subcortical structures such as the amygdala, they are much less abundant outside the cortex, and their early appearance in Down's syndrome would be consistent with a primary cortical locus for Alzheimer-type changes.

Conclusions

The co-localization of aluminium and silicon at the centre of the senile plaque core and the elevated levels of these elements in NFT-bearing neurones is a common factor of these two important neuropathological features. A key question is whether aluminium or silicon play an essential role in the pathophysiological processes which underly SDAT. Rudelli et al. (1984) have proposed that amyloid is the initiating factor in the formation of plaques, at least in subcortical white matter, where stellate or globular amyloid deposits were observed in the absence of terminal neuritic elements. While it is improbable that focal concentrations of aluminium and silicon cause cellular degeneration by a simple direct action, their presence may reflect a more subtle derangement involving some form of dystrophic mineralization such as that implicated in the Parkinsonian-dementia complex of Guam. In the latter, an environmental deficiency of calcium and magnesium appears to produce a hyperparathyroid state which leads to concomitant deposition of aluminium and calcium in neurones. Present evidence would at least warrant a serious epidemiological study of the incidence of SDAT in different geographical populations to determine the relevance of such environmental factors. As the Parkinsonian-dementia complex may develop long after individuals have migrated from the high-risk environment (Garruto et al. 1980), a similar study of SDAT would need to encompass environmental factors pertaining to the early years of life.

Acknowledgements. The authors thank M. Willis and G. Staines of the Scanning Electron Microscope Service Unit of the University of Necastle upon Tyne for expert assistance. D. Mantle provided help with the fluorescamine assays, and J. Russell (Macaulay Soil Research Institute, Aberdeen) is thanked for providing infrared analysis and imogolite samples. G. Blessed and A. Fairbairn provided clinical assessment of cases used in this study. We are grateful to D. Hinds for secretarial assistance.

References

Bigl V, Arendt T, Tennstedt A, Arendt A (1984) Different degeneration pattern in sub-divisions of the nucleus basalis in SDAT correlates with predominance in neuritic plaque formation in cortical target areas. In: Vizi ES, Magyar K (eds) Regulation of transmitter function. Academiai Kiado, Budapest, pp 271–274

Blessed G, Tomlinson BE, Roth M (1968) The association between quantitative measures of dementia and of senile change in the cerebral grey matter of elderly subjects. Brit J Psychiatry 114:797–801

Bloxham CA, Perry EK, Perry RH, Oakley AE, Edwardson JA, Candy JM (1985) Neuropathological and neurochemical correlates of Alzheimer-type and Parkinsonian dementia. In: Iversen SD (ed) Psychopharmacoloy: recent advances and future prospects. Oxford University Press, Oxford

Boegman RJ, Bates LA (1984) Neurotoxicity of aluminium. Can J Physiol Pharmacol 62:1010–1014

Bowen DM, Davison AN, Francis PT, Neary D, Palmer AM (1984) Alzheimer's disease: importance of acetylcholine and tanglebearing cortical neurones. In: Wurtman RJ, Corkin SH, Growdon JH (eds) Alzheimer's disease: advances in basic research and therapies: proceedings of the 3rd meeting of the International Study Group on the Treatment of Memory Disorders Associated with Aging. Zurich, Switzerland, pp 9–27

Bullamore JR, Wilkinson R, Gallagher JC, Nordin BEC, Marshall DH (1970) Effect of age on calcium absorption. Lancet II:535–537

Burger PC, Vogel FS (1973) The development of the pathological changes of Alzheimer's disease and senile dementia in patients with Down's syndrome. Ann J Pathol 73:457–476

Candy JM, Oakley AE, Atack J, Perry RH, Perry EK, Edwardson JA (1984) New observations on the nature of senile plaque cores. In: Vizi ES, Magyar K (eds) Regulation of transmitter function. Akademiai Kiado, Budapest, pp 301–304

Candy JM, Oakley AE, Klinowski J, Carpenter TA, Perry RH, Atack JR, Perry EK, Blessed G, Fairbairn A, Edwardson JA (1985) Presence of aluminosilicates in senile plaques in the cerebral cortex in Alzheimer's disease. Submitted to Nature

Cann CE, Prussin SG, Gordon GS (1979) Aluminium uptake by the parathyroid glands. J Clin Endocrinol Metab 49:543–545

Crapper DR (1976) Functional consequences of neurofibrillary degeneration. In: Terry RD, Gershon S (eds) Neurobiology of aging. Raven, New York, pp 405–432

Crapper DR, Krishman SS, Dalton AJ (1973) Brain aluminium distribution in Alzheimer's disease and experimental neurofibrillary degeneration. Science 180:511–513

Crapper DR, Krishman SS, Quittkat S (1976) Aluminium, neurofibrillary degeneration and Alzheimer's disease. Brain 99:67–80

Cross AJ, Crow TJ, Ferrier IN, Johnson JA, Bloom SR, Corsellis JAN (1984) Serotonin receptor changes in dementia of the Alzheimer type. J Neurochem 43:1574–1581

Duckett S, Galle P (1976) Mise en évidence de l'aluminium dans les plaques séniles de la maladie d'Alzheimer: étude de la microsonde de castaing. CR Acad Sci (Paris) 292:393–395

Duckett S, Galle P (1980) Electron microscope microprobe studies of aluminium in the brains of cases of Alzheimer's disease and ageing patients. J Neuropathol Exp Neurol 39:350 (Abstract)

Farmer VC, Adams MJ, Fraser AR, Palmieri F (1983) Synthetic imogolite: properties, synthesis and possible applications. Clay Miner 18:459–472

Garruto RM, Gajdusek DC, Chen KM (1980) Amyotrophic lateral sclerosis among Chamarro migrants from Guam. Ann Neurol 8:612–619

Garruto RM, Fukatsu R, Yanagihara R, Gajdusek DC, Hook G, Fiori CE (1984) Imaging of calcium and aluminium in neurofibrillary tangle-bearing neurones in parkinsonism – dementia of Guam. Proc Natl Acad Sci USA 81:1875–1879

Glenner GG, Eanes ED, Bladen HA, Linke RP, Termine JD (1974) β-pleated sheet fibrils: a comparison of native amyloid with synthetic protein fibrils. J Histochem Cytochem 22:1141–1158

Hardy J, Adolfson R, Alafuzoff I, Bucht G, Marcusson J, Nyberg P, Perdahl E, Wester P, Winblad B (1985) Transmitter deficits in Alzheimer's disease. Neurochem Int (to be published)

Karlik SJ, Eichhorn GL, Lewis PN, Crapper Dr (1980) Interaction of aluminium species with deoxyribonucleic acid. Biochemistry 19:5991–5998

McDermott JR, Smith AI, Iqbal K, Wisniewski HM (1979) Brain aluminium in aging and Alzheimer's disease. Neurology 29:809–814

Malik MN, Meyers LA, Iqbal K, Sheikh AM, Scotto L, Wisniewski HM (1981) Calcium-activated proteolysis of fibrous proteins in central nervous system. Life Sci 29:795–802

Marsden CD (1982) Basal ganglia disease. Lancet II:1141–1147
Marquis JK, Black EG (1984) Aluminium activation and inactivation of bovine caudate acetylcholinesterase. Bull Environ Contam Toxicol 32:704–710
Mayor GH, Remedi RF, Sprague SM, Lovell KL (1980) Central nervous system manifestations of oral aluminium: effect of parathyroid hormone. Neurotoxicology 1:33–42
Nikaido T, Austin J, Trueb L, Rinehart R (1972) Studies in ageing of the brain. II. Microchemical analyses of the nervous system in Alzheimer patients. Arch Neurol 27:549–554
Oakley AE, Perry RH, Candy JM, Perry EK (1981) Elecron microscopic appearances and implications of neuropeptide fibrillary forms. Neuropeptides 2:1–11
Perl DP, Brody AR (1980) Alzheimer's disease: X-ray spectrometric evidence of aluminium accumulation in neurofibrillary tangle-bearing neurones. Science 208:297–299
Perry EK, Perry RH (1980) The cholinergic system in Alzheimer's disease. In: Robert PJ (ed) Biochemistry of dementia. John Wiley, Chichester, pp 135–183
Perry RH, Blessed G, Perry EK, Tomlinson BE (1980) Histochemical observations on cholinesterase activities in the brains of elderly normal and demented (Alzheimer-type) patients. Age Ageing 9:9–16
Perry EK, Oakley AE, Candy JM, Perry RH (1981) Properties and possible significance of substance P and insulin fibrils. Neurosci Lett 25:321–325
Perry RH, Candy JM, Perry EK, Irving D, Blessed G, Fairbairn AF, Tomlinson BE (1982) Extensive loss of choline acetyltransferase activity is not reflected by neuronal loss in the nucleus of Meynert in Alzheimer's disease. Neurosci Lett 33:311–315
Perry RH, Candy JM, Perry EK (1983a) Some observations and speculations concerning the cholinergic system and neuropeptides in Alzheimer's disease. In: Katzman R (ed) Banbury Report 15: Biological Aspects of Alzheimer's Disease. Cold Spring Harbor Laboratory, pp 351–361
Perry RH, Tomlinson BE, Candy JM, Blessed G, Foster JF, Bloxham CA, Perry EK (1983b) Cortical cholinergic deficit in mentally impaired Parkinsonian patients. Lancet II:789–790
Perry EK, Curtis M, Dick DJ, Candy JM, Atack JR, Bloxham CA, Blessed G, Fairbairn A, Tomlinson BE, Perry RH (1985) Cholinergic correlates of cognitive impairment in Parkinson's disease: comparisons with Alzheimer's disease. J Neurol: Neurosurg Psychiatry 48:413–421
Petit TL, Biederman GB, McMullen PA (1980) Neurofibrillary degeneration, dendritic dying back and learning memory deficits after aluminium administration: implications for brain aging. Exp Neurol 67:152–162
Prusiner SB (1982) Novel proteinaceous infectious particles cause scrapie. Science 216:136–144
Prusiner SB (1984) Some speculations about prions, amyloid and Alzheimer's disease. N Eng J Med 310:661–663
Rossor MN, Emson PC, Iversen LL, Mountjoy CR, Roth M (1984) Patterns of neuropeptide deficits in Alzheimer's disease. In: Wurtman RJ, Corkin SH, Growdon JH (eds) Alzheimer's disease: advances in basic research and therapies: proceedings of the 3rd meeting of the International Study Group on the Treatment of Memory Disorders Associated with Aging. Zurich, Switzerland, pp 29–37
Rudelli RD, Ambler MW, Wisniewski HM (1984) Morphology and distribution of Alzheimer neuritic (senile) and amyloid plaques in striatum and diencephalon. Acta Neuropathol 64:273–281
Rushton C (1978) Vitamin D hydroxylation in youth and old age. Age Ageing 7:91–95
Siegel N, Haug A (1983) Aluminium interaction with calmodulin. Evidence for altered structure and function from optical and enzymatic studies. Biochim Biophys Acta 744:36–45
Tomlinson BE (1982) Plaques, tangles and Alzheimer's disease. Psychol Med 12:449–459
Tomlinson BE, Blessed G, Roth M (1968) Observations on the brains of nondemented old people. J Neurol Sci 7:331–356
Westermark P, Grimelius L, Polak JM, Larsson L-I, Van Noarden S, Wilander E, Pearse AGE (1977) Amyloid in polypeptide hormone-producing tumours. Lab Invest 37:212–215
Wiske PS, Epstein S, Bell NH, Queener SF, Edmondson J, Johnston CC (1979) Increase in immunoreactive parathyroid hormone with age. N Eng J Med 300:1419–1421

Biochemical Changes in Alzheimer's Disease: A Comment

A. N. Davison[1]

Neuronal Loss and Tangle Formation

Alzheimer's disease is characterized by an acquired global impairment of higher cortical functions which affects short-term memory in particular. There is evidence that these behavioural abnormalities are probably related to pathologic changes in the limbic system, especially in the hippocampus and amygdala. However, the discovery that patients afflicted with Alzheimer's disease suffer a substantial loss of subcortical and brain stem neurons has emphasised the importance of cortical abnormalities, for fibres from neurons in this region project widely to the neocortex. The reduction in choline acetyltransferase (ChAT) activity in this part of the brain (Whitehouse et al. 1982) and the diminished synthesis of acetylcholine by resting and stimulated brain synaptosomes (Sims et al. 1983) can be ascribed to the loss of cortical presynaptic cholinergic terminals in the nucleus basalis (Fig. 1).

However, other pathologic changes are also apparent in the cortex. Using antibody to neurofilament protein as an index of nerve cells, Rasool et al. (1984) found a 20%–30% loss of neurons and dendrites in the brains of patients with Alzheimer's disease. Morphometric analysis shows a loss of about 40% of large neurons (those larger than 90 μ^2) from the midfrontal and superior temporal regions (Terry et al. 1981). Terry and his colleagues further showed that the concentration of neuritic plaques does not correlate significantly with brain weight, cortical thickness or cell counts. It was therefore of interest when Wilcock et al. (1982) found that both the reduction in ChAT activity and the severity of the dementia correlate well with the number of neurofibrillary tangles in the cortex. Neurofibrillary changes are much more severe in younger subjects with Alzheimer's disease than in elderly patients (Wisniewski and Iqbal 1980). This suggests that tangle formation is a feature of a more aggressive disease process occurring in the younger patients. Paired helical filaments have been described in other dementing disorders such as the Guam Parkinsonian complex, Parkinson's disease, dementia pugilistica and Down's syndrome.

1 Department of Neurochemistry, Institute of Neurology, The National Hospital, Queen Square, London WC1N 3BG, UK

Senile Dementia of the Alzheimer Type
Ed. by J. Traber and W. H. Gispen

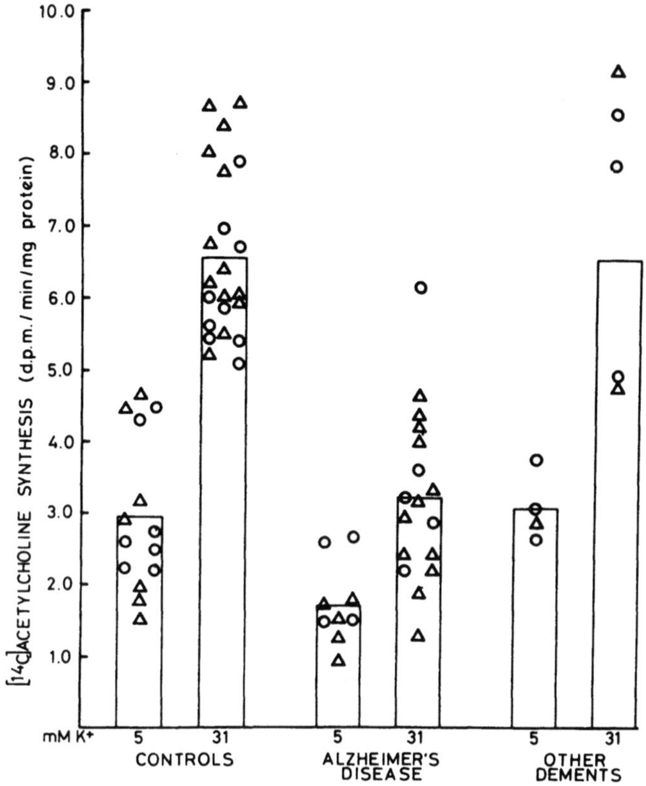

Fig. 1. Acetylcholine synthesis in fresh brain tissue preparations. Synthesis was measured in the presence of 5 m*M* or 31 m*M* K^+ with radioactive glucose as substrate. Synaptosomes were prepared from temporal neocortex (△) and frontal neocortical (○) biopsies. (For details, see Sims et al. 1983; reprinted here with the permission of the authors and the Journal of Neurochemistry)

Biochemical Changes in the Cortex of Alzheimer Patients

Glucose Metabolism

Further evidence of cortical pathology comes from imaging techniques and data on cerebral blood flow. Hypometabolism of glucose is commonly found in the cortex of Alzheimer patients, the parietal and temporal lobes being particularly affected. Positron emission tomography using labelled fluoro-2-deoxy-D-glucose shows evidence of focal cortical metabolic changes (Benson et al. 1983; Foster et al. 1983), as summarised in Table 1. This information may be related to histologic finding which suggest that Alzheimer's disease results in damage to and eventual loss of large pyramidal neurons in the neocortex. Examination of glycolytic enzyme activity in the brain of Alzheimer patients shows that enzyme activity may decrease significantly in the temporal cortex. Aldolase and phosphohexoisomerase are decreased by about half, phosphoglycerate mutase by a third, glyceraldehyde-3-phosphate dehydrogenase and pyruvate kinase to 20% of control values

Table 1. Cortical metabolism in Alzheimer patients as shown by positron emission tomography using ^{18}F-deoxyglucose

Region:	Mean glucose uptake (mg/100 mg/min)			
	Frontal	Parietal	Temporal	Occipital
Controls ($n=5$)	7.4±0.8	7.9±0.8	6.5±0.6	6.9±0.7
Alzheimer patients ($n=17$)	5.8±0.3	4.0±0.3	4.8±0.3	4.8±0.3

IQ scores of the patients with Alzheimer's disease were 35% below controls, and they showed a mean reduction in cortical glucose metabolism of 30%. The posterior parietal lobes and superior temporal cortex were most affected (Chase et al. 1983; Foster et al. 1983)

(Bowen et al. 1979; Meier-Ruge et al. 1980). An apparently large decrease in phosphofructokinase activity also occurs. In the frontal and occipital cortex of Alzheimer patients, the activity of the pyruvate dehydrogenase complex is reduced to 20%–30% of control activity. This loss occurs even in histologically normal tissue, but another mitochondrial enzyme (glutamate dehydrogenase) is not affected (Sheu et al. 1984; Sorbi et al. 1983).

Unfortunately, this interesting data is confounded by pre- and postmortem conditions to which many of the glycolytic enzymes are susceptible. Thus, it is necessary to study glucose metabolism and enzyme activity in fresh tissue samples. When this is done, a different picture emerges. Increased production of $^{14}CO_2$ from labelled glucose can be observed in biopsy tissue prisms taken from the neocortex of Alzheimer patients (Sims et al. 1983). Moreover, adenylate energy charge is unaltered in the tissue, although there is a reduction in the nucleotide pool that is possibly related to the loss of presynaptic terminals. One of several possible explanations for the increased CO_2 production and the reduction in adenine nucleotides could be uncoupled oxidative phosphorylation.

Protein Synthesis

In early studies (Bowen et al. 1977) on whole temporal lobe taken from postmortem Alzheimer patients, a reduction in total protein and a loss of RNA were reported. A possible defect in protein synthesis was indicated by the work of Mann and his associates (Mann et al. 1981), who have described considerable reductions in nuclear and nucleolar volume, together with a loss of cytoplasmic RNA in patients with Alzheimer's disease. A diminished capability for protein synthesis in cortical tissue associated with translational defects in mRNA has been described by Sajdel-Sulkowska and Marotta (1984).

Neurotransmitters

As a result of a collaborative study between Bowen and Neary (Manchester Royal Infirmary) and Mann (University of Manchester), new data is emerging

Table 2. High-affinity choline uptake in samples of neocortex obtained through diagnostic craniotomy from demented patients and neurosurgical controls as compared with other presynaptic cholinergic markers in the same demented patients

	Tissue prisms (in 31 mM K^+)		Homogenate
	Choline uptake (% controls)	Acetylcholine synthesis (% controls)	Choline acetyltransferase activity (% controls)
Patients with Alzheimer's disease	52[a]	59[a]	43[a]
Other demented patients	89	101	84

Choline uptake was determined using a low concentration (0.82 μM) of ^{3}H-choline. Acetylcholine synthesis was measured with glucose ^{14}C (ul) [Bowen et al. (1983); Sims et al. (1983)]
[a] Significant changes

from the analysis of neocortical biopsy samples. The specimens are obtained from patients who have been subjected to extensive clinical and psychometric assessments. With tissue samples obtained by diagnostic craniotomy, it became possible for Bowen and his colleagues to carry out a systematic search for neurotransmitter systems in the cortex which might be affected. The experiments investigating the synthesis of acetylcholine from glucose indicate reduced synthetic capability with impaired choline uptake in histologically identified Alzheimer cases (Table 2, Sims et al. 1983). This is probably due to a loss of presynaptic cholinergic terminals, since it is unlikely that the loss of cholinergic interneurons is primarily responsible for such changes. Animal experiments indicate that damage to subcortical afferent cholinergic pathways leads to a substantial decrease in cortical ChAT activity (Wenk et al. 1980; Bowen et al. 1983).

Our previous studies on postmortem cortical tissue showed, when allowance was made for premortem artefacts, that glutamate decarboxylase activity remains unaltered in Alzheimer's disease. This was confirmed when biopsy samples were analysed. Since glutamate decarboxylase is responsible for gamma-aminobutyric acid (GABA) synthesis, it acts as a marker for GABA interneurons and suggests that these are unimpaired. Indeed, evoked release of putative amino acid transmitters does not seem to be reduced in Alzheimer's disease (Table 3) and, apart

Table 3. Potential amino acid transmitter nerve ending markers in Alzheimer's disease

Brain region and marker	Alzheimer's disease (% controls)
Neocortex obtained through neurosurgery	
K^+-evoked release from tissue prisms	
Glutamate	141
Aspartate	117
Gamma-aminobutyrate	108
Glutamate decarboxylase activity	97

(After Smith et al. 1983)

Table 4. Biochemical parameters in Alzheimer's disease and control as assayed from caudate nucleus samples

Variable measured	Controls	Alzheimer's disease patients
Caudate nucleus weight (g)	3.06 ± 0.43	2.67 ± 0.43[b]
Total protein (mg/caudate)	380 ± 94	281 ± 42[b]
ChAT activity (nmol/mg/min)	297 ± 119	118 ± 77[b]
Total dopamine (pmol/mg)	150.0 ± 44.0	99.9 ± 47.9[b]
Total serotonin (pmol/mg)	25.0 ± 11.0	20.9 ± 12.0
Noradrenaline (pmol/mg)	2.4 ± 1.2	2.3 ± 1.1
^{3}H glutamate binding		
0.3 μM (pmol/mg membrane protein)	10.3 ± 6.5	16.8 ± 6.8[a]
1.0 μM (pmol/mg)	22.0 ± 8.4	28.6 ± 11.8

The results are the means ±SD (per mg total protein, except where stated otherwise) for 12–13 control and 13–15 Alzheimer's disease samples. Asterisks identify significant differences from control values: [a] $P<0.02$; [b] $P<$at least 0.01 (after Pearce et al. 1984)

from possibly increased glutamate and aspartate concentrations, the content of other amino acids in the cortex is unaltered (Perry et al. 1984).

The neurotransmitter affected by Alzheimer's disease in terminals from descending projections emanating from the large pyramidal cortical neurons is unknown. Such cortical afferent fibres are often glutamergic Fonnum 1984). Cortical ablation in the rat reduces kainic acid neurotoxicity and receptor binding in the striatum, suggesting that glutamate-containing fibres project to the striatum (Biziere and Coyle 1979). Furthermore, up to 4 weeks after frontal cortical ablation in the rat, a significant reduction in glutamate concentrations is found in the striatum on the ipsilateral side (Hassler et al. 1982). Acetylcholine and monoamine transmitters are not affected. Thus, it is most likely that glutamate is the transmitter of the corticostriatal fibres. This hypothesis is supported by data from a study of biochemical changes in the caudate nucleus observed in postmortem cases of Alzheimer's disease (Pearce et al. 1984).

The increased specific binding of L-^{3}H glutamate to membranes of the caudate nucleus in the brains of Alzheimer patients (Table 4), which is directly related to the cortical tangle score, provides evidence that Alzheimer's disease produces a change in glutamergic neurotransmission. Hemidecortication of rats results in an elevated binding of L-^{3}H glutamate to striatal membranes, possibly reflecting the development of supersensitivity (Roberts et al. 1982). Thus, it is possible that the positive relationship between the number of tangles in the neocortex and values for glutamate binding reflects a change in glutamate receptors in the caudate nucleus, resulting from dysfunction of descending tracts from glutamergic perikarya in the neocortex.

In a study by Pearce et al. (1984) on Alzheimer's disease striatum, it is unclear whether the reduction in ChAT activity of the caudate nucleus is caused by a loss of whole cholinergic cells. The neurotoxic effects of kainic acid in rat striatum include the loss of ChAT activity and markers of GABA interneurons as well as the loss of ^{3}H-kainic acid binding sites (Biziere and Coyle 1979, London and Coyle

1979; Vincent and McGeer 1979). ^{3}H-Kainic acid binding in the caudate nucleus of patients with Alzheimer's disease is similar to control values (Pearce and Bowen 1984). Moreover, the concentration of GABA is unchanged (Rossor et al. 1982). Thus, neurons intrinsic to the caudate nucleus seem by most criteria to be relatively intact in Alzheimer's disease. The atrophy of the caudate nucleus and the diminished ChAT activity remain unexplained.

Conclusion

The loss of ascending projections from certain subcortical and brain stem nuclei is a partial explanation for the neurotransmitter deficiencies in the cortex and other brain areas typical of Alzheimer's disease. Diminished cortical noradrenergic and serotonergic functions may, like the cholinergic system and the nucleus basalis be related to cell loss from the locus ceruleus and tangle formation in the raphe nucleus. There is the possibility that Alzheimer's disease may be a syndrome, with differences between early-onset and late-onset cases (Bowen et al. 1979; Rossor et al. 1984). Another complication comes from recent work on Parkinson's disease that indicates cell loss from the nucleus basalis and cholinergic abnormalities in the absence of neuritic plaques (Perry et al. 1983). Finally, little is known about the aetiology of Alzheimer's disease and other degenerative disorders of the mature brain. This still remains an outstanding problem.

References

Benson DF, Kuhl DE, Hawkins RA, Phelps ME, Cummings JL, Tsai SY (1983) The fluorodeoxy glucose 18F scan in Alzheimer's disease and multi-infarct dementia. Arch Neurol 40:711–14

Biziere K, Coyle JT (1979) Effects of cortical ablation on the neurotoxity and receptor binding of kainic acid in striatum. J Neurosci Res 4:383–393

Bowen DM, Smith CB, White P, Flack RHA, Carrasco LH, Gedye JL, Davison AN (1977) Chemical pathology of cellular change in post-mortem brains. II. Quantitative estimation of cellular changes in post-mortem brains. Brain 100:427–453

Bowen DM, Spillane JA, Curzon G, Meier-Ruge W, White P, Goodhardt MJ, Iwangoff P, Davison AN (1979) Accelerated ageing or selective neuronal loss as an important cause of dementia? Lancet I:11–14

Bowen DM, Allen SJ, Benton JS, Goodhardt MJ, Haan EA, Palmer AM, Sims NR, Smith CCT, Spillane JA; Esiri MM, Neary D, Snowdon JS, Wilcock G, Davison AN (1983) Biochemical assessment of serotonergic and cholinergic dysfunction and cerebral atrophy in Alzheimer's disease. J Neurochem 41:266–272

Chase TN, Foster NL, Mansi L (1983) Alzheimer's disease and the parietal lobe. Lancet II:225

Fonnum F (1984) Glutamate: a neurotransmitter in mammalian brain – a short review. J Neurochem 42:1–11

Foster NL, Chase TN, Fedio P, Patronas NJ, Brooks RA, Di Chiro G (1983) Alzheimer's disease: focal cortical changes shown by positron emission tomography. Neurology 33:961–965

Hassler R, Huag P, Nitsch C, Kim JS, Paik K (1982) Effect of motor and premotor cortex ablation on concentrations of amino acids, monoamines and acetylcholine and on the ultrastructure in rat striatum. A confirmation of glutamate as the specific cortico-striatal transmitter. J Neurochem 38:1087–1098

London ED, Coyle JT (1979) Specific binding of 3H kainic acid to receptor sites in rat brain. Mol Pharmacol 15:492–505

Mann DMA, Neary D, Yates PO, Lincoln J, Snowden JS, Stanworth P (1981) Alterations in protein synthetic capability of nerve cells in Alzheimer's disease. J Neurol Neurosurg Psychiatry 44:97–103

Meier-Ruge W, Iwangoff P, Reichlmeier K, Sandoz P (1980) Neurochemical findings in the aging brain. In: Goldstein M (ed) Ergot compounds and brain function: neuroendocrine and neuropsychiatric. Raven, New York, pp 323–328

Pearce BR, Bowen DM (1984) 3H Kainic acid binding and choline acetyltransferase activity in Alzheimer's dementia. Brain Res 310:376–378

Pearce BR, Palmer AM, Bowen DM, Wilcock GK, Esiri MM, Davison AN (1984) Neurotransmitter dysfunction and atrophy of the caudate nucleus in Alzheimer's disease. Neurochem Pathol 2:221–232

Perry RH, Tomlinson BE, Candy JM, Blessed G, Foster JF, Bloxham CA, Perry EK (1983) Cortical cholinergic deficit in mentally impaired Parkinsonian patients. Lancet II:789–790

Perry EK, Atack JR, Perry RH, Hardy JA, Dodd PR, Edwardson JA, Blessed G, Tomlinson BE, Fairbairn AF (1984) Intralaminar neurochemical distributions in human midtemporal cortex: comparison between Alzheimer's disease and the normal. J Neurochem 42:1402–1410

Rasool CG, Rogers SJ, Drachman DA (1984) Neuron and neurite loss in Alzheimer's disease. Trans Amer Soc Neurosci 10:273 (abstract)

Roberts PJ, McBean GJ, Sharif NA, Thomas EM (1982) Striatal glutamergic functions: modifications following specific lesions. Brain Res 235:83–91

Rossor MN, Garrett NJ, Johnson AL, Mountjoy CQ, Roth M, Iversen LL (1982) A postmortem study of the cholinergic and GABA systems in senile dementia. Brain 105:313–330

Rossor MN, Iversen LL, Reynolds GP, Mountjoy CQ, Roth M (1984) Neurochemical characteristics of early and late onset types of Alzheimer's disease. Br Med J 288:961–964

Sajdel-Sulkowska EM, Marotta CA (1984) Alzheimer's disease brain: alterations in RNA levels and in a ribonuclease-inhibitor complex. Science 225:947–949

Sheu RKF, Kim YT, Blass JP, Weksler M (1984) Decreased pyruvate dehydrogenase complex activity in histologically normal Alzheimer brain. Soc Neurosci 10:884 (abstract)

Sims NR, Bowen DM, Allen SJ, Smith CCT, Neary D, Thomas DJ, Davison AN (1983) Presynaptic cholinergic dysfunction in patients with dementia. J Neurochem 40:503–509

Smith CCT, Bowen DM, Sims NR, Neary D, Davison AN (1983) Amino acid release from biopsy samples of temporal neocortex from patients with Alzheimer's disease. Brain Res 264:138–141

Sorbi S, Bird ED, Blass JP (1983) Decreased pyruvate dehydrogenase complex activity in Huntington and Alzheimer Brain. Ann Neurol 13:72–78

Terry RD, Peck A, DeTeresa R, Schechter R, Horoupian DS (1981) Some morphometric aspects of the brain in senile dementia of the Alzheimer's type. Ann Neurol 10:184–192

Vincent SR, McGeer EG (1979) Kainic acid binding to membranes of striatal neurons. Life Sci 24:265–270

Wenk H, Bigl V, Meyer U (1980) Cholinergic projections from magnocellular nuclei of the basal forebrain to cortical areas in rats. Brain Res 2:295–316

Whitehouse PJ, Price DL, Struble RG, Clark AW, Coyle JT, Delong MR (1982) Alzheimer's disease and senile dementia: loss of neurons in the basal forebrain. Science 215:1237–1239

Wilcock GK, Esiri MM, Bowen DM, Smith CCT (1982) Alzheimer's disease: correlation of cortical choline acetyltransferase activity with the severity of dementia and histological abnormalities. J Neurol Sci 57:407–417

Wisniewski HM, Iqbal K (1980) Ageing of the brain and dementia. Trends Neurosci 3:226–228

The Nature of Neurofibrillary Tangles*

B. H. ANDERTON[1], M. C. HAUGH[1], J. KAHN[2], C. MILLER[1], A. PROBST[3], and J. ULRICH[3]

Introduction

Dementia of the Alzheimer type (ATD), both presenile and senile, has a characteristic brain histopathology comprising neurofibrillary tangles (NFT), senile plaques, granulovacuolar bodies and Hirano bodies. Alzheimer-type NFT are also found in several other diseases, including Down's syndrome, postencephalitic Parkinson's disease, dementia pugilistica, subacute sclerosing panencephalitis, Parkinson-dementia complex and Hallevorden-Spatz syndrome (Wisniewski et al. 1979). In ATD, NFT are found in certain cortical and subcortical neuronal perikarya and consist of aggregates of abnormal fibres.

Ultrastructurally, most of these fibres have the appearance of filaments (approximately 10–13 nm in diameter) helically twisted about each other in pairs (Kidd 1963; Wisniewski et al. 1976). These twisted filaments are now commonly referred to as paired helical filaments (PHF). PHF are also found in smaller aggregates in the degenerating neurites of the senile plaque (Gonatas et al. 1967; Kidd 1963, 1964; Terry et al. 1964). Some NFT also contain straight filaments approximately 15 nm in diameter (Hirano et al. 1968; Okamoto et al. 1982; Oyanagi 1974; Shibayama and Kitoh 1978; Yagishita eet al. 1981). Straight 15 nm filaments are found as a predominant component of Pick bodies, another type of intraneuronal fibrous accumulation characteristic of Pick's disease (Rewcastle et al. 1968; Towfighi 1982; Brion et al. 1973; Wisniewski et al. 1972). It is therefore assumed that, in those diseases exhibiting NFT and Pick bodies, the cytoskeleton of many neurones is abnormal.

Three different fibrous organelles are the major constituents of the cytoskeleton. These are microtubules 24 nm in diameter, 6–7-nm microfilaments and 10-nm intermediate filaments (Anderton 1981, 1982; Lazarides 1980, 1982). In neurones, the intermediate filaments are represented by neurofilaments which, because of their diameter, led to the early suggestion that they may be the principal component of PHF (Kidd 1963). However, the chemical composition of NFT and the molecular identity of PHF is far from resolved, in spite of numerous immunochemical and biochemical investigations.

---

* This work was supported by the Medical Research Council and The Wellcome Trust

1 Department of Immunology, St. George's Hospital Medical School, University of London, Cranmer Terrace, London SW17 ORE, UK

2 Department of Neuropathology, Institute of Psychiatry, University of London, De Crespigny Park, Denmark Hill, London SE5 8AF, UK

3 Department of Neuropathology, Institute of Pathology, University of Basel, Schönbeinstraße 40, CH-4056 Basel, Switzerland

Senile Dementia of the Alzheimer Type
Ed. by J. Traber and W. H. Gispen

Characterisation of NFT

Isolation and Chemical Properties

Fractions enriched in PHF were first isolated by Iqbal and colleages and reported to contain a protein of mol. wt. 50,000 not present in equivalent fractions from control brain (Iqbal et al. 1974, 1975). More recently, Selkoe and colleagues have shown that NFT are resistant to the usual protein-denaturing and -solubilizing agents, such as sodium dodecyl sulphate (SDS), urea or guanidium hydrochloride, and have exploited this property to enrich for NFT (Selkoe et al. 1982a). These SDS-insoluble NFT retain their overall morphology and, ultrastructurally, are composed of PHF. This insolubility makes further analysis by conventional protein chemistry difficult; for example, the enriched, SDS-insoluble NFT fraction will not enter a SDS-polyacrylamide gel. In contrast, Iqbal et al. (1984) have reported that, although many NFT are resistent to protein denaturants, others are readily solubilized in SDS. The proportion of resistant NFT to those which are solubilized varies from case to case of ATD. This group also claimed that the SDS-insoluble NFT, which are composed of PHF bundles, can be induced to break down and yield polypeptides resolvable on SDS gels by prolonged extraction in SDS and sonication. The major polypeptides produced are of 57,000 and 62,000 mol. wt., with several minor components smaller than 57,000 mol. wt. These solubilized proteins were found to possess a tendency to reaggregate even in SDS. Thus, the solubility properties of PHF are complex and probably need further definition. The identities of the 57,000 and 62,000 mol. wt. proteins remain to be established. Neurofilaments are composed of a polypeptide triplet with individual mol. wts. of approximately 200,000, 150,000 and 70,000. The PHF proteins of mol. wt. 57,000 and 62,000 are therefore not normal neurofilament polypeptides, nor have they been found to comigrate with tubulin or actin, the principal structural proteins of microtubules and microfilaments (Iqbal et al. 1984). Certain neurofilament-related antigens present in NFT also exhibit complex solubility properties (see "Antibody Staining of NFT" and "Treatment of NFT with Hydrolytic Enzymes").

Cross-Linking of Neurofilaments

The apparent total resistance to denaturants exhibited by at least some PHF led Selkoe and colleagues to suggest that the constituent proteins may be covalently cross-linked by bonds other than disulphide (Selkoe et al. 1982a). They proposed that neurofilaments might be cross-linked by an ε-(γ-glutamyl)-lysine peptide bond catalyzed by a transglutaminase, a widely distributed enzmye (Chung 1972). The cross-link produced is the most common for a variety of cross-linked proteins other than the lysine-lysine bond found in collagen.

Transglutaminase requires calcium ions as a cofactor and, in vitro, either cross-link protein substrates to form insoluble polymers or can be assayed more conveniently by the incorporation of radiolabelled or fluorescently labelled lysine analogues of low mol. wt. into protein substrates. Selkoe et al. (1982b) have detected transglutaminase activity in a soluble fraction of human brain and, using this crude supernatant, have investigated whether neurofilament polypeptides are substrates for the enzyme. In their assay the crude fraction failed to incorporate any detectable amounts of the fluorescent lysine analogue, dansylcadaverine, into any neurofilament polypeptides. However, myelin basic porotein, which was present in their preparations, was labelled. Whilst this observation indicates that myelin basic protein was the only transglutaminase substrate present, the cross-linked insoluble polymer formed after incubation did apparently stain with some neurofilament antibodies. To resolve this anomaly and further elucidate the role of transglutaminase in NFT formation, we have reinvestigated the potential of neurofilaments to act as a substrate for transglutaminase as well as whether NFT themselves are substrates.

Transglutaminase was purified from guinea pig liver, since this is the richest known source of the enzyme. Immunochemical, chromatographic and reaction kinetic studies indicate it to be the same enzyme as that found in brain (Chung 1972). The enzyme ran as a single major band on SDS gels, demonstrating that the preparation was approximately 95% pure (Fig. 1, track g). Neurofilaments were isolated from rat and human brain as a Triton X100-insoluble fraction (Wood and Anderton 1981) and from bovine spinal cord by the method of Delacourte et al. (1980). Triton X100-insoluble neurofilaments also contain glial fibrillary acidic protein (GFAP, the intermediate filament protein of astrocytes and some vimentin (the intermediate filament protein of mesenchymal cells). Neurofilaments isolated by the Delacourte method are approximately 60% pure and contain much less GFAP and vimentin; this protocol probably yields one of the purest preparations possible without resorting to denaturing conditions. Incubation of this neurofilament preparation with transglutaminase, Ca^{++} and high concentrations of the fluorescent lysine analogue, dansylcadaverine (which competitively inhibits cross-linking), followed by separation by SDS polyacrylamide gel electrophoresis (PAGE) shows labelling of all three neurofilament proteins (Fig. 1). This clearly demonstrates that neurofilament polypeptides are substrates for transglutaminase. Lowering the concentration of dansylcadaverine in the reaction mixture, thus permitting cross-linking, results in a corresponding decrease in the amount of neurofilament proteins and a concomitant increase in the quantities of fluorescent cross-linked material remaining at the top of the stacking gel (Fig. 1). Similar results were obtained with rat and human brain neurofilament preparations. Thus, with the limitations of the best native neurofilament preparations available, each of the neurofilament triplet polypeptides is a substrate for transglutaminase, and all three of the neurofilament polypeptides are capable of becoming ε-(γ-glutamyl)-lysine–cross-linked in vitro into an insoluble polymer.

We tested whether the SDS-insoluble NFT would act as a substrate by incubating them with high concentrations of dansylcadaverine and purified transglutaminase. Following incubation, the preparations were viewed under the fluorescence microscope, but no NFT were seen to be stained above background (Fig. 2). Thus, it appears that the SDS-insoluble NFT are not substrates for transglutaminase. This implies that, if transglutaminase plays a role in insolubilizing NFT by cross-linking the constituent proteins, then all available glutamine side chains must already participate in cross-links.

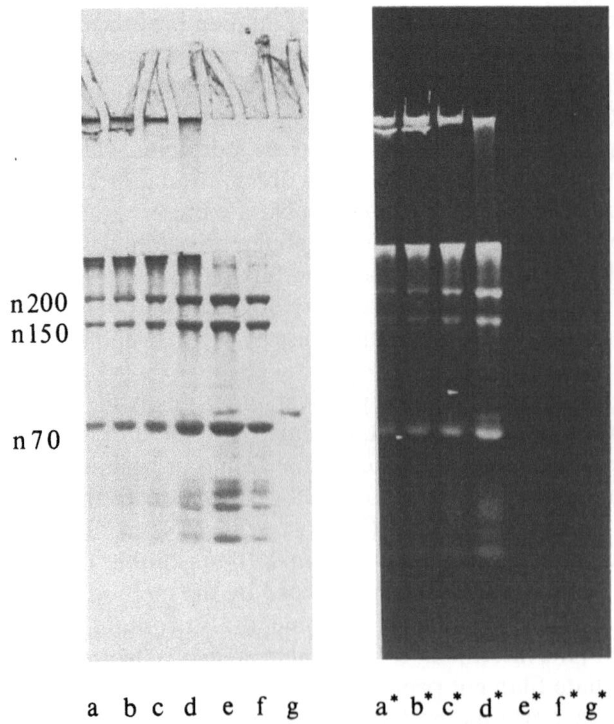

Fig. 1. Neurofilaments as a substrate for transglutaminase. Bovine spinal cord neurofilaments (75 μg per incubation) (Delacourte et al. 1980) were incubated for 2 h at 37 °C with 6.7 μg of purified guinea pig liver transglutaminase and dansyl cadaverine at 0.5 m*M* (*a, a**), 1 m*M* (*b, b**), 2 m*M* (*c, c**) and 5 m*M* (*d, d**, *e, e**) in a total volume of 100 μl containing 50 m*M* TRIS-HCl pH 7.5, 40 μg/ml leupeptin and either 5 m*M* $CaCl_2$ (*a, a*, b, b*, c, c*, d, d**) or 5 m*M* EDTA as a control (*e, e**); incubations were stopped by boiling in SDS sample buffer and 15 μl of each loaded on a 10% w/v polyacrylamide SDS gel. *Track f, f** contained a sample of unincubated neurofilaments. *Track g, g** contained a sample of the purified transglutaminase. *Tracks a–g* represent the Coomassie blue-stained gel and *tracks a*–g** are of the same gel viewed under UV illumination. The results show that Ca^{2+} is required for transglutaminase activity and that all three neurofilament polypeptides are substrates. As the competing dansylcadaverine concentration is reduced, a larger proportion of the neurofilaments become cross-linked. The band corresponding to the transglutaminase also becomes incorporated into the cross-linked product. (*n200, n150, n70,* neurofilament polypeptides)

Antibody Staining of NFT

Immunohistochemical studies indicate that NFT may contain microtubule-associated antigens (Grundke-Iqbal et al. 1979; Nukina and Ihara 1983; Perry et al. 1984; Yen et al. 1981), vimentin antigens (Yen et al. 1983) and neurofilament antigens (Fig. 3) (Anderton et al. 1982; Autilio-Gambetti et al. 1983; Elovaara et al. 1983; Forno et al. 1983; Gambetti et al. 1980, 1983; Ihara et al. 1981; Johnson 1984; Perry et al. 1984; Rasool et al. 1984a, 1984b). However, several groups of workers have noted that some antisera and monoclonal antibodies to neurofilaments do not stain NFT in situ (Gambetti et al. 1980; Kahn et al. 1980; Yen et

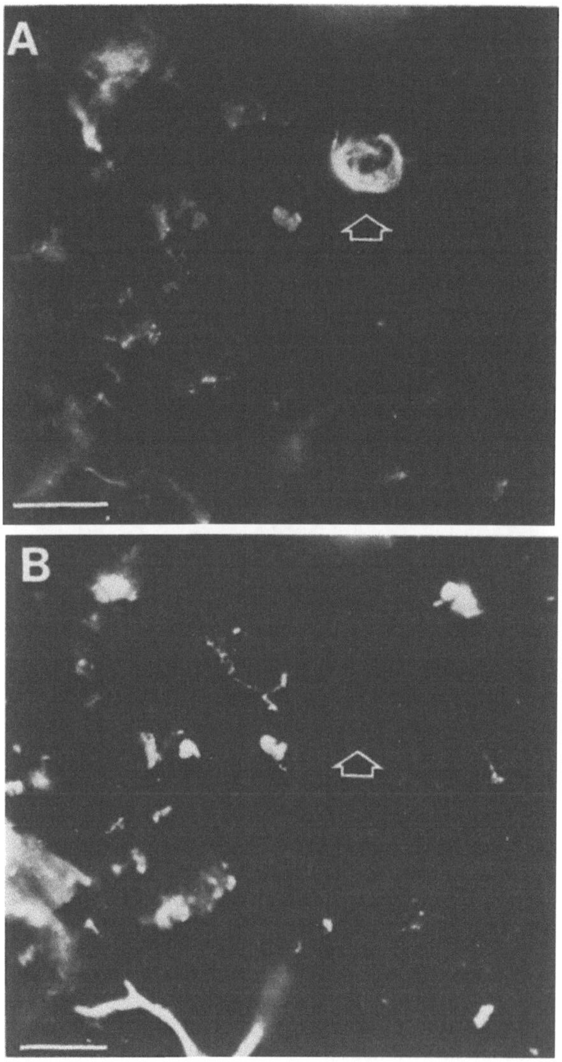

Fig. 2 A, B. SDS-insoluble NFT are not a substrate for transglutaminase. Preparations of SDS-insoluble NFT (Rasool et al. 1984 a) were air-dried onto microscope slides. 1.6 μg of purified transglutaminase in 50 μl of 50 m*M* TRIS-HCl pH 7.5, 5 m*M* $CaCl_2$, 40 μg/ml leupeptin and 5 m*M* dansylcadaverine was incubated for 2 h at 37 °C as a drop on the slides. Slides were washed in 50 m*M* TRIS HCl, pH 7.5 and then in acidified alcohol (85% ethanol: 15% acetic acid), followed by phosphate-buffered saline (PBS). Slides were blocked with 10% v/v normal goat serum and incubated with anti-PHF serum (dil 1:50) (Ihara et al. 1983). After being washed in PBS, they were incubated in rhodamine-conjugated goat anti-rabbit immunoglobulins, washed and mounted. The same field viewed in the fluorescence microscope (**A**) with rhodamine filter system for anti-PHF–labelled structures and (**B**) with Leitz filter system A for dansylcadaverine–labelled structures. In (**B**) some amorphous material and capillaries are labelled with dansylcadaverine, but the NFT, which is stained with anti-PHF in (**A**) (*arrow*) is unlabelled with dansyl-cadaverine. (*Scale bar*, 20 μm)

al. 1981; Probst et al. 1983). One interpretation of these findings is that, while neurofilaments are a component of NFT, the neurofilament structure is modified during NFT formation such that certain epitopes are lost or masked. Certainly, one neurofilament monoclonal antibody, RT97, appears to decorate all of the fibres in the NFT in situ as seen by electron microscopy (Kahn et al. 1984). However, the absence of labelling by some neurofilament antibodies cannot simply be the result of individual neurofilaments twisting about each other and preventing access by gross steric hindrance, since the same pattern of selective antibody staining of Pick bodies, which contain straight filaments, has been observed (Table 1) (Probst et al. 1983). These two disease therefore appear to manifest a similar aberration in neurofilament structure.

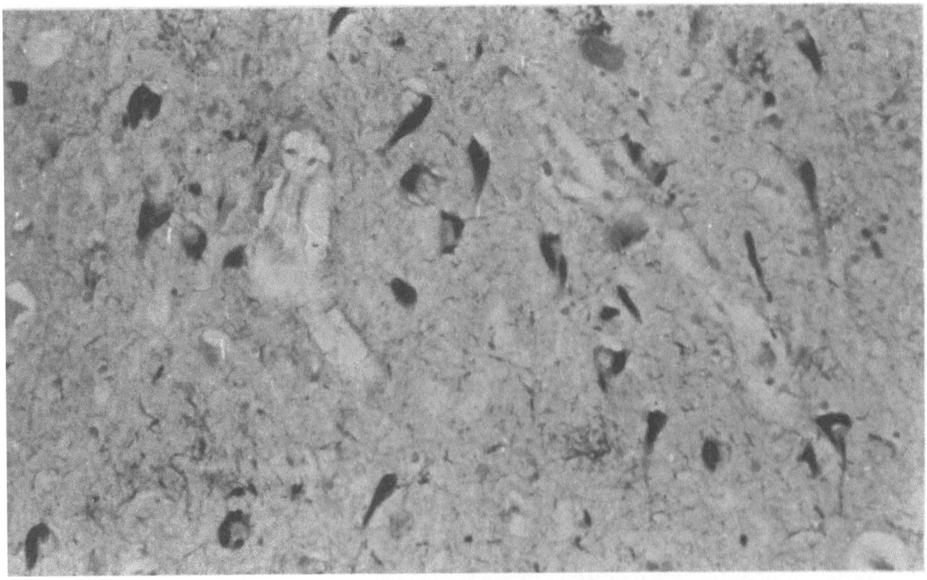

Fig. 3. Immunostaining of NFT in situ by neurofilament antibodies. The section was stained using an indirect peroxidase method to visualise the reaction. The photograph shows staining by Mab BF10 (ascitic fluid dil 1:1000) which recognises the 150,000-mol.-wt. neurofilament polypeptide. Similar staining is found with RT97 and 8D8, which both recognise the 200,000-mol.-wt. neurofilament polypeptide

Two laboratories have now reported that polyclonal and monoclonal antibodies have been produced using SDS-insoluble, purified PHF as immunogen. These antibodies label NFT in situ including SDS-insoluble NFT, but do not react with neurofilaments, microtubules or any other identifiable normal cellular constituent (Grundke-Iqbal et al. 1984; Ihara et al. 1983; Wang et al. 1984). These anti-PHF antibodies recognize "inherent" NFT antigens, which may arise

Table 1. Immunostaining of NFT and Pick bodies by neurofilament antibodies

	NFT	Pick bodies	Neuro-filaments	Principal neurofilament antigen (mol. wt.)
Monoclonal antibodies				
BF10	+	+	+	150000
RT97	+	+	+	200000
147	–	–	+	200000
Polyclonal antisera				
anti-200K	–	–	+	200000
anti-150K	–	–	+	150000

through several factors: they may be newly generated structures stemming from grossly abnormal alterations of normal proteins (e.g. modified neurofilaments), they may be proteins which are not expressed in normal healthy neurones, the genes for which have become derepressed, or they may be a component of an extraneous agent, such as a virus.

We have previously compared two neurofilament antibodies, RT97 and BF10, which label NFT in situ with the anti-PHF of Selkoe and colleagues (Rasool et al. 1984a). The monoclonal antibodies and the PHF antiserum gave identical staining patterns on NFT in tissue sections. However, whereas the anti-PHF labelled all the SDS-insoluble NFT, only a minority were strongly stained by the monoclonal antibodies; the majority were stained only very lightly or were barely distinguishable above background. Somewhat more NFT were stained with the monoclonal antibodies in preparations prepared in TRIS-saline, the isolation procedure being less harsh than the SDS treatment, but again, many more were stained by the anti-PHF. Thus, it would appear that the RT97 and BF10 epitopes present in NFT are extracted relatively easily on isolation and that most of the SDS-insoluble cores of PHF are denuded of these particular neurofilament antigens. However, this is not so for all these SDS-insoluble NFT, since some 5% were still strongly stained with neurofilament antibodies after all normal neurofilaments in axonal segments had been completely solubilized.

Recently, we have isolated another monoclonal antibody, 8D8, which is also directed against the neurofilament polypeptide of mol. wt. 200,000, gives a typical neurofilament staining pattern on sections of brain and stains NFT in situ. However, this antibody does stain SDS-insoluble NFT which are also labelled with anti-PHF serum (Fig. 4). Thus, this 8D8 neurofilament epitope is not easily lost from NFT when they are isolated and appears to be incorporated into the denaturant-resistant core, as are the "inherent" PHF antigens.

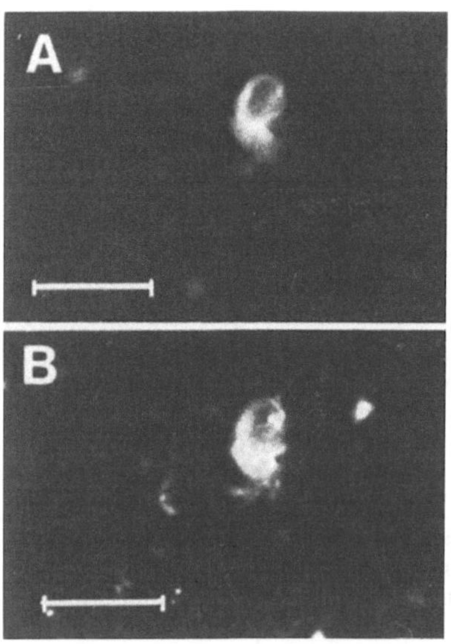

Fig. 4. Double-labelling of SDS-insoluble NFT with **A** Mab 8D8 and **B** rabbit anti-PHF serum. Aliquotes of the SDS-insoluble NFT preparation (Rasool et al. 1984a) were air-dried onto a microscope slide and incubated overnight with 8D8 tissue culture supernatant (dil 1:1) and anti-PHF serum (dil 1:50). After washing, the samples were incubated further with rhodamine-conjugated goat anti-rabbit immunoglobulins and fluorescein-conjugated goat anti-mouse immunoglobulins. After washing and mounting, the slides were viewed in the fluorescence microscope. (*Scale bar*, 20 μm)

Treatment of NFT with Hydrolytic Enzymes

Sternberger and Sternberger (1983) have reported that treatment of sections from brain with alkaline phosphatase can alter the staining pattern obtained with different neurofilament antibodies. We have now discovered that several of our monoclonal antibodies are directed against phosphorylated epitopes and that phosphatase treatment of either unfixed frozen or fixed sections results in diminished staining of normal neurofilaments by monoclonal antibodies RT97, BF10 and 147; the former two also stain NFT, whereas 147 is a neurofilament antibody which does not recognize NFT (Anderton et al. 1982). In contrast, alkaline phosphatase treatment does not appear to result in diminnished NFT staining by BF10, but does induce weak staining of occasional NFT by monoclonal antibody 147 (Fig. 5; Table 2). Thus, in NFT, the BF10 epitope seems to be unavailable to alkaline phosphatase. The positive staining of some NFT by monoclonal antibody 147 after enzyme treatment leads us tentatively to suggest that NFT may contain this 147 epitope. The NFT must be a substrate for alkaline phosphatase such that removal of phosphate makes some 147 epitope accessible to the anti-

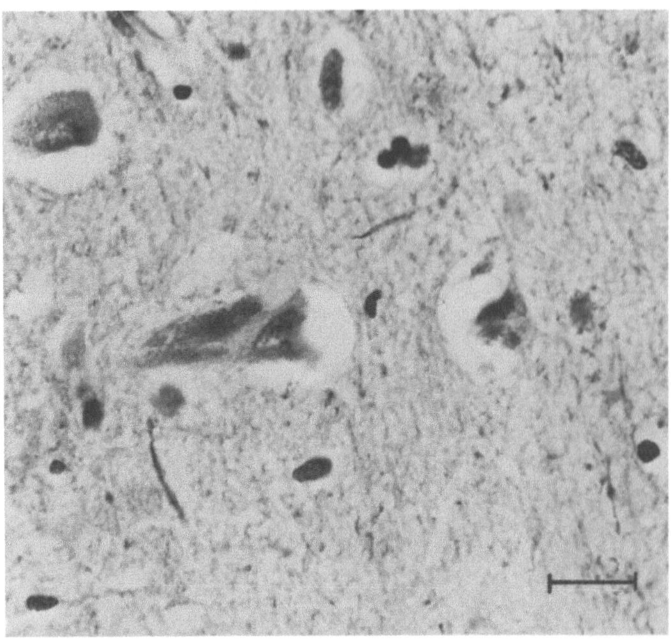

Fig. 5. A neurofilament epitope can be revealed on some NFT following alkaline phosphate treatment. A section of fixed hippocampus from an ATD brain was incubated with alkaline phosphatase (100 μg/ml in 0.2 *M* TRIS-HCl pH 8.0) for 2.5 h at 37 °C prior to an overnight incubation with Mab 147 (ascitic fluid dil 1:1000). The reaction was visualised using a biotin-avidin-peroxidase system (Vectastain ABC kit). Occasional NFT were found to be lightly stained by Mab 147; one such NFT is shown here. Mab 147, which recognises the 200,000-mol.-wt. neurofilament polypeptide, does not normally stain NFT. Controls in this experiment, i.e. incubation with buffer alone or alkaline phosphatase in sodium phosphate (phosphate inhibits alkaline phosphatase) prior to immunostaining with Mab 147 resulted in no staining of NFT. (*Scale bar*, 20 μm)

Table 2. Effects of alkaline phosphatase treatment on axonal neurofilament and NFT immunostaining by antineurofilament antibodies

Treatment	Antibody	Frozen cerebellum	Frozen hippocampus		Fixed hippocampus	
		NF	NF	NFT	NF	NFT
Untreated	RT97	+	+	+	+	+
	BF10	+	+	+	+	+
	147	+	+	−	+	−
Alkaline phosphatase (100 µg/ml) 2.5 h at 37 °C	RT97	+	↓	↓	↓	↓
	BF10	↓	+	+	+	+
	147	↓	↓↓	−	+	−[a]
Alkaline phosphatase (100 µg/ml) 18.0 h at 37 °C	RT97	↓	↓↓	↓	↓	↓
	BF10	↓	↓[b]	+	↓	+
	147	↓	↓↓	−[a]	↓	−[a]

Histological sections from an ATD brain were treated with alkaline phosphatase (EC 3.1.3.1) under the conditions indicated, followed by immunocytochemical staining with the antineurofilament antibodies shown. The reaction was visualised by Vectastain ABC system. The decreased intensity of staining (↓) was judged relative to the untreated sections.
NF, axonal neurofilament staining; NFT, perikaryal neurofibrillary tangle staining
[a] Small numbers of slightly positive NFT were seen
[b] Decreased intensity of staining was observed after 32 h incubation with alkaline phosphatase

body; the 147 epitope may also be attacked by the enzyme, since only weak staining was obtained with the antibody.

Finally, we have found that, when SDS-insoluble NFT are treated with trypsin, more NFT are stained by monoclonal antibody RT97 (Fig. 6). This suggests that the RT97 epitope is still present in the SDS-insoluble NFT, but is masked. This result is consistent with the observation of Rasool et al. (1984b) that incu-

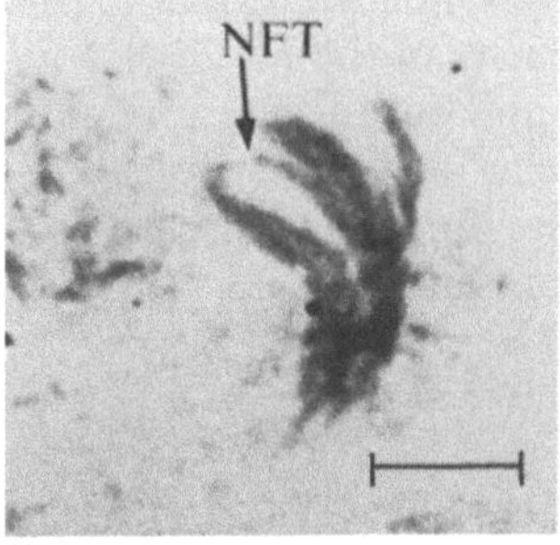

Fig. 6. Immunostaining by Mab RT97 of trypsin-treated SDS-isolated NFT. Aliquots of the SDS-insoluble NFT preparation (Rasool et al. 1984a) were air-dried onto microscope slides. These were incubated with 40 µg/ml trypsin in 50 m*M* TRIS-HCl pH 7.6 containing 0.3 *M* NaCl and 20 m*M* $CaCl_2$ for 10 min at 37 °C, followed by immunostaining with Mab RT97 (ascitic fluid dil 1:500). The reaction was visualised with Vectastain ABC kit. Without the trypsin treatment, only about 5% of the NFT were found to be weakly stained; occasionally, more strongly stained NFT were found. (Results not shown; see Rasool et al. 1984a.) However, after trypsin treatment, many more NFT were found to be strongly stained. (*Scale bar,* 10 µM)

bation of SDS-insoluble NFT in aqueous medium at room temperature for 3 weeks also produces staining by RT97 of larger numbers of SDS-insoluble NFT.

Conclusions

The molecular composition of NFT still remains to be established. However, some progress has been made, and there is now greater interlaboratory agreement over their properties than existed only a few years ago.

Certainly, NFT have unusual solubility properties, and it is now accepted that many are highly insoluble. Further work is required to establish what proportion of NFT in a given case of ATD are insoluble in denaturants as well as whether there is significant variation among cases of ATD in the solubility properties of the NFT. The molecular events which give rise to this insolubility are not at all understood. Transglutaminase-catalysed cross-linking remains a possibility, and neurofilaments are a potential substrate.

Neurofilaments probably contribute to NFT, since there are many independent and corroborative reports that neurofilament antibodies label NFT. However, the neurofilaments are structurally modified and, certainly, some neurofilament ross-reactive epitopes present in NFT are readily extractable from most, but not all NFT. Three observations suggest that additional, hidden neurofilament epitopes are present in NFT: phosphatase-induced staining of occasional NFT in situ by monoclonal antibody 147; trypsin-induced increased staining of SDS-insoluble NFT by monoclonal antibody RT 97; increased staining of SDS-insoluble NFT by RT97 after prolonged incubation in aqueous media. One neurofilament monoclonal antibody, 8D8, still stains SDS-insoluble NFT. Thus, the possibility that the PHF are indeed grossly abnormal neurofilaments deserves further examination. We should not dismiss the possibility that the unique "inherent" epitopes present in the SDS-insoluble PHF core which are the antigens for the anti-PHF antibodies may be determinants generated by the aberrant metabolism of neurofilaments. Finally, a complicating factor is the heterogeneity of the NFT; this appears to apply to the solubility properties and is also apparent in the expression of neurofilament antigenic epitopes. Whether this is due to intrinsic chemical differences or reflects temporal changes as NFT accumulate during the disease progression can only be the subject of speculation for the present.

Acknowledgements. We thank D. J. Selkoe for the gift of rabbit anti-PHF serum.

References

Anderton BH (1981) Intermediate filaments: a family of homologous structures. J Muscle Res Cell Motil 2:141–166

Anderton BH (1982) The neuronal cytoskeleton: proteins and pathology. In: Smith WT, Cavanagh JB (eds) Recent advances in neuropathology, vol 2. Livingstone, Edinburgh, pp 29–51

Anderton BH, Breinburg D, Downes MJ, Green PJ, Tomlinson BE, Ulrich J, Wood JN, Kahn J (1982) Monoclonal antibodies show that neurofibrillary tangles and neurofilaments share antigenic determinants. Nature 298:84–86

Autilio-Gambetti L, Gambetti P, Crane RC (1983) Paired helical filaments: relatedness to neurofilaments shown by silver staining and reactivity with monoclonal antibodies. Banbury reports 15: Biochemical aspects of Alzheimer's disease. Cold Spring Harbour Laboratory, Cold Spring Harbour, pp 117–124

Brion S, Mikol J, Osimaras A (1973) Recent findings in Pick's disease. In: Zimmermann HM (ed) Progress in neuropathology, vol 2. Grune and Stratton, New York, pp 421–452

Chung SI (1972) Comparative studies on tissue transglutaminase and factor XIII. Ann NY Acad Sci 202:240–255

Delacourte A, Filliatreau G, Boutteau F, Biserte G, Schrevel J (1980) Study of the 10 nm filament fraction isolated during the standard microtubule preparation. Biochem J 191:543–546

Elovaara I, Paetau A, Lehto V-P, Dahl D, Virtanen I, Palo J (1983) Immunocytochemical studies of Alzheimer neuronal perikarya with intermediate filament antisera. J Neurol Sci 62:315–326

Forno LS, Strefling AM, Sternberger LA, Sternberger NH, Eng LF (1983) Immunocytochemical staining of neurofibrillary tangles and of the periphery of Lewy bodies with a monoclonal antibody to neurofilaments. J Neuropathol Exp Neurol 42:342

Gambetti P, Velasco ME, Dahl D, Bignami A, Roessmann U, Sindely SP (1980) Alzheimer neurofilament tangles: an immunohistochemical study. In: Amaducci L, Davison AN, Antuono P (eds) Aging of the brain and dementia (aging, vol 13). Raven, New York

Gambetti P, Autilo-Gambetti L, Perry G, Shecket G, Crane RC (1983) Antibodies to neurofibrillary tangles of Alzheimer's disease raised from human and animal neurofilament fractions. Lab Invest 49:430–435

Gonatas NK, Anderson W, Evangelista I (1967) The contribution of altered synapses in the senile plaque: an electron microscope study in Alzheimer's dementia. J Neuropathol Exp Neurol 26:25–39

Grundke-Iqbal K, Johnson AB, Wisniewski HM, Terry RD, Iqbal K (1979) Evidence that Alzheimer neurofibrillary tangles originate from neurotubules. Lancet I:578–580

Grundke-Iqbal K, Iqbal K, Tung Y-C, Wisniewski HM (1984) Alzheimer paired helical filaments: immunochemical identification of polypeptides. Acta Neuropathol 62:259–267

Hirano A, Dembitzeer HM, Kurland LT, Zimmermann HM (1968) The fine structure intraganglionic alterations. Neurofibrillary tangles, granulovacuolar bodies and "rod-like" structures as seen in Guam amyotrophic lateral sclerosis and parkinsonism-dementia complex. J Neuropathol Exp Neurol 27:167–182

Ihara Y, Nukina N, Sugita H, Toyokura Y (1981) Staining of Alzheimer's neurofibrillary tangles with antiserum against 200K components of neurofilament. Proc Jap Acad 57(B):152–156

Ihara Y, Abraham C, Selkoe DJ (1983) Antibodies to paired helical filaments in Alzheimer's disease do not recognise normal brain proteins. Nature 304:727–730

Iqbal K, Wisniewski HM, Shelanski ML, Brostoff S, Liwnicz BH, Terry RD (1974) Protein changes in senile dementia. Brain Res 77:337–343

Iqbal K, Wisniewski HM, Grundke-Iqbal I, Korthals JK, Terry RD (1975) Chemical pathology of neurofibrils. Neurofibrillary tangles of Alzheimer's presenile-senile dementia. J Histochem Cytochem 23:563–569

Iqbal K, Zaidi T, Thompson CH, Merz PA, Wisniewski HM (1984) Alzheimer paired helical filaments: bulk isolation, solubility, and protein composition. Acta Neuropathol 62:167–177

Johnson AB (1984) On the relation of neurofilaments (NF) and Alzheimer neurofibrillary tangles (NFT). J Neuropathol Exp Neurol 43:347

Kahn J, Green PG, Thorpe R, Anderton BH (1980) Immunohistochemistry of neurofilaments in Alzheimer's disease. J Clin Exp Gerontol 2:199–210

Kahn J, King T, Anderton BH, Oyanagi S, Haga S, Ishii T (1984) Immuno-electron microscopy of rat neurofilaments and Alzheimer type neurofibrillary tangles. Neuropathol Appl Neurobiol 10:306

Kidd M (1963) Paired helical filaments in electron microscopy of Alzheimer's disease. Nature 197:192–193

Kidd M (1964) Alzheimer's disease – an electron microscopical study. Brain 87:307–320
Lazarides E (1980) Intermediate filaments as mechanical integrators of cellular space. Nature 283:249–256
Lazarides E (1982) Intermediate filaments: a chemically heterogeneous, developmentally regulated class of proteins. Annu Rev Biochem 51:219–250
Nukina N, Ihara Y (1983) Immunocytochemical study on senile plaques in Alzheimer's disease. I. Preparation of an anti-microtubule-associated proteins (MAPs) antiserum and its specificity. Proc Japan Acad 59B:284–287
Okamoto K, Hirano A, Yamaguchi H, Hirai S (1982) The fine structure of eosinophilic stages of Alzheimer's neurofibrillary tangles. Clin Neurol (Tokyo) 22:840–846
Oyanagi S (1974) On ultrastructure of the aging structure of the brain. Brain Nerve (Tokyo) 26:637–653
Perry G, Rizzuto N, Autilio-Gambetti L, Gambetti P (1984) Ultrastructural localization of cytoskeletal markers on Alzheimer's paired helical filaments. J Neuropathol Exp Neurol 43:346
Probst A, Anderton BH, Ulrich J, Kohler R, Kahn J, Heitz PU (1983) Pick's disease: an immunocytochemical study of neuronal changes. Monoclonal antibodies show that Pick bodies share antigenic determinants with neurofibrillary tangles and neurofilaments. Acta Neuropathol 60:175–182
Rasool CG, Abraham C, Anderton BH, Haugh M, Kahn J, Selkoe DJ (1984a) Alzheimer's disease: immunoreactivity of neurofibrillary tangles with anti-neurofilament and anti-paired helical filament antibodies. Brain Res 310:249–260
Rasool CG, Abraham C, Selkoe DJ (1984b) Alzheimer's disease: exposure of neurofilament immunoreactivity in SDS-insoluble pair helical filaments. Brain Res 322:194–198
Rewcastle NB, Ball CB, Ball MJ (1968) Electron microscopic structure of the "inclusion bodies" in Pick's disease. Neurology 18:1205–1213
Selkoe DJ, Ihara Y, Salazar FJ (1982a) Alzheimer's disease: insolubility of partially purified paired helical filaments in sodium dodecyl sulphate and urea. Science 215:1243–1245
Selkoe DJ, Abraham C, Ihara Y (1982b) Brain transglutaminase: in vitro crosslinking of human neurofilament proteins into insoluble polymers. Proc Natl Acad Sci USA 79:6070–6074
Shibayama H, Kitoh J (1978) Electron microscopic structure of the Alzheimer's neurofibrillary changes in a case of atypical senile dementia. Acta Neuropathol 41:229–234
Sternberger LA, Sternberger NH (1983) Monoclonal antibodies distinguish phosphorylated and nonphosphorylated forms of neurofilaments in situ. Proc Natl Acad Sci USA 80:6126–6130
Terry RD, Gonatas NF, Weiss M (1964) Ultrastructural studies in Alzheimer's presenile dementia. Am J Pathol 44:269–297
Towfighi J (1972) Early Pick's disease. Acta Neuropathol 21:224–231
Wang GP, Grundke-Iqbal I, Kascsak RJ, Iqbal K, Wisniewski HM (1984) Alzheimer neurofibrillary tangles: monoclonal antibodies to inherent antigen(s). Acta Neuropathol 62:268–275
Wisniewski HM, Coblentz J, Terry RD (1972) Pick's disease. A clinical and ultrastructural study. Arch Neurol 26:97–108
Wisniewski HM, Narang HK, Terry RD (1976) Neurofibrillary tangles of paired helical filaments. J Neurol Sci 27:173–181
Wisniewski K, Jervis GA, Moretz RC, Wisniewski HM (1979) Alzheimer neurofibrillary tangles in diseases other than senile dementia and presenile dementia. Ann Neurol 5:288–294
Wood JN, Anderton BH (1981) Monoclonal antibodies to mammalian neurofilaments. Biosci Rep 1:263–268
Yagishita S, Itoh Y, Nan W, Amano N (1981) Reappraisal of the fine structure of Alzheimer's neurofibrillary tangles. Acta Neuropathol 54:239–246
Yen S-H, Gaskin F, Terry RD (1981) Immunocytochemical studies of neurofibrillary tangles. Am J Pathol 104:77–89
Yen S-H, Gaskin F, Fu SM (1983) Neurofibrillary tangles in senile dementia of the Alzheimer type share an antigenic determinant with intermediate filaments of the vimentin class. Am J Pathol 113:373–381

Brain Plasticity and Trophic Factors

Trophic Factors in Brain Aging and Disease*

S. H. Appel, K. Ojika, Y. Tomozawa, and R. Bostwick [1]

Introduction

Success in treating and preventing infection and vascular disease has led to a significant increase in the number of people over the age of 65. This increase in the elderly population has focused attention on normal changes of the aging brain and the chronic disorders that may develop during the aging process. Clearly, such disorders are not inevitable consequences of aging, but they are present to a greater extent in aged individuals. The two common conditions which fall into this category are parkinsonism and Alzheimer's disease. Both of these devastating diseases of the nervous system are degenerative disorders of unknown origin. In each, multiple etiologies, including viral or immunologic causes, have been implicated but never proven. Both conditions reflect pathologic changes in relatively limited pathways within the central nervous system. In Alzheimer's disease and, to a much lesser extent, Parkinson's disease, changes are noted which are known to occur in healthy older individuals. Thus, both conditions may represent accelerated aging of specific neuronal pathways. In order to understand the quantitative alterations in the brain of patients with these disorders, it is necessary to define the extent to which normal individuals demonstrate alterations in the number of neurons, in microscopic pathology, and in neurotransmitter metabolism during the aging process.

Brain Changes During Normal Aging

Numerous studies have suggested that shrinkage of the brain and development of atrophy commonly accompany aging. However, such findings cannot be considered definitive because each of the studies may have several flaws (Katzman and Terry 1983). One of the major problems in conducting such investigations is the large variation in normal brain size. Others include the failure to determine whether the brain may have come from patients with mild dementia or the extent of ventricular enlargement when measurements of cerebral volume are made (Davis and Wright 1977). Brody (1955) demonstrated no increase in cortical thickness of five different brain areas in a 95-year-old individual as compared with younger individuals. Other studies have similarly found no evidence of an age-related de-

* Supported in part by grants from the Harkins Foundation and the Robert J. Kleberg, Jr., and Helen C. Kleberg Foundation

1 Department of Neurology, Baylor College of Medicine, Houston, Texas 77030, USA

Senile Dementia of the Alzheimer Type
Ed. by J. Traber and W. H. Gispen

crease in cortical width (Colon 1973; Henderson et al. 1980). Corsellis suggested that, in the first 50 years, thre is a greater loss of gray matter than white, whereas in the subsequent 50 years, there is a greater loss of white matter than gray. Katzman and Terry (1983) suggest that such findings might be explained by the loss of small cortical neurons before the age of 50 and the loss of large neurons with long myelinated axons after the age of 50. Clearly, more work is needed to document brain shrinkage and atrophy in aging. Perhaps computerized axial tomography and nuclear magnetic resonance imaging of the brain will permit a detailed evaluation of these factors and a more accurate estimate of the extent and location of brain atrophy during the aging process.

In the human brain, neuronal cell loss with increasing age has been well-documented. However, different areas of the brain are by no means uniformly susceptible. In the classic study of Brody comparing brains taken from individuals aged 70–95 years with the brains of individuals aged 16–21 years there was a 68% decrease in neurons of the precentral gyrus, a 51% decrease in neurons of the superior temporal gyrus, and a 66% decrease in visual striate cortex, while no significant decrement was noted in the postcentral gyrus. Brody (1970) noted a 48% neuronal cell loss from the fifth to ninth decade in neurons of the superior frontal gyrus. Henderson et al. (1980) found a similar 40%–50% decrement of both small and large neurons at age 90 as compared with age 20 in all areas, including the postcentral gyrus.

Using cytoarchitectonic areas as a reference point, Colon (1973) noted an overall loss of 44% of neurons in areas 4, 10, 17, and 25 by the eighth decade, as compared with the third decade, while Shefer (1972) noted a 20%–30% loss in area 10 of the frontal polar cortex, area 6 of the premotor cortex, and area 21 of the association cortex in the temporal lobe. These data suggest that neuronal cell loss may be minimal in primary cortices and more extensive in association cortices.

All areas of the hippocampal formation demonstrated age-related neuronal cell loss of approximately 20%–30% (Ball 1977; Dam 1979; Kemper 1984). However, several cranial nerve nuclei maintained neuronal populations throughout the normal life span, while other subcortical, brainstem, and cerebellar loci exhibited highly selective neuronal loss. The age-related neuronal loss in the substantia nigra was approximately 50% by the ninth and tenth decades (McGeer et al. 1977), whereas the age-related neuronal loss in the locus ceruleus was 30%–40% in the eighth to ninth decades as compared with the end of the fifth decade. Within the cerebellum, Purkinje's cell loss increased at a linear rate (Hall et al. 1975), while dentate cell exhibited no evidence of age-related loss (Heidary and Tomasch 1969). Unfortunately, no information is available as to the age-related loss of neurons in the nucleus basalis of Meynert or the medial septal nuclei. Nevertheless, data are available with regard to neurotransmitter-synthetic enzymatic changes accompanying aging which suggest an age-related loss in these nuclei.

Microscopic Lesions

Five specific microscopic lesions are of pertinence both to normal aging and the chronic disorders of aging such as parkinsonism and Alzheimer's disease. These lesions include neurofibrillary tangles, senile or neuritic plaques, granulovacuolar degeneration, Hirano bodies, and corpora amylacea. The incidence of corpora amylacea is not accentuated in disease, but these lesions do appear more frequently as a function of age. They are intra-astrocytic spheroids which appear in the subpial and subependymal region and consist of polysaccharides and proteins (Stam and Roukema 1973).

The neurofibrillary tangle is an intraneuronal fibrillary structure composed of paired helical filaments (PHF) 10 nm in diameter, with a periodic twist every 80 nm (Terry et al. 1964). The structures are best elucidated with silver stains and consist of darkly stained thick bands which become twisted and whorled, displacing the nucleus and distorting the cell body. They are relatively insoluble, perhaps because of their cross-linking (Selkoe et al. 1982). These tangles may be associated with focal deposits of aluminum located within the nuclei of the neurons rather than in the cytoplasmic tangles themseves. The neurofibrillary tangle, although unique to man, is not specific to the aging brain. It is found in Alzheimer's disease, Down's syndrome, Parkinson-dementia complex of Guam, postencephalitic parkinsonism, subacute sclerosing panencephalitis, tuberous sclerosis, Hallervorden-Spatz syndrome, as well as in the "punch-drunk" syndrome (Iqbal et al. 1977). The etiology is unknown. Furthermore, it is unknown whether the neurofibrillary tangle is composed of normal neuronal constituents or a mixture of normal and abnormal constituents. Evidence on the one hand suggests that antibodies to neurofilament proteins may cross-react with neurofibrillary tangles (Dahl et al. 1982; Gambetti et al. 1983), whereas on the other hand (Wang et al. 1984) no reactivity with neurofilament proteins is noted with eight different monoclonal antibodies raised against neurofibrillary tangles. Increasing numbers of neurofibrillary tangles are commonly found in Sommer's sector (CA1) of the hippocampus and in the subiculum and the entorhinal cortex with increasing age. Neurofibrillary tangles are far less common in the neocortex at any age (Kemper 1978). In patients 60 years of age and older, neurofibrillary tangles are a frequent finding, present in the locus ceruleus of almost half the patients (Forno 1969), and in the substantia nigra of 10%.

Senile plaques consist of a spherical mass of degenerating neurites and reactive cells. The typical plaque consists of a central core of amyloid surrounded by reactive astrocytes, microglia, and degenerating neuronal processes. The senile plaque occurs as an age-related change in both animals and man in the neocortex and the hippocampus, with a special predilection for the parahippocampal and fusiform gyri. The nature of the amyloid in senile plaques as well as that found in the vessel of patients with Alzheimer type senile dementia has been a topic of considerable controversy. Immunocytochemical studies have suggested the presence of immunoglobulin L-chains in the corona of the amyloid or within its substance. Other evidence has suggested that the amyloid may be derived from complexes of peptide hormones and a variety of mucopolysaccharides and/or glycoproteins. These constituents may originate in cells which have their origin in the neural crest and have been named amine precursor uptake and decarboxylation (APUD) cells. More recently, the studies of Prusiner et al. (1983) have suggested that amyloid in senile plaques may reflect proteinaceous particles of scrapie virions. If so, scrapie is present in almost all normal, aged individuals. Just as the nature and the derivation of the amyloid in vessels is unknown, the relation of plaque amyloid to the amyloid found in vessel walls is equally uncertain.

Granulovacuolar degeneration is most commonly noted in Sommer's sector of the hippocampus. It consists of an intraneuronal, membrane-bound vesicle with a central, electron-dense granule. It is not unique to either aging or Alzheimer's disease, having been reported in progressive supranuclear palsy, Down's syndrome, tuberous sclerosis, and parkinsonism-dementia complex of Guam. It occurs with increasing concentration and frequency with advancing age.

Another microscopic finding in aged brains is the Hirano body, which consists of an eosinophilic intracytoplasmic inclusion measuring up to 15 μm in diameter. Located predominantly in neurons of Sommer's sector of the hippocampus, it has a crystalline or paracrystalline pattern. It appears with increasing frequently after the sixth decade. A higher incidence of Hirano bodies can occur in Alzheimer's disease, but it has also been noted in other conditions where granulovacuolar degeneration is seen, such as kuru in man and scrapie in mice. Another intraneuronal cytoplasmic eosinophilic inclusion is the Lewy body, which is seen in aged individuals without Parkinson's disease, especially in the locus ceruleus, but also in the substantia nigra or the dorsal motor nucleus of the vagus. In idiopathic parkinsonism, the number of Lewy bodies increases markedly.

Neurotransmitter Metabolism

Wide variation in neurotransmitter levels has been reported to be a function of aging. The possible presence of clinical abnormalities in the brains of the apparently "normal" patients studied may play an important role in accounting for such differences, as well as a number of technical pitfalls, such as length of the interval between death and autopsy. The clinical state of the patient prior to death is, however, perhaps the major cause of variation. Since acetylcholine is rapidly hydrolized in postmortem tissue, levels of this transmitter are unavailable. The enzyme which synthesizes acetylcholine, choline acetyltransfeerase (ChAT), is stable in autopsied brain and has been studied repeatedly. Levels of ChAT have been noted to decrease significantly in the hippocampus and temporal neocortex as a function of age, while remaining stable in the caudate and putamen (Davies 1978). The concentration of dopamine declines with normal aging, at least in the caudate. Furthermore, tyrosine hydroxylase and DOPA decarboxylase decrease with age in the striatum, substantia nigra, and amygdala (McGeer 1978). These changes may well reflect the neuronal loss in the substantia nigra and the locus ceruleus occurring as a function of aging. Monoamine oxidase, on the other hand, has been noted to increase with age (Robinson et al. 1972). However, despite the loss of neurons in the locus ceruleus, Grote et al. (1974), found no change in the enzyme dopamine beta-hydroxylase in the striatum during aging. The effects of aging on serotonin and its synthetic enzymes have not been well studied. Glutamic acid decarboxylase, which synthesizes gamma-aminobutyric acid (GABA), decreases with advancing age, especially in the thalamus, but not in those areas where levels of ChAT and tyrosine hydroxylase diminish.

Theories of Cellular Aging

No acceptable theory is available to explain this nonrandom loss of neurons, the microscopic changes of senile plaques, the amyloid deposition of vessels, the neurotransmitter changes, or the appearance of neurofibrillary tangles, granulovacuolar degeneration, Hirano bodies, and Lewy bodies. Current hypotheses of the cellular basis of aging include the coding of aging in DNA, aging-related alterations in DNA repair, and a progressive degeneration in the accuracy of protein synthesis. In addition, a number of cellular changes caused by exogenous factors may result in an increased number of free radicals, a cross-linkage of macromolecules, or the presence of autoimmune attack. As none of these explanations has been experimentally verified, our search continues. As long as the study of normal cellular aging fails to provide meaningful clues, insight may perhaps come from the study of pathologic alterations which differ quantitatively rather than qualitatively from those characterizing the normal aging process. Alzheimer's disease provides the best example of such changes. However, given the age-related alterations in the dopaminergic system noted above, Parkinson's disease may be considered in a similar way. Thus, an understanding of the molecular changes in neurons occurring in both Alzheimer's disease and parkinsonism may provide significant insight into the mechanism of aging changes in the brains of normal individuals.

Pathologic Brain Changes

Parkinson's Disease

Parkinson's disease is a disorder of older individuals for which the mean age of onset is 67 years. It is characterized by resting tremor, rigidity, akinesia, and a loss of postural reflexes. It may begin insidiously and proceed gradually with tremor and gait changes, ending many years later with severe disability resulting for the most part from progressive akinesia and postural instability. The availability of pharmacologic therapy prolongs the life span of an increasing number of patients, who may develop dementia. The primary pathologic abnormality is neuronal degeneration in the zona compacta of the substantia nigra. Other pathologic changes may occur, including atrophy of the cerebral cortex. Pathologically, Lewy bodies are present in both nigral neurons and in the locus ceruleus in concentrations considerably more dense than those of age-matched brains. The loss of nigral cells leads to a marked impairment of the nigra-striatal pathway and a reduction of the dopaminergic synaptic input to the caudate and putamen. Of importance is the fact that little diminution is noted in the dopaminergic receptors within the striatum, thus suggesting that the presynaptic neuron is impaired while the postsynaptic neuron remains intact. Although high concentrations of Lewy bodies are present in pigmented nuclei, they may also be found in nonpigmented nuclei, predominantly in monoaminergic cell bodies such as the peripheral autonomic ganglia. The etiology of this disorder is unknown.

Alzheimer's Disease

Alzheimer's disease is a disorder of the later decades of life characterized by diffuse deterioration of mental function, primarily in thought and memory and secondarily in feeling and conduct. The diagnosis depends on ruling out such secondary causes of loss of memory and impaired cognitive function as depression, multiple infarcts, intracranial mass lesions, infections, or toxic and metabolic disorders. However, even when such secondary causes are ruled out, the clinical symptoms of the remaining patients do not comprise a discrete homogenous entity. As a result, it is difficult to understand how any single process could cause such devastation and leave as few clues.

The brains of patients with Alzheimer's disease and senile dementia of the Alzheimer type are characterized by a profusion of senile plaques, neurofibrillary tangles, granulovacuolar degeneration, and Hirano bodies. No single one of these features is specific to Alzheimer's disease, but their presence is vastly increased in Alzheimer's disease as compared with age-matched controls. In patients with both senile dementia and Alzheimer's disease, there is a more significant loss of neurons than in age-matched controls. In addition, there is extensive compromise of neurons in the nucleus basalis of Meynert (Whitehouse et al. 1982), in the diagonal band of Broca, and to a lesser extent, in the medial septal nucleus. All of these constitute a basal forebrain cholinergic system with widespread projections to the amygdala, hippocampus, and cortex. Thus, patients with either presenile Alzheimer's disease or senile dementia of the Alzheimer type undergo neuronal losses in numbers that are several times higher than those noted in the same areas of normal brains belonging to age-matched controls. In the case of the amygdala, the neuronal loss of Alzheimer's disease occurs in areas that fail to show age-related cell losses. In Alzheimer's disease, the density of neurofibrillary tangles from primary cortices to the respective primary and secondary association cortices increases progressively; neurofibrillary tangles are most prevalent in the multimodal association area, which is reciprocally related to the limbic neocortex and to the hippocampal complex.

Biochemical changes in the brains of patients with Alzheimer's disease are quite distinct most important ones being a reduction in ChAT and acetyl cholinesterase and a decrease in the synthesis of acetylcholine. These biochemical data suggest a major loss of cholinergic nerve terminals in the cerebral cortex and the hippocampus and correlate with the degeneration of cholinergic neurons in the nucleus basalis. Of interest is the fact that cholinergic receptors in the cortex and hippocampus are normal. Thus, the primary defect appears to involve the presynaptic neurons, leaving the postsynaptic cell relatively intact.

Transmitter depletion is not confined to acetylcholine or the enzymes that synthesize or degrade acetylcholine. A diminution in serotonin uptake has been reported in biopsied cerebral cortex (Bowen 1983), where approximately 70% depletion was noted, with comparatively little change in imipramine binding or indoleamines (Bowen 1983). In selected Alzheimer patients, especially those with degeneration of the substantia nigra and extrapyramidal tract signs, concentrations of dopamine and dopamine metabolites may be decreased. However, when Alzheimer patients show no involvement of the substantia nigra, then no alterations in dopaminergic metabolites are noted (Yates et al. 1978). A significant reduction in the concentration of norepinephrine in patients with senile dementia was reported by Adolfsson et al. (1979), while a 40% reduction of dopamine-beta-hydroxylase activity was found in the cerebral cortex of patients with senile dementia of the Alzheimer type (Cross 1981). Both of these observations may relate to a loss of about 80% of the locus ceruleus neurons observed in a select group of patients with Alzheimer's disease. This group is predominantly female and of a younger mean age at death than patients afflicted with senile dementia of the Alzheimer type who show less depopulation of neurons in structure (Bonderaff et al. 1982).

The fact that neurotransmitter alterations vary in different Alzheimer's disease populations has raised considerable doubt about the primacy of the cholinergic changes. However, number of factors reinforce the importance of the cholinergic system: (a) the ability of inhibitors of the cholinergic network to impair performance in healthy young adults, (b) the similarity of memory impairment noted for both healthy aged individuals and those with senile dementia of the Alzheimer type (Drachman 1983), (c) the normal age-dependent depletion of cholinergic metabolic activity (Davies 1978), (d) the depletion of acetylcholine synthesis in the early stages of Alzheimer's disease (Bowen 1983), and (e) the marked alteration in cholinergic activity throughout the spectrum of Alzheimer's disease. In contrast, evidence supporting the primacy of other neurotransmitter-specific networks is far less compelling. When adrenergic drugs of dopaminergic agonists and antagonists are administered, they do not influence Alzheimer's symptomatology. The hallmark of Alzheimer's disease, namely impairment of memory, is not characteristic of the manipulation of the dopaminergic, noradrenergic, serotonergic, or gabaergic systems. However, it is of interest that manipulation of the noradrenergic system does have an effect on long-term potentiation, a hippocampal synaptic model of memory (Hopkins and Johnson 1984).

Neuropeptides have also been extensively examined in Alzheimer's disease, although their role in the normal aging process has not been investigated to the same extent. Of all the neuropeptides examined to date, only somatostatin appears to undergo significant change in Alzheimer's disease (Davies et al. 1980). Unlike cholinergic activity, which is largely derived from neurons projecting from the subcortex and the nucleus basalis of Meynert to the cortex or from the medial septal region to the hippocampus, somatostatin is unaffected by lesions in the subcortical areas. Thus, somatostatin is likely to be present in intrinsic cortical and hippocampal neurons. None of the other peptides present in large numbers of cortical and hippocampal neurons, such as cholecystokinin or vasoactive intestinal peptide, are altered in Alzheimer's disease.

Etiology of Parkinson's Disease and Alzheimer's Disease

The pathologic expression of both Alzheimer's disease and parkinsonism is a marked increase in age-related changes beyond what is normally seen in the brain of any aged individual. Thus, these two disorders are not simply an acceleration of aging, but reflect specific disease processes. Nevertheless, one cannot exclude the possibility that both normal aging and these two degenerative diseases of the nervous system are based on a common denominator. Our understanding of degenerative disease has led to the insight that both the changes in aging and in disease may result from alterations in limited pathways. Thus, abnormalities in cholinergic, dopaminergic, noradrenergic, and possibly even serotonergic projections may give rise to diffuse dysfunction. The viability of each of these projection systems may depend upon retrogressive neurotrophic factors (Appel 1981). Thus, an impairment in retrograde trophic effects from the striatum may alter the presynaptic neurons of the substantia nigra. In normal aging, there would be a gradual depletion of such hormones and subsequent loss of dopaminergic input to the striatum. With disease, there would be an accentuation of this retrograde trophic factor loss, either through toxic factors, immunologic attack against the neurotrophic factors or their receptors, or other mechanisms. The common denominator would be a diminution in retrograde trophic function, with different etiologic factors giving rise to the heterogeneous clinical expression of parkinsonism.

Similar impairment in retrograde trophic effects could explain the gradual depletion of cholinergic activity in normal aging and the marked aggravation of this process in senile dementia of the Alzheimer type. A number of disease processes, including antibodies directed against specific cholinergic neurotrophic factors or their receptors, toxins, viruses, or other agents would be responsible for such impairment in different cases. Similarly, in young patients with Alzheimer's disease, impairment of the retrograde trophic effects may be present in several systems, including the dopaminergic, noradrenergic, serotonergic, and cholinergic systems. Thus, the normal aging process would be associated with an age-related depletion of specific neurotrophic factors, together with nonrandom loss of neurons, altered neuronal morphology, and specific neurotransmitter changes. Alzheimer's disease would be associated with a marked depletion of trophic effects due to a specific disease process such as immune attack.

Trophic Factors

The most cogent support for the existence of trophic factors comes from recent advances in developmental neurobiology which document the importance of target cells for the survival, growth, and differentiation of innervating neurons. In the peripheral autonomic nervous system, nerve growth factor (NGF) can be demonstrated to influence neuronal viability and maturation in vivo and in vitro (Bradshaw 1978). Although in vivo demonstrations of the retrograde effect on the motor system or in other central nervous system pathways are not available, Hamburger's experiments on the chick lumbar cord motor neuron survival are plausibly explained by the availability of muscle-derived retrograde neurotrophic effects (Holliday and Hamburger 1976). If the chick limb is removed in ovo, motor neuron death is enhanced; if a limb is added, diminution in cell death results. Studies by Oppenheim and his colleagues suggest the diminution in muscle activity or blockade of the muscle nicotonic acetylcholine receptor would also decrease motor neuron cell death (Pittman and Oppenheim 1978).

Within the central nervous system, the phenomenon of retrograde transneuronal degeneration (Torch et al. 1977) provides circumstantial evidence for the existence of retrograde trophic factors. Such retrograde degeneration is noted in the limbic system, i.e., in the medial mamillary nucleus of the ventral tegmental nucleus, following lesions of the limbic cortex or cerebral cortex (Cowan 1970). It also has been demonstrated in pyramidal cells of the precentral cortex following limb amputation or in the inferior olivary nucleus following damage to cerebral or Purkinje's cells. Lesions of the occipital visual cortex have been noted to give rise to changes in retinalganglion cells, optic nerve, and lateral geniculate bodies, presumably secondary to retrograde transneuronal degeneration. Such a process may take from days to several years in experimental animals.

Neurotrophic Effects in the Nigral-Striatal System

Our laboratory has examined the effect of striatal extracts on substantia nigra tissue in culture as a means of monitoring and purifying neurotrophic factors. Both explant and dissociation cultures are obtained from 14-day old rat embryos at a time when the mesencephalic dopaminergic neurons are postmitotic, but have not yet innervated their striatal target. Explants can be cultured in Sato's defined media (Bottenstein and Sato 1979) or in 4% heat-inactivated horse serum and monitored for several weeks. The dopaminergic activity monitored by ^{3}H-dopamine uptake of dissociated mesencephalic neurons is enhanced by coculturing with striatum. Furthermore, activity can be enhanced by membrane fractions of corpus striatum or by heat-inactivated horse serum. The ability of striatal membrane constituents to enhance dopaminergic activity was previously reported by Prochiantz et al. (1979, 1981). Our own studies demonstrate that soluble striatal factors, predominantly peptides smaller than 2,000 daltons, may also enhance survival of dopaminergic neurons in culture and may enhance neurite density, the uptake of ^{3}H dopamine, and the appearance of positive histofluorescence for dopamine. Other tissues, such as skeletal muscle and liver and cerebellum, do not appear to have a similar effect on dopaminergic activity of mesencephalic cultures.

Neurothrophic Effects in the Septal-Hippocampal System

As a means of monitoring the effect of trophic factors in a central cholinergic system, we have cultured medial septum tissue and assayed morphological and cholinergic-enhancing effects of hippocampal extracts. Explants of medial septal tissues are obtained from the brains of 16-day embryonic albino Sprague-Dawley rats. Explants are grown either in Sato's defined media or in inactivated horse serum. Sato's defined media require hippocampal membranes to document an effect of hippocampal supernatant on cholinergic activity. However, serum can substitute for the membrane component in vitro, leaving the stimulating effect of hippocampal supernatant intact. The addition of hippocampal supernatant results in a substantial increase in the length and density of neuritic outgrowth after 3 days in vitro. Within the same period, both acetylcholine synthesis and choline acetyltransferase activity are enhanced, a state which continues for at least 8 days, by which time a three- to fourfold increase is noted (Ojika and Appel 1984). Other types of tissues, such as cerebellum, spinal cord, muscle, liver, and kidney, do not produce the same effect. NGF cannot reproduce the effects of hippocampal extract, nor can antibodies to NGF diminish its activity. The supernatant activity resides primarily in a peptide fraction of less than 2,000 daltons. Cholecystokinin, vasoactive intestinal peptide, and somatostatin have no effects on the morphological or cholinergic activities of cultured medial septal neurons.

Discussion

The cause of gradual depletion of neurons within the brain; the appearance of senile plaques, neurofibrillary tangles, Hirano bodies, and granulovacuolar degeneration; and the loss of neurotransmitters is unknown. Our own thesis is that, in both normal aging and diseases such as parkinsonism and Alzheimer's disease, there is a loss of neurotrophic hormones elaborated or stored in the synaptic target of the affected neurons land exerting a specific retrograde effect. These neurotrophic hormones are of vital importance to the survival of neurons during development, and their absence results in an increase in cell death during this period. Further depletion of "developmental" or "maintenance" neurotrophic hormones during the aging process could result in the brain changes noted above. Any process which depletes neurotrophic hormones or interferes with their retrograde action on presynaptic receptors may result in gradual neuronal failure. A depletion of factors may accompany normal aging and result in gradual neuronal loss. A more specific process associated with either autoimmunity against the neurotrophic factors or their receptors or with other toxins could cause a catastrophic depletion with significant clinical devastation. Both Parkinson's disease and Alzheimer's disease would then be formally analogous to such major endocrinopathies as thyroiditis, juvenile diabetes, and Addison's disease. In juvenile diabetes, for example, antibodies against insulin or the insulin receptor may be a major cause of lifelong clinical disability. Similar immunologic alterations would give rise to Hashimoto's struma. In addition, inborn errors of metabolism, nutritional deficiencies, or other etiologies can give rise to a depletion of thyroid hormone. The common denominator is a depletion of the hormone or the inability of hormone to react with its receptor, such as that caused by antireceptor antibodies in diabetes and resulting in altered receptor function.

The primary difference between conventional, well-known neurotransmitters and neurotrophic factors is the fact that the latter probably exert their effects over periods ranging from weeks to months rather than over shorter intervals. Thus, the nervous system not only seems to possess the capacity for intercellular communication over short periods, but also appears to retain the important long-term anterograde and retrograde intercellular communication characteristic of the endocrine system. The changes associated with both normal aging and the devastations noted in Alzheimer's disease and parkinsonsim may occur for periods ranging from many months to many years prior to the onset of clinical manifestations and be attributable to a lengthy process such as immune attack.

At the present time data to prove our hypothesis are insufficient. However, the explosion of information increasing our understanding of trophic factors and their intercellular effects may permit an adequate test of this hypothesis in the near future.

References

Adolfsson R, Gottfries CG, Roos BE (1979) Changes in the brain catecholamines in patients with dementia of Alzheimer type. Br J Psychiatry 135:216–223

Appel SH (1981) A unifying hypothesis for the cause of amyotrophic lateral sclerosis, parkinsonism and Alzheimer's disease. Ann Neurol 10:499

Ball MJ (1977) Neuronal loss, neurofibrillary tangles and granulovacuolar degeneration in the hippocampus with aging and dementia. Acta Neuropathol 37:111–118

Bondareff W, Mountjoy CQ, Roth M (1982) Loss of neurons of origin of the adrenergic projection to cerebral cortex (*nucleus locus ceruleus*) in senile dementia. Neurology 32:164

Bottenstein JE, Sato GH (1979) Growth of a rat neuroblastoma cell line in serum-free supplemented medium. PNAS 76:514–517

Bowen DM (1983) Biochemical assessment of neurotransmitter and metabolic dysfunction and cerebral atrophy in Alzheimer's disease. In: Katzman R (ed) Banbury report 15, biological aspects of Alzheimer's disease. Coldspring Harbor, New York, pp 219

Bradshaw RA (1978) Nerve growth factor. Annu Rev Biochem 47:191

Brody H (1955) Organization of the cerebral cortex. III. A study of aging in the human cerebral cortex. J Comp Neurol 102:511

Brody H (1970) Structural changes in the aging nervous system. In: Blumenthal HT (ed) Regulating role of the nervous system in aging. Karger, Basel (Interdisciplinary topics in gerontology, vol 7

Colon EJ (1973) The cerebral cortex in presenile dementia – a quantitative analysis. Acta Neuropathol 23:281–290

Cowan WM (1970) Anterograde and retrograde transneuronal degeneration in the central and peripheral nervous system. In: Nauta WJ, Ebbson SD (eds) Contemporary research methods in neuroanatomy. Springer, Berlin Heidelberg New York, p 217

Cross AJ, Crow TJ, Perry EK, Perry RH, Blessed G, Tomlinson BE (1981) Reduced dopamine beta-hydroxylase of Alzheimer's disease. Br Med J 282:93–94

Dahl D, Selkoe DJ, Poro RT, Bignami A (1982) Immunostaining of neurofibrillary tangles in Alzheimer's senile dementia with neurofilament anti-sera. J Neurosci 2:113–119

Dam AM (1979) The density of neurons in the human hippocampus. Neuropathol Appl Neurobiol 5:249–264

Davies P (1978) Loss of choline acetyltransferase activity in normal aging and in senile dementia. Adv Exp Med Biol 113:251

Davies P, Katzman R, Terry RD (1980) Reduced somatostatin-like immunoreactivity in cerebral cortex from cases of Alzheimer's disease and Alzheimer's senile dementia. Nature 288:279–280

Davis PJM, Wright EA (1977) A new method for measuring cranial cavity volume and its application to the assessment of cerebral atrophy at autopsy. Neuropathol Appl Neurobiol 3:341

Drachman DA (1983) Aging and dementia: insights from the study of anti-cholinergic drugs. In: Katzman R (ed) Banbury report 15, biological aspects of Alzheimer's disease. Coldspring Harbor, New York, p 363

Forno LS (1969) Concentric hyalin intraneuronal inclusions of Lewy type in the brains of elderly persons (50 incidental cases): relationship to parkinsonism. J Am Geriatr Soc 17:557–575

Gambetti P, Autilio-Gambetti L, Perry GG, Shecket G, Crane RC (1983) Antibodies to neurofibrillary tangles of Alzheimer's disease raised from human and animal neurofilament fractions. Lab Invest 49:430–435

Grote SS, Moses SG, Robins E, Hudgens RW, Croninger AB (1974) A study of selected catecholamine-metabolizing enzymes: a comparison of depressive suicides and alcoholic suicides with controls. J Neurochem 23:791–802

Hall TC, Miller AKH, Corsellis JAN (1975) Variation in human Purkinje cell population according to age and sex. Neuropathol Appl Neurobiol 1:267–292

Heidary H, Tomasch J (1969) Neuron numbers in perikaryon areas in the human cerebral nuclei. Acta Anat 74:290–296

Henderson G, Tomlinson BE, Gibson PH (1980) Cell counts in human cerebral cortex in normal adults throughout life using an image-analyzing computer. J Neurol Sci 46:113-136

Hollyday M, Hamburger V (1976) Reduction of the naturally occurring motor neuron loss by enlargement of the periphery. J Comp Neurol 170:311–320

Hopkins WF, Johnston D (1984) Frequency-dependent noradrenergic modulation of long-term potentiation in the hippocampus. Science 226:350–352

Iqbal K, Wisniewski HM, Grundke-Iqbal I, Terry RD (1977) Neurofibrillary pathology: an update. In: Nandy K, Sherwin I (eds) The aging brain in senile dementia. Plenum, New York

Katzman R, Terry RD (1983) The neurology of aging. Davis, Philadelphia

Kemper K (1984) Neuroanatomical and neuropoathological changes in normal aging and in dementia. In: Albert ML (ed) Clinical neurology of aging. Oxford University Press, Oxford, pp 9–52

Kemper T (1978) Senile dementia: a focal disease in the temporal lobe. In: Nandy K (ed) Senile dementia: a biochemical approach. Elsevier, New York, pp 105–113

McGeer EG (1978) Aging and neurotransmitter metabolism in human brain. In: Katzman R, Terry RD, Bick KL (eds), Alzheimer's disease: senile dementia and related disorders. Raven, New York, pp 427–440

McGeer PL, McGeer EG, Suzuki PS (1977) Aging in extrapyramidal function. Arch Neurol 34:33–35

Ojika K, Appel SH (1984) Neurotrophic effects of hippocampal extracts on medial septal nucleus in vitro. PNAS 81:2567–2571

Pittman R, Oppenheim R (1978) Neuromuscular blockading increases motor neuron survival during normal cell death in the chick embryo. Nature 271:364

Prochiantz A, di Porzio, Kato A, Berger B, Glowinski J (1979) In vitro maturation of mesencephalic dopaminergic neurons from mice embryos is enhanced in the presence of their striatal target cells. PNAS 76:5387–5391

Prochiantz A, Daquet M-C, Herbet A, Glowinski J (1981) Specific stimulation of in vitro maturation of mesencephalic dopaminergic neurones by striatal membranes. Nature 293:570–572

Prusiner SB, McKinley MP, Bowman KA, Bolton DC, Bendheim PE, Groth DS, Glenner GG (1983) Scrapie prions aggregate to form amyloid-like birefringent rods. Cell 35:349–358

Robinson DS, Nies A, Davis JN, Bunney WE, Davis JM, Colburn RW, Bourne HR, Shaw DM, Coppen AJ (1972) Aging, monoamines and monoamine oxidase levels. Lancet 1:290–291

Selkoe DJ, Ihara Y, Salazar FJ (1982) Alzheimer's disease: an insolubility of partially purified paired helical filaments in sodium dodecyl sulfate and urea. Science 215:1243–1245

Shefer VF (1972) Absolute number of neurons and thickness of the cerebral cortex during aging, senile and vascular dementia and Pick's and Alzheimer's disease. Zh Nevropat Psikhiatr Korsakov 72:1024–1029

Stam FC, Roukema PA (1973) Histochemical and biochemical aspects of *corpora amylacea*. Acta Neuropathol 25:95

Terry RD, Gonatas NK, Weiss M (1964) Ultrastructural studies in Alzheimer's presenile dementia. Am J Pathol 44:269–281

Torch WC, Hirano A, Solomon S (1977) Anterograde transneuronal degeneration in the limbic system: clinical-anatomic correlation. Neurology 27:1157
Wang GP, Grundke-Iqbal I, Kascsak RJ, Iqbal I (1984) Alzheimer neurofibrillary tangles: Monoclonal antibodies to inherent antigens. Acta Neuropathol 62:268–275
Whitehouse PO, Price DL, Struble RG, Clark AW, Coyle JT, Delon MR (1982) Alzheimer's disease and senile dementia: Loss of neurons in the basal forebrain. Science 215:1237
Yates CM, Allison Y, Simpson J, Malone AF, Gordon A (1978) Dopamine in Alzheimer's disease and senile dementia. Lancet 2:851

Melanocortin Peptides and Neural Plasticity

P. M. EDWARDS and W. H. GISPEN[1]

Introduction

The term melanocortin peptides is used to describe peptides related to the pituitary hormones, adrenocorticotrophic hormone (ACTH) and melanophore-stimulating hormones (α- and β-MSH). The amino acid sequences of these hormones, together with other biologically active peptides such as β-endorphin, are contained within a common precursor, proopiomelanocortin (POMC) (Fig. 1).

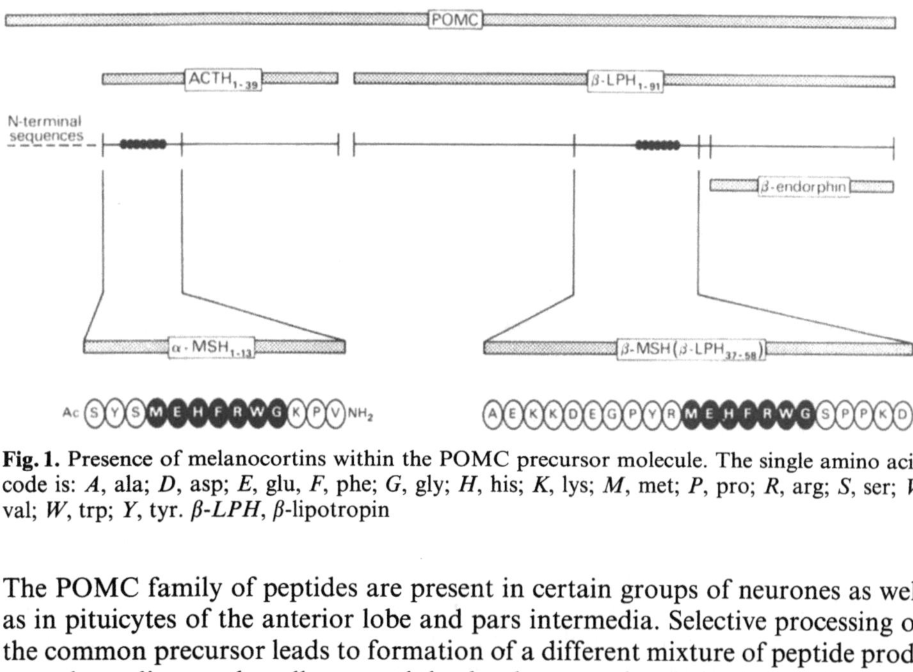

Fig. 1. Presence of melanocortins within the POMC precursor molecule. The single amino acid code is: *A*, ala; *D*, asp; *E*, glu, *F*, phe; *G*, gly; *H*, his; *K*, lys; *M*, met; *P*, pro; *R*, arg; *S*, ser; *V*, val; *W*, trp; *Y*, tyr. *β-LPH*, β-lipotropin

The POMC family of peptides are present in certain groups of neurones as well as in pituicytes of the anterior lobe and pars intermedia. Selective processing of the common precursor leads to formation of a different mixture of peptide products, depending on the cell type and the developmental and physiological state of the animal.

The influence of melanocortin peptides on neuronal function was first suggested from observation of the effects of pituitary removal coupled with melanocortin hormone replacement therapy. Melanocortin hormones have been shown to enhance performance in behavioural tests requiring learning and memory (De

1 Division of Molecular Neurobiology, Rudolf Magnus Institute for Pharmacology and Departm. of Physiological Chemistry, Institute of Molecular Biology Padualaan 8, 3584 CH Utrecht, The Netherlands

Senile Dementia of the Alzheimer Type
Ed. by J. Traber and W. H. Gispen

Wied and Jolles 1982), regenerative ability following axon damage (Bijlsma et al. 1984), impulse transmission at the neuromuscular junction (Strand and Smith 1980), brain protein synthesis (Dunn and Schotman 1981), and foetal brain development (Swaab and Martin 1981). The spectrum of melanocortin actions suggests that such peptides may possess neurotrophic activity and be involved in interactions between neurones and their postsynaptic targets.

Neural plasticity, the ability of the nervous system to modify the coupling between input and output signals, implies both alteration in the efficiency of impulse transmission across existing synapses and the growth and formation of new synapses. Melanocortin peptides appear to possess the attributes of putative agents involved in both types of plastic alterations. The mediation of both short-term functional effects and long-term trophic influences by a single agent is observed in the effects of many peptide hormones on their peripheral target cells.

In considering the role of melanocortin peptides on neural plasticity, emphasis is placed here on the trophic actions. Further, the significance of peptides derived from sources other than the pituitary and the POMC precursor is explored.

Effects of Melanocortins on Developing Nerves

There have been few studies on the influence of melanocortins on the developing central nervous system. Swaab and Martin (1981) indicated that MSH is physiologically important in normal foetal development and has a trophic influence on several organs, including the brain. Neonatal peptide treatment also accelerates eye-opening (Van der Helm-Hylkema and De Wied 1976) and alters certain adult behavioural parameters (Beckwith et al. 1977). Trophic actions of ACTH on cultured embryonic chick cortical cells have been reported (Daval et al. 1983), but we have been unable to demonstrate such effects in a variety of tissue culture systems (P. M. Edwards and M. Schmidt 1984, unpublished observations).

The developing neuromuscular junction is sensitive to two distinct classes of POMC-derived peptides, melanocortins and β-endorphin. β-Endorphin has been shown to be present in immature, but not adult, motor neurones (Haynes et al. 1982). This peptide inhibits the catalytic activity of the junction-specific 16S form of muscle acetylcholinesterase (AChE) and exerts more complex modulations of the synthesis and distribution of this enzyme (Haynes et al. 1984). The timing of β-endorphin expression and its action on the muscle AChE suggest a physiological role in the function of the immature neuromuscular junction (Haynes and Smith 1984). Electrophysiological studies have shown that the immature neuromuscular junction is highly sensitive to melanocortins (Smith and Strand 1981). The observed increase in amplitude of muscle contraction and delay in the onset of fatigue were suggested to be predominantly of neurogenic origin. The combined effects of β-endorphin on muscle AChE and melanotropins on the nerve terminal would serve to facilitate neuromuscular transmission, and this could have implications for the stabilisation of newly formed synaptic contacts (Haynes and Smith 1984).

Effects of Melanocortins on Regeneration

Peripheral Nervous System

Crush lesion of the rat sciatic nerve results in degeneration of the distal portion of the nerve and loss of sensory and motor functions in the hind paw. Re-establishment of normal function, assessed experimentally by toe-spreading or a foot-flick reflex, is dependent on the regenerative outgrowth of axons from the damaged nerve and the formation of synaptic connections with appropriate target muscle and sensory receptor cells. Treatment of rats with melanocortin peptides accelerates the return of normal function in this experimental model (Bijlsma et al. 1984; Strand and Kung 1980). Studies on the potency of different peptide structures (Bijlsma et al. 1983 b) and in adrenalectomised rats (Strand and Kung 1980) showed that the peptide effect is independent of anti-inflammatory and corticotrophic actions.

Faster recovery from sciatic nerve crush is only observed in rats treated with peptides during the first week following the lesion (Fig. 2), the period during which the outgrowth of axons is initiated. Later treatment, during the period of synaptogenesis, does not accelerate the return of the foot-flick response. The critical period for effective treatment suggests that melanocortins are involved in the initial regenerative sprouting response to injury. This is corroborated by histological demonstration of a larger number of regenerating fibres in melanocortin-treated rats, which is most marked at early times after the lesion (Bijlsma et al. 1983 a). Measurement of the numbers of regenerating fibres at different distances along the nerve and times after the lesion indicated that melanocortins alter the sprouting response rather than the rate of fibre outgrowth.

In addition to the early effects on the number of regenerating axons, continuous treatment with melanocortins results in other modulations of the repair pro-

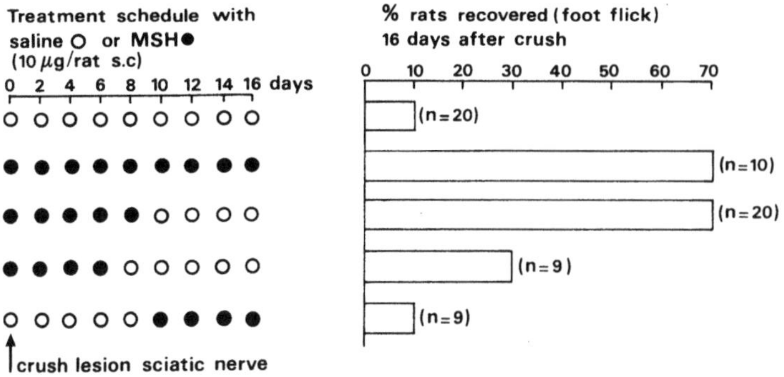

Fig. 2. Acceleration of recovery of sensorimotor function by early α-MSH treatment. Return of sensorimotor function was judged by the reappearance of reflex withdrawal of the hind paw from a hot-air stimulus. Tests were performed on alternate days prior to peptide dosing. All rats were recovered on day 24. Analysis of variance, followed by a supplemental *t*-test, on the time course of recovery indicated a significant difference ($P<0.05$) between the saline group and all day-0–commencing MSH groups

cess. The postrecovery decrease in sciatic nerve fibres (related to degeneration of axons that either failed to make synaptic connections or lost their connections during the elimination of polyinnervation of muscle fibres) is prevented by melanocortin treatment (Bijlsma et al. 1983 a). Such peptides also have a beneficial effect on the pattern of muscle innervation and on nerve-muscle transmission during regeneration of motor performance (Strand and Kung 1980; Saint-Côme et al. 1982).

These late peptide effects were all observed in rats that had been treated with melanocortins from the time of the initial axon lesion. They could be consequential to early peptide actions, either on the sprouting response as described above or on the loss of central dendritic connections, a rapid reaction to sciatic nerve crush which has not been studied in melanocortin-treated animals. However, the foot-flick parameter used to demonstrate the early critical period of melanocortin sensitivity would not have measured the subtle changes that might be expected from alterations in the patterns of synaptic connectivity. Melanocortins may also be exerting late effects either by direct trophic actions analogous to the early sprouting stimulation or secondary to effects on synaptic efficiency. Gonzalez and Strand (1981) have demonstrated that, in hypophysectomised adult rats, melanocortins modify neuromuscular transmission (an effect on neural plasticity of the short-term functional type).

Central Nervous System (CNS)

The regenerative capacity of the central nervous system is very poor compared with that of the peripheral nervous system. Early studies on the effect of melanocortins on recovery from CNS lesions gave conflicting results (Berry et al. 1979). The access of peripherally administered peptides to the site of injury may be limited by the blood-brain barrier (Wilson et al. 1984) and the degree of vascular alterations caused by the injury. Peptides with full endocrine activity were used, since the rationale behind the treatment was reduction of reactive scar tissue believed to limit CNS regeneration. Studies on the peripheral nervous system have subsequently shown that the immunosuppressant and corticotrophic activities of these peptides are not involved in the trophic response and may have disturbed the final outcome. More recent studies, using a noncorticotrophic peptide analogue, have indicated a beneficial effect on behavioural parameters during recovery from septal lesions (Isaacson and Poplawsky 1983). However, it is not yet possible to say whether these effects are due to a trophic action on regenerative processes, such as are observed in the peripheral nervous system. In a histological study of CNS regeneration, Fertig et al. (1971) found that treatment with ACTH during the first week following injury was as effective as long-term treatment in increasing the number of regenerating fibres. This suggests that mechanisms of peptide action in the CNS are analogous to those occurring in the peripheral nervous system.

Physiologic Source of Neurotrophic Melanocortins

Tissue Source

Experimental evidence has shown that circulating peptides, derived either from the pituitary or injected into the animal, can modify nerve outgrowth and synaptic efficiency. Pituitary peptides may be important in providing a maintenance level of trophic support and in facilitating plastic mechanisms as part of a general response to stress. In the immature nervous system, melanocortins derived from neuronally synthesised POMC may be an important additional source of trophic melanocortins. The transient expression of POMC-derived peptides at certain periods of development in motor nerves is an indication of the physiological significance of this source of peptides (Haynes and Smith 1984). The POMC peptides are not present in mature peripheral nerves and have been shown in only a restricted number of central nerves in adult animals.

Functionally relevant neurotrophic actions in the mature nervous system would be predicted to involve agents generated close to the sensitive targets and in response to appropriate stimuli (nerve damage or persistent synaptic activation). Circulating peptides are unlikely to have other than a permissive role in such processes. Damage to nerves in the central and peripheral nervous system leads to a reactive, localised sprouting response. Trophic factors that can enhance cell survival and stimulate outgrowth in vivo and in tissue culture are formed at injury sites in both central and peripheral nerve tissue (Politis and Spencer 1983; Schonfeld et al. 1984; Nieto-Sampedro et al. 1984). Extracts of degenerating peripheral nerve contain a peptidergic neurotrophic agent that stimulates and directs peripheral nerve outgrowth in vivo (Politis and Spencer 1983). Such extracts also contain an agent that causes melanophore dispersion in an in vitro bioassay, suggesting the presence of MSH-like activity (Edwards et al. 1984a). Extracts of control, nondegenerating, nerves do not contain either neurotrophic (Politis and Spencer 1983) or detectable melanotropic (Edwards et al. 1984a) activity. These observations suggest that MSH-like peptides may be generated in the region of nerve damage and contribute to the physiological stimulus leading to local sprouting.

Polypeptide Source

The POMC precursor is not normally present in adult peripheral nerves and, although there is some evidence that the POMC peptides may be re-expressed in damaged nerves (M. E. Smith and L. W. Haynes 1984, personal communication), it seems unlikely that they would be formed in distal axons traumatically separated from the nerve cell body.

Studies with anti-MSH antisera have revealed that the neurofilament (NF) proteins constitute a potential source of MSH-like peptide fragments. Dräger et al. (1983) originally demonstrated that an antiserum to α-MSH reacted with neurofilaments in tissue sections and with one, referred to here as NF150 because of its approximate mobility in sodium dodecyl sulphate (SDS) gels, of the triplet NF proteins separated on SDS gels. We have confirmed the cross-reactivity of anti-α-MSH serum with NF150 using two-dimensional separation combined with immunoblotting (Edwards et al. 1984b).

The whole of the MSH sequence is probably not represented in the NF150 sequence, since only a minority of MSH antisera cross-react with the protein (J. Verhaagen et al. 1984, unpublished observations). However, absorption with different peptide fragments have shown that NF150–cross-reacting sera recognise sequences within the 1–10 region of ACTH that has been shown to be responsible for the neurotrophic actions of ACTH (J. Verhaagen et al. 1984, unpublished observations; Bijlsma et al. 1983b).

Breakdown of the ultrastructurally recognisable neurofilaments and selective proteolytic cleavage of the constituent proteins are well-known early events in peripheral axon degeneration (Schlaepfer and Micko 1978; Schlaepfer et al. 1984). Interestingly, these processes are much slower and less complete in central nerves (Bignami et al. 1981; Soifer et al. 1981), which regenerate poorly. The loss of the

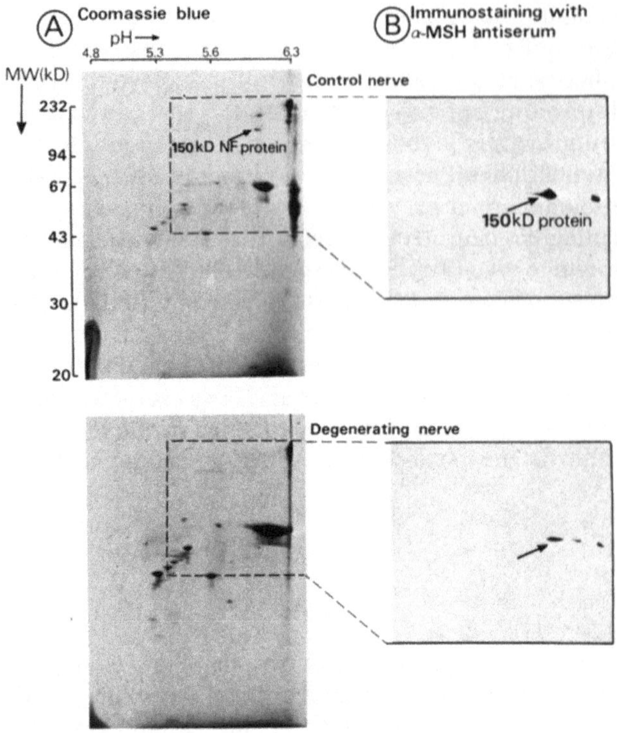

Fig. 3 A, B. Decrease in 150 kD NF protein and comigrating MSH-immunoreactivity in degenerating rat sciatic nerve. Portions (1.5 cm) of control nerve or degenerating nerve 8 days after sciatic nerve crush were homogenised in an SDS/urea medium to extract total proteins. Two-dimensional separation of proteins was carried out as described by Edwards et al. (1984c). The protein pattern is shown in **A**. Identical gels were transferred electrophoretically on to nitrocellulose and incubated with anti-α-MSH antiserum (Immuno Nuclear Corporation). Bound antibody was visualised using a peroxidase-conjugated secondary antibody

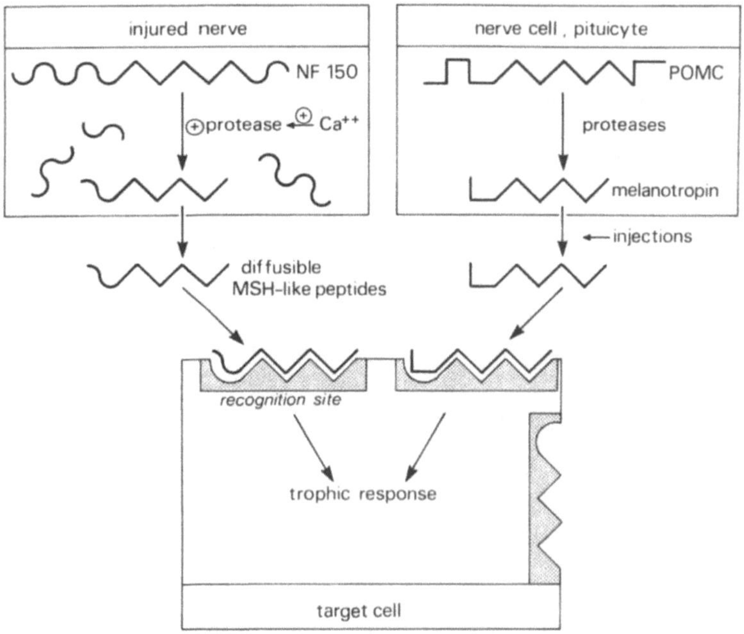

Fig. 4. Model of the proposed multiple origins of MSH-like peptides exerting a common neurotrophic action

NF150 protein in degenerating portions of crushed sciatic nerve are shown (Fig. 3) by the loss of protein staining and immunostaining with anti-MSH antiserum. It is generally believed that the neurofilament breakdown observed in degenerating nerve tissue is the result of activation of protease(s) by an increase in local calcium concentrations. Neurofilament proteins are highly susceptible to the calcium-activated neutral protease (CANP) activated by relatively high (m*M*) concentrations of calcium (Kamakura et al. 1981; Schlaepfer and Hasler 1979). Furthermore, proteolytic modification of NF proteins in situ has been shown to be dependent on endogenous calcium concentrations (Nixon et al. 1983). However, the involvement of other enzymes cannot be excluded. It has recently been shown, for instance, that NF proteins are also highly susceptible to brain cathepsin D (Nixon and Marotta 1984).

In conclusion, we have postulated (Fig. 4) that MSH-like peptides, generated by injury-induced proteolysis of the NF150 protein, are responsible for the melanotropic and neurotrophic activities found in extracts of degenerating nerves. This scheme is the first attempt to link the actions of functionally relevant biological extracts with pharmacological agents used to stimulate nerve outgrowth.

Perspectives

The ability of melanocortins to stimulate outgrowth of peripheral nerve axons following injury has been unequivocally demonstrated and a hypothesis linking this observation to physiological responses to injury has been proposed. The possibility that more subtle adaptive changes rely on similar mechanisms cannot yet be assessed. However, the ability of melanocortins to facilitate adaptive behavioural responses (De Wied and Jolles 1982) and to alleviate some of the behavioural deficits associated with aging suggest that such peptides may play a role in synaptic plasticity of this type.

The enzyme CANP, which may play a critical role in the peripheral nerve response to injury, has been implicated in other neuronal events related to plasticity. Lynch and coworkers have suggested that changes in synaptic efficiency associated with long-term potentiation and memory are initiated by calcium-induced proteolysis of postsynaptic membrane proteins, leading to increased glutamate receptor binding (Lynch and Baudry 1984). Diminished presynaptic sensitivity to calcium leading to reduced synaptic plasticity has been proposed to play a role in behavioural deficits characteristic of brain aging (Landfield 1983). At the neuromuscular junction, a role for CANP in the elimination of excess nerve terminals has been indicated (O'Brien et al. 1984). In this instance, disruption of neurofilaments in the nerve terminals is connected with a degenerative rather than a trophic action.

We have proposed that NF150 proteolysis may generate trophic MSH-like peptides in degenerating nerve tracts, and an analogous process occurring in nerve terminals is plausible. Such a process would result in activity-dependent local formation of trophic peptides. The accumulation of highly abnormal forms of NF proteins (Anderton, this volume) in the neurofibrillary tangles of the brains of individuals with senile dementia of the Alzheimer type is suggestive of disturbed metabolism of NF proteins in this disease. Nerve fibres containing melanocortins derived from the classic POMC precursor would be less dependent on electrical activity for survival, a characteristic of obvious advantage in the developing nervous system. Thus, the melanocortins are seen (Fig. 4) as deriving from several tissue and polypeptide sources; the relative importance of different sources will vary depending on the functional, pathological and developmental status of the nerve.

Acknowledgements. The authors wish to thank the many colleagues of the Institute of Molecular Biology, the Rudolf Magnus Institute, the Physiological Chemistry Department and the Academic Hospital, without whose work this paper would not have been written.

References

Beckwith BE, Sandman CA, Hothersall D, Kastin AJ (1977) Influence of neonatal injections of α-MSH on learning, memory and attention in rats. Physiol Behav 18:63–71

Berry M, Knowles J, Willis P, Riches AC, Morgans GP, Steers D (1979) A reappraisal of the effects of ACTH on the response of the central nervous system to injury. J Anat 128:859–871

Bignami A, Dahl D, Nguyen BT, Crosby CJ (1981) The fate of axonal debris in Wallerian degeneration of rat optic and sciatic nerves. Electron microscopy and immunofluorescence studies with neurofilament antisera. J Neuropathol Exp Neurol 40:537–550
Bijlsma WA, Jennekens FGI, Schotman P, Gispen WH (1983a) Stimulation by ACTH4–10 of nerve fiber regeneration following sciatic nerve crush. Muscle Nerve 6:104–112
Bijlsma WA, Schotman P, Jennekens FGI, Gispen WH, de Wied D (1983b) The enhanced recovery of sensorimotor function in rats is related to the melanotropic moiety of ACTH/MSH neuropeptides. Eur J Pharmacol 92:231–236
Bijlsma WA, Jennekens FGI, Schotman P, Gispen WH (1984) Neurotrophic factors and regeneration in the peripheral nervous system. Psychoneuroendocrinology 9:199–215
Daval JL, Louis JC, Gerard MJ, Vincendon G (1983) Influence of adrenocorticotropic hormone on the growth of isolated neurons in culture. Neurosci Lett 36:299–304
De Wied D, Jolles J (1982) Neuropeptides derived from pro-opio cortin: behavioral, physiological and neurochemical effects. Physiol Rev 62:976–1059
Dräger UC, Edwards DL, Kleinschmidt J (1983) Neurofilaments contain α-melanocyte-stimulating hormone (α-MSH)-like immunoreactivity. Proc Natl Acad Sci USA 80:6408–6412
Dunn AJ, Schotman P (1981) Effects of ACTH and related peptides on cerebral RNA and protein synthesis. Pharmacol Ther 12:353–372
Edwards PM, van der Zee CEEM, Verhaagen J, Schotman P, Jennekens FGI, Gispen WH (1984a) Evidence that the neurotrophic actions of α-MSH may derive from its ability to mimick the actions of a peptide formed in degenerating nerve stumps. J Neurol Sci 64:333–340
Edwards PM, Schrama LH, Spierings T, Verhaagen J, Schotman P, Gispen WH (1984b) Presence of melanotropic activity in degenerating nerve extracts. Possible connection with generation of neurotrophic factors by neurofilament protein breakdown. Neurosci Lett [Suppl] 18:S89
Edwards PM, Spierings T, Verhaagen J, Terlou M (1984c) A quantitative micromethod for 2-dimensional analysis of proteins in whole tissue extracts. Neurosci Lett [Suppl] 18:S331
Fertig A, Kiernan JA, Seyan SSAS (1971) Enhancement of axonal regeneration in the brain of the rat by corticotrophin and triiodothyronine. Exp Neurol 33:372–385
Gonzales ER, Strand FL (1981) Neurotropic action of MSH/ACTH4-10 on neuromuscular function in hypophysectomized rats. Peptides [Suppl 11] 2:107–113
Haynes LW, Smith ME (1984) The actions of proopiomelanocortin peptides at the developing neuromuscular junction. Trends Pharmacol Sci 5:165–168
Haynes LW, Smyth DG, Zakarian S (1982) Immunocytochemical localisation of lipotropin C-fragment (β-endorphin) in the developing rat spinal cord. Brain Res 232:115–128
Haynes LW, Smith ME, Smyth DG (1984) Evidence for the neurotrophic regulation by collagen-tailed acetylcholinesterase in immature skeletal muscle by β-endorphin. J Neurochem 42:1542–1551
Isaacson RL, Poplawsky A (1983) An ACTH4-9 analog (Org 2766) speeds recovery from septal hyperemotionality in the rat. Behav Neural Biol 39:52–59
Kamakura K, Ihara Y, Sugita H, Toyokura Y (1981) Inhibition by E-64-c of neurofilament degeneration induced by calcium ions. Biomed Res 2:327–329
Landfield PW (1983) Mechanisms of altered neural function during aging. Dev Neurol 7:51–71
Lynch G, Baudry M (1984) The biochemistry of memory: a new and specific hypothesis. Science 224:1057–1063
Nieto-Sampedro M, Whittemore SR, Needels DL, Larson J, Cotman CW (1984) The survival of brain transplants is enhanced by extracts from injured brain. Proc Natl Acad Sci USA 81:6250–6254
Nixon RA, Marotta CA (1984) Degradation of neurofilament proteins by purified human brain cathepsin D. J Neurochem 43:507–516
Nixon RA, Brown BA, Marotta CA (1983) Limited proteolytic modification of a neurofilament protein involves a proteinase activated by endogenous levels of calcium. Brain Res 275:384–388
O'Brien RAD, Ostberg AJC, Vrbova G (1984) Protease inhibitors reduce the loss of nerve terminals induced by activity and calcium in developing rat soleus muscles in vitro. Neuroscience 12:637–646

Politis MJ, Spencer PS (1983) An in vivo assay of neurotropic activity. Brain Res 278:229–231
Saint-Côme C, Acker GR, Strand FL (1982) Peptide influences on the development and regeneration of motor performance. Peptides 3:439–449
Schlaepfer WW, Hasler MH (1979) Characterization of the calcium-induced disruption of neurofilaments in rat peripheral nerve. Brain Res 168:299–309
Schlaepfer WW, Micko S (1978) Chemical and structural changes of neurofilaments in transected rat sciatic nerve. J Cell Biol 78:369–378
Schlaepfer WW, Lee C, Trojanowski JQ, Lee VMY (1984) Persistence of immunoreactive neurofilament protein breakdown products in transected rat sciatic nerve. J Neurochem 43:857–864
Schonfeld AR, Heacock AM, Katzman R (1984) Enhancement of central cholinergic sprouting by prior injury: correlation with endogenous trophic content of hippocampus. Brain Res 321:377–380
Smith CM, Strand FL (1981) Neuromuscular response of the immature rat to ACTH/MSH 4–10. Peptides 2:197–206
Soifer D, Iqbal K, Czosnek H, de Martini J, Sturman JA, Wisniewski HM (1981) The loss of neuron-specific proteins during the course of Wallerian degeneration of optic and sciatic nerve. J Neurosci 5:461–470
Strand FL, Kung TT (1980) ACTH accelerates recovery of neuromuscular function following crushing of peripheral nerve. peptides 1:135–138
Strand FL, Smith CM (1980) LPH, ACTH, MSH and motor systems. Pharmacol Ther 11:509–533
Swaab DF, Martin JT (1981) Functions of α-melanotropin and other opiomelanocortin peptides in labour, intrauterine growth and brain development. Peptides of the pars intermedia. Ciba Found Symp 81:196–217
Van der Helm-Hylkema H, de Wied D (1976) Effect of neonatally injected ACTH and ACTH analogues on eye-opening of the rat. Life Sci 18:1099–1104
Wilson JF, Anderson S, Snook G, Llewellyn KD (1984) Quantification of the permeability of the blood-CSF barrier to α-MSH in the rat. Peptides 5:681–685

Brain Plasticity and Aging

S. Hoyer and L. Frölich[1]

Introduction

The prevalence of most of the cerebral disorders in middle and old age has become obvious. Illnesses such as brain infarction, Parkinson's disease, and the dementias, to mention only the most important ones, appear most frequently in later life. In addition to the burden they impose on the affected individuals and their families, such disorders consume socioeconomic resources. Both medical practice and research are challenged to alleviate disabilities originating in the diseased brain and to elucidate their underlying causes. To do this, it would seem necessary to determine whether aging per se inevitably leads to cerebral disorders such as those mentioned or whether such brain disorders occur in middle and old age independently of normal brain aging processes. Several findings support the view that normal cerebral aging is distinct from cerebral disorders of later life, particularly dementia (for review, see Hoyer 1982b). For the normal brain, however, it has been possible to demonstrate certain differences between adulthood and senescence relating to mental capacities such as intelligence (Baltes and Schaie 1976; Baltes and Willis 1982; Horn and Cattell 1976; Horn and Donaldson 1976) and biological processes such as morphological and biochemical events (for review, see Hoyer 1982a). It is therefore necessary to define the normal ranges of brain functions as they relate to age and to evaluate the effects of stress conditions on brain functions in later life in order to study the plasticity of the aging brain.

It has been well-documented that rats may be designated as aged when their strain has a 50% survival rate and when their survival curve is more or less rectangular. In male Wistar rats, this deflection point has been found to occur at the age of 24 months (Hollander et al. 1983). Thus, adulthood in this strain is reached at the age of 12 months and senescence at 24 months. In this study these two ages were compared under both normal and well-defined stress conditions such as severe arterial hypoxemia and complete cerebral ischemia.

It is well-established that, under physiologic conditions, the healthy adult brain oxidizes glucose only to obtain energy (Gibbs et al. 1942; Gottstein et al. 1963; Hoyer 1970; Siesjö 1978). It would therefore seem reasonable to relate the biological plasticity of the aging brain to variations in its glycolytic and oxidative glucose catabolism and in its energy production.

1 Department of Pathochemistry and General Neurochemistry, University of Heidelberg, D-6900 Heidelberg, FRG

Senile Dementia of the Alzheimer Type
Ed. by J. Traber and W. H. Gispen

Normal Cerebral Aging

Earlier, we reported our findings demonstrating that cortical concentrations of glucose, glucose-6-phosphate, fructose-1,6-phosphate, pyruvate, lactate, malate, creatine phosphate, and adenosine triphosphate (ATP) show a general tendency to decrease with age, whereas adenosine diphosphate (ADP) levels increase. This pattern was demonstrated as exponential fit curves (Hoyer 1983). However, among different age groups, the changes vary to a remarkable extent. Glucose, fructose-1,6-phosphate, and ATP drop starting at the age of 6–12 months, whereas concentrations of pyruvate, malate, and creatine phosphate diminish between 12 and 24 months of age (Ulfert et al. 1982).

These results are in agreement with studies which show a gradual decrease in oxidative processes in the cortex of rats beginning at the age of 12 month and continuing to between 18 and 28 months onward (Peng et al. 1977) and a reduction in glucose oxidation in 2-year-old rats (Patel 1977). These findings also seem to be supported by the findings that the activities of hexokinase and phosphofructokinase are not reduced in rat brain cortex between 12 and 24 months of age (Iwangoff et al. 1980); that no differences exist in the enzyme activities of pyruvate carboxylase, citrate synthase and nicotine adenine dinucleotide (NAD)-isocitrate dehydrogenase in the brain cortex of 1- and 2-year-old rats (Patel 1977); and that the enzyme activities of lactate dehydrogenase, pyruvate dehydrogenase and NAD^+-malate dehydrogenase do not change in the brain cortex of rats between the ages of 3 months and 2 years. In contrast, fumarase decreases significantly during this time (Leong et al. 1981). These findings may suggest that glucose and energy metabolism in rat brain cortex is only slightly diminished between 12 and 24 months of age.

Aging and Stress Conditions

Arterial Hypoxemia

In severe arterial hypoxemia with a mean arterial PO_2 of 21 mmHg, significant increases in brain cortical concentrations of glucose, glucose-6-phosphate (only in the 1-year old group), fructose-1,6-phosphate, dihydroxyacetone phosphate, pyruvate, lactate, malate, ADP, and AMP, as well as significant reductions in creatine phosphate and ATP were observable in both age groups, as compared with the respective controls. These findings may indicate activation of the flux-controlling enzymes hexokinase, phosphofructokinase, and pyruvate kinase after severe arterial hypoxemia lasting 15 min (Fig. 1). In young mature rats, similar findings were reported by Bachelard et al. (1974) and Norberg and Siesjö (1975). That the oxidative metabolism in the tricarboxylic acid cycle may also be involved is obvious through the slight changes in citrate and α-ketoglutarate quantities and the significant increase in malate concentrations. The former may indicate reduced activity of the pyruvate dehydrogenase complex (Gibson and Blass 1976).

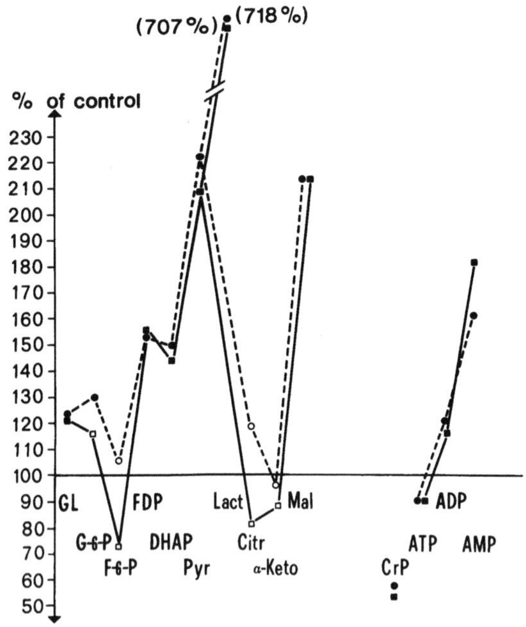

Fig. 1. Metabolites of glycolysis and the tricarboxylic acid cycle and energy-rich compounds in the brain cortex of 1- and 2-year-old rats after profound arterial hypoxemia (PO_2 20–25 mmHg) lasting 15 min. The 100% level corresponds to the respective control groups. *Filled symbols* represent statistically significant variations ($\alpha \leqq 0.05$). (○---○, hypoxemia in 1-year-old animals; □——□, hypoxemia in 2-year-old animals; GL, glucose; G-6-P, glucose-6-phosphate; F-6-P, fructose-6-phosphate; FDP, fructose-1,6-phosphate; fructose diphosphate; DHAP, dihydroxyacetone phosphate; Pyr, pyruvate; Lact, lactate; Citr, citrate; α-Keto, α-ketoglutarate; Mal, malate; CrP, creatine phosphate; ATP, adenosine triphosphate; ADP, adenosine diphosphate; AMP, adenosine monophosphate)

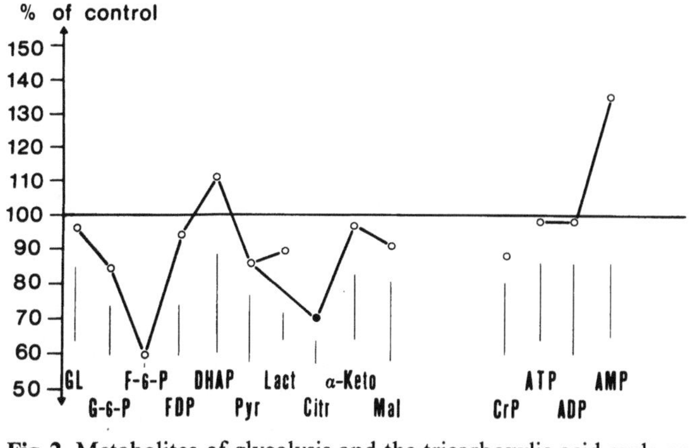

Fig. 2. Metabolites of glycolysis and the tricarboxylic acid cycle and energy-rich compounds in the brain cortex of 1- and 2-year-old rats after profound arterial hypoxemia lasting 15 min (PO_2 20–25 mmHg). The 100% level corresponds to the 1-year-old hypoxemia group. *Filled symbols* represent statistically significant variations ($\alpha \leqq 0.05$). Abbreviations defined in Fig. 1

However, it is also evident that metabolic adaptation to hypoxemic stress conditions tends to become somewhat slower with age, a finding which the significantly reduced citrate concentration makes particularly obvious. Thus, the metabolic capacity to meet severe hypoxemic stress may diminish with age (Fig. 2). This also holds true for hypoxic ischemia, where the increase in cerebral blood flow has been found to be less marked in aged than in young animals (Hoffman 1984).

Ischemia

Complete cerebral ischemia depleted substrate concentrations of glucose, oxaloacetate, ATP, and creatine phosphate, and severely reduced those of pyruvate, citrate, α-ketoglutarate, and malate. In contrast, levels of fructose-1,6-phosphate, succinate, and adenosine monophosphate (AMP) rose in both age groups (Fig. 3). In principle, similar results had been obtained from other studies of young mature animals (Benzi et al. 1979; Folbergrova et al. 1974; Ljunggren et al. 1974a, b). There were, however, some significant differences between the two age groups studied concerning the substrates glucose, fructose-1,6-phosphate, lactate, succinate, malate, ADP, and AMP.

In 1-year-old rats, glucose concentration was depleted to 4% but decreased to only 14% in the aged group, as compared with the respective controls. The pro-

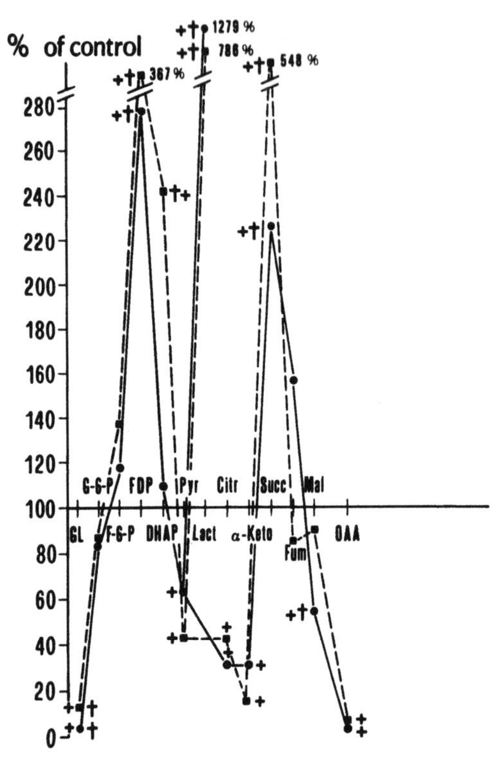

Fig. 3. Cerebral gray matter concentrations of glycolytic and tricarboxylic-acid-cycle intermediates after complete cerebral ischemia lasting 15 min in 1-year-old (●) and 2-year-old (■) rats. The 100% level corresponds to the respective control groups. †, statistically significant variation between age groups; +, statistically significant variation from respective controls ($2P \leq 0.05$). (Succ, succinate; Fum, fumarate; OAA, oxaloacetate; other abbreviations defined in Fig. 1)

nounced diminution of the two glucose concentrations may be attributed to a facilitation of the phosphofructokinase step, an explanation which is also corroborated by the increased fructose-1,6-phosphate concentration. At first sight, the significantly enhanced fructose-1,6-phosphate level in the 2-year-old group as compared with the 1-year-old animals suggests an increased glycolytic flux due to higher levels of enzyme activity. On the other hand, as mentioned above, no differences in the activity of phosphofructokinase between 1- and 2-year-old rats were observable (Iwangoff et al. 1980), although a significant decrease of about 30% in phosphofructokinase activity was noted between 3 months and 2 years of age (Leong et al. 1981). Other researchers have found similar decreases of more than 50% in elderly humans (Meier-Ruge et al. 1980), so that reasons other than the activation of the phosphofructokinase step alone must be taken into consideration to explain the large ischemia-induced rise in fructose-1,6-phosphate concentrations in aged animals. The ostensibly smaller increases in the activity of phosphofructokinase suggest a slight activation of the glycolytic flux and thus a less severe diminution in glucose concentration as was found in the aged rats during ischemia. Provided glycolytic flux is not greatly accelerated in aged ischemic brain cortex as compared with that of young adults, a less pronounced increase in pyruvate levels may be expected. In our study, the pyruvate concentration was found to be about 20% less for 2-year-old than for 1-year-old animals. The smaller amount of ischemia-induced lactate formation in the 2-year-old group might seem to be at least partially attributable to this reduction in quantities of pyruvate. Nevertheless, during ischemia, lactate formation from pyruvate by means of lactate dehydrogenase is extremely elevated because of the depletion of NAD^+ and the accumulation of NADH and H^+, which favors lactate production (Nilsson et al. 1975).

With respect to the drop in concentrations of pyruvate during ischemia, its further metabolic degradation might be also of significance. In mammalian tissue, including the brain, pyruvate is metabolized to acetyl CoA, the formation of which is controlled by the multienzyme pyruvate dehydrogenase complex. Acetyl CoA enters the tricarboxylic acid cycle, the flux of which is known to be regulated by means of isocitrate dehydrogenase. In the heart, it has been shown that these two enzymes are inhibited when NADH accumulates (Bremer 1969; La Noue et al. 1970). It may be assumed that this also holds true for the brain, so that pyruvate might be expected to accumulate first, and the tricarboxylic acid cycle to be emptied of its intermediates. However, the sum of the carbon skeletons of the tricarboxylic acid cycle did not change during ischemia in 1-year-old rats and even increased significantly in the 2-year-old group. An anaplerotic reaction, unproven in the mammalian brain as yet, might therefore be considered responsible.

In invertebrates, phosphoenolpyruvate (PEP) may be carboxylated to oxaloacetate by means of PEP carboxykinase, of which the optimal activity occurs at a pH of between 5.0 and 6.0. In reversal reactions to aerobic tissues, the oxaloacetate thus formed was found to be converted to succinate via malate and fumarate (Hochachka and Mustafa 1972; Saz 1971), and succinate accumulated as an end product of anaerobic glucose breakdown. The formation of oxaloacetate is associated with the gain of inosine triphosphate (ITP) and guanosine triphosphate (GTP) respectively. A further advantage of the reductive reactions in the tricarboxylic acid cycle may be seen in the role of NADH and the generation of NAD when malate is formed from oxaloacetate and in the activity of flavine adenine dinucleotide (FADH) and the generation of FAD when succinate is formed from fumarate. It is tempting to hypothesize that, provided oxidative metabolism in mammalian tissue is completely blocked when complete ischemia occurs, the phylogenetically highly developed oxidative pathway switches to a phylogenetically primitive one. This reaction allows the formation of at least some energy-rich compounds, thus reducing to some extent the tissue damage caused by energy failure. At present, the question of why succinate formation was found to be significantly higher in aged than in adult animals remains unresolved. If the amount of succinate reflects the degree of anaplerosis, the question of whether this is of benefit or not becomes all the more pertinent, since the role of ITP and GTP in the brain is poorly understood.

Ljunggren et al. (1974b) calculated a brain tissue pH of 6.5 after complete ischemia of 10 min. This is obviously due to a marked increase in lactic acid production. Although the activity of PEP carboxykinase may remain close to its optimum under ischemic conditions, it should be emphasized that the metabolic pathway discussed above has been proven for invertebrates, but not yet for mammalian brain.

The ischemia-induced depletion of ATP and creatine phosphate was found to be extreme in both age groups. ATP levels diminished to 6% and 9% respectively, compared with controls. Under aerobic conditions, ATP formation by means of glycolysis amounts to 5% as related to the total ATP formation derived from the breakdown of glucose. In ischemia, where oxidative ATP generation ceases ATP formation might be maintained in both age groups by the (increased) glycolytic flux alone. The insignificantly greater amounts of ATP noted in 2-year-old ischemic animals are assumed to be functionally meaningless (Fig. 4).

Although changes in glucose breakdown may only be minor in normal cerebral aging of animals between 1 and 2 years of age, ischemia-induced and age-

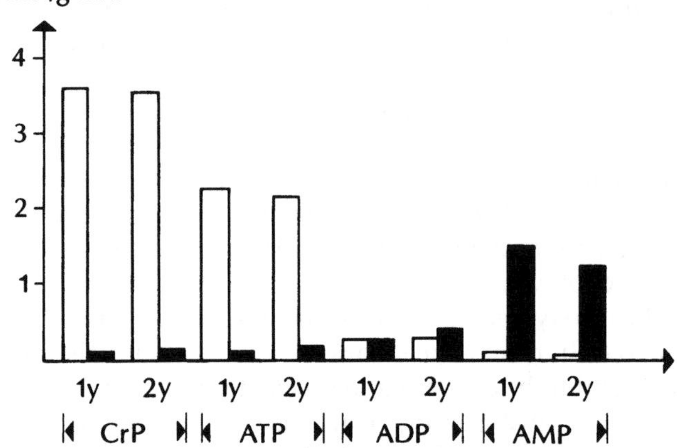

Fig. 4. Concentration of creatine phosphate (CrP) and the adenine nucleotides ATP, ADP, and AMP in the brain cortex of 1- and 2-year-old rats. (□, control; ■, after a 15-min complete cerebral ischemia; abbreviations defined in Fig. 1)

related variations such as those found in glycolysis lead to the tentative conclusion that the aging brain may be less capable of coping with stress conditions such as ischemia. In short, the biological plasticity of the aging brain may be reduced with age. However, this reduction seems to be slight, suggesting that severe tissue damage can be avoided.

References

Bachelard HS, Lewis LD, Ponten U, Siesjö BK (1974) Mechanisms activating glycolysis in the brain in arterial hypoxia. J Neurochem 22:395–401

Baltes PB, Schaie KW (1976) On the plasticity of intelligence in adulthood and old age: where Horn and Donaldson fail. Am Psychologist 31:720–725

Baltes PB, Willis SL (1982) Plasticity and enhancement of intellectual functioning in old age. In: Craik FIM, Trehub EE (eds) Aging and cognitive processes. Plenum, New York, pp 353–389

Benzi G, Arrigoni E, Marzatico F, Villa RF (1979) Influence of some biological pyrimidines on the succinate cycle during and after cerebral ischemia. Biochem Pharmacol 28:2545–2550

Bremer J (1969) Pyruvate dehydrogenase, substrate specificity and product inhibiton. Eur J Biochem 8:535–540

Folbergrova J, Ljunggren B, Norberg K, Siesjö BK (1974) Influence of complete ischemia on glycolytic metabolites, citric acid cycle intermediates, and associated amino acids in the rat cerebral cortex. Brain Res 80:265–279

Gibbs EL, Lennox WG, Nims LF, Gibbs FA (1942) Arterial and cerebral venous blood. Arterial-venous differences in man. J Biol Chem 144:325–332

Gibson GE, Blass JP (1976) Impaired synthesis of acetylcholine in brain accompanying mild hypoxia and hypoglycemia. J Neurochem 27:37–42

Gottstein U, Bernsmeier A, Sedlmeyer I (1963) Der Kohlenhydratstoffwechsel des menschlichen Gehirns. I. Untersuchungen mit substratspezifischen enzymatischen Methoden bei normaler Hirndurchblutung. Klin Wochenschr 41:943–948

Hochachka PW, Mustafa T (1972) Invertebrate facultative anaerobiosis. Science 178:1056–1060

Hoffman WE, Pelligrino D, Miletich DJ, Albrecht RF (1984) Cerebrovascular and metabolic response of the aged rat to hypoxia. In: Fieschi C, Lenzi GL, Loeb CW (eds) Effects of aging on regulation of cerebral blood flow and metabolism. Karger, Basel, pp 8–16

Hollander CF, van Zwieten MJ, Zurcher C (1983) The aged animal. In: Gispen WH, Traber J (eds) Aging of the brain. Elsevier, Amsterdam, pp 187–196

Horn JL, Cattell RB (1976) Age differences in fluid and crystallized intelligence. Acta Psychol (Anst) 26:107–129

Horn JL, Donaldson G (1976) On the myth of intellectual decline in adulthood. Am Psychologist 31:701–719

Hoyer S (1970) Der Aminosäurenstoffwechsel des normalen menschlichen Gehirns. Klin Wochenschr 48:1239–1243

Hoyer S (1982a) The young-adult and normally aged brain. Its blood flow and oxidative metabolism. A review – part I. Arch Gerontol Geriatr 1:101–116

Hoyer S (1982b) The abnormally aged brain. Its blood flow and oxidative metabolism. A review – part II. Arch Gerontol Geriatr 1:195–207

Hoyer S (1983) Circulation and oxidative metabolism in the normally and abnormally aging brain. In: Gispen WH, Traber J (eds) Aging of the brain. Elsevier, Amsterdam, pp 151–165

Iwangoff P, Enz A, Armbruster R, Emmenegger H, Pataki A, Sandoz P (1980) Der Einfluß von Alter. Zeitspanne bis zur postmortalen Isolierung des Gewebes sowie der Agonie auf einige glykolytische Enzyme in autoptischen Gehirnproben des Menschen. akt gerontol 10:203–212

La Noue K, Nicklas WJ, Williamson JR (1970) Control of citric acid cycle activity in rat heart mitochondira. J Biol Chem 245:102–111

Leong SF, Lai JCK, Lim L, Clark JB (1981) Energy-metabolizing enzymes in brain regions of adult and aging rats. J Neurochem 37:1548–1556

Ljunggren B, Norberg K, Siesjö BK (1974a) Influence of tissue acidosis upon restitution of brain energy metabolism following total ischemia. Brain Res 77:173–186

Ljunggren B, Schutz H, Siesjö BK (1974b). Changes in energy state and acid-base parameters of the rat brain during complete compression ischemia. Brain Res 73:277–289

Meier-Ruge W, Hunziker O, Iwangoff P, Reichlmeier K, Schultz U (1980) Effect of age on morphological and biochemical parameters of the human brain. In: Stein DC (ed) The psychobiology of aging: problems and perspectives. Elsevier, Amsterdam, pp 297–317

Nilsson B, Norberg K, Siesjö BK (1975) Biochemical events in cerebral ischaemia. Br J Anasth 47:751–760

Norberg K, Siesjö BK (1975) Cerebral metabolism in hypoxic hypoxia. I. Pattern of glycolysis; a re-evaluation. Brain Res 86:31–44

Patel MS (1977) Age-dependent changes in the oxidative metabolism in rat brain. J Gerontol 32:643–646

Peng MT, Peng YI, Chen FN (1977) Age-dependent changes in the oxygen consumption of the cerebral cortex, hypothalamus, hippocampus, and amygdaloid in rats. J Gerontol 32:517–522

Saz HJ (1971) Facultative anaerobiosis in the invertebrates: Pathways and control systems. Am Zoologist 11:125–135

Siesjö BK (1978) Brain energy metabolism. Wiley, Chichester

Ulfert G, Schmidt U, Hoyer S (1982) Glucose and energy metabolism of rat cerebral cortex during aging. In: Hoyer S (ed) The aging brain. Physiological and pathophysiological aspects. Exp Brain Res [Suppl] 5:102–111

Animal Models

Parallels and Contrasts Between Scrapie and Dementia of the Alzheimer Type and Ageing: Strategies and Problems for Experiments Involving Life Span Studies

H. Fraser and P. A. McBride[1]

Introduction

Scrapie is a naturally occurring, lethal degeneration of the nervous system of adult sheep, caused by an unconventional, virus-like agent the nature of which has yet to be resolved. Recently, several parallels between experimental models of scrapie in mice and Alzheimer's disease (AD) have been drawn. Each has a slowly progressing unremitting course and produces lesions confined to the CNS which are largely degenerative, with little evidence of inflammation. Some scrapie models in mice produce pathological features which are highly characteristic of AD, in particular, argyrophilic amyloid plaques and selective neuronal degeneration in the hippocampus (Bruce 1984; Bruce and Dickinson 1982; Bruce and Fraser 1975; Fraser and Bruce 1973; Hyman et al. 1984; Scott and Fraser 1984).

Serial passage of scrapie isolates in mice has led to the identification of some 15 different strains of scrapie. Strains of scrapie are distinguished on the basis of highly repeatable incubation period characteristics in particular mouse genotypes as well as on characteristic patterns of pathological change (Dickinson and Fraser 1977; Fraser 1979). Scrapie research requires rigorous experimental control and economy of design to which workers from other fields may find it difficult to submit. There are no easy options with scrapie research – the disease, although infectious, has no specific immunological expression and does not cause homeostatic responses – which means that there have been no in vitro methods for its study, no laboratory tests to monitor its progress and no biochemical indices of any primary molecular disorganisation. Recently, one clue has emerged which may lead to some significant advance in understanding the disease process – the discovery by Merz, Somerville and their colleagues of fibrillar structures, called scrapie-associated fibrils (SAF), in detergent- and enzyme-treated brain or spleen homogenates (Merz et al. 1981, 1983 b). Complementary work by Diringer, who has confirmed the findings, has suggested some correlation between SAF and levels of infectivity in scrapie brain. Diringer's study has confirmed the work of Prusiner and his group, who succeeded in identifying an SAF-associated, microheterogeneous protein resistant to proteinase, with a molecular weight of 27,000–30,000, which may turn out to be not just a product of the disease process, but more closely associated with the structure of the disease agent itself (Diringer et al. 1983; McKinley et al. 1983).

1 AFRC & MRC Neuropathogenesis Unit, West Mains Road, Edinburgh EH9 3JF, UK

Senile Dementia of the Alzheimer Type
Ed. by J. Traber and W. H. Gispen

These groups have produced antibodies to antigens in the SAF preparations (Bendheim et al. 1984; Diringer et al. 1984), an accomplishment which may provide a long-sought probe making it possible to study some aspects of the pathogenesis of scrapie with conventional immunological methods. However, this will depend on identifying the specificity of the antibodies concerned: many years of painstaking work in several centres have previously failed to demonstrate either the antigenicity of scrapie agents or specific immunological responses in infected animals (Collis and Kimberlin 1983; Gardiner and Marucci 1969; Porter et al. 1973). It will therefore be necessary to account for this ready demonstration of antigen in light of past failures to demonstrate antigenicity of scrapie tissues. It has even been suggested by Prusiner that the 27,000-to-30,000-MW, microheterogeneous protein represents the infectious agent (Prusiner 1984), despite the lack of evidence that the purified protein is infectious. At is simplest, the microheterogeneity of this protein might simply reflect no more than differences in neural targetting of lesions, which is a well-known distinction among strains of scrapie agent (Dickinson and Fraser 1977; Fraser 1979).

Recently, it has been speculated that the infectious agent aggregates to form the amyloid fibrils of the argyrophilic plaques of some scrapie models, a notion that has been extrapolated to account for Alzheimer senile plaques. The congophilia of β-pleated sheet structures such as amyloid, paired helical filaments (of neurofibrillary tangles) and SAFs is the only basis for this speculation. This confuses rather than clarifies the subject because it has been shown that these structures are morphologically distinguishable even when more than one of these types of fibril occur in the same brain (Merz et al. 1983a).

Methods of Study

Primary and subsequent passage has been undertaken, using various routes of infection, source materials, doses and dilutions in inbred mice. Mouse strains carry alternative alleles of a gene *Sinc* which controls scrapie replication (Dickinson and Fraser 1977). Most mice carry the s7 allele, including the C57BL, RIII, VL and C3H strains, but the VM inbred strain carries the opposite one, the p7 allele. Homozygous s7 mice undergo a "short" incubation period with the ME7-group of scrapie agents, whereas homozygous p7 mice have a long incubation period. The s7s7 to p7p7 ranking is reversed in the case of the 22A-group of scrapie strains. To designate these alternatives, the terms "nonrestrictive" and "restrictive" are used respectively for the short and long models. In the latter case, it is known that some of the delay can occur at the initiation of the early infective event. Terminal scrapie status can occur from around 130 days up to or beyond life span. For example, intracerebral injection of an ME7-group strain of scrapie (such as 22C or 79A) at high doses (10^4 $ICLD_{50}$) into *Sinc*^{s7} mice produces incubation periods of around 150–180 days, whereas injection, particularly by peripheral routes, of low doses of agent into restrictive host genotypes, e.g. injection of ME7 into *Sinc*^{p7} genotype or of a 22A-group strain into a *Sinc*^{s7} genotype, leads to very much longer incubation periods.

There are good grounds for regarding certain scrapie varieties as "wild-type" strains (Bruce and Dickinson 1984): certain ones have long incubation periods (over 300 days) even when injected a high doses into nonrestrictive hosts. In this sort of work, many mice have to be observed until senility; this is especially true in experiments to establish infectivity estimates because end-point dilution techniques are necessary. This is also the case in primary transmission attempts, where the biological properties of any "new" strains isolated in field-derived inocula from sheep are completely unknown. In some series of primary transmissions, the success rate has been as low as 20% within the limits set by the lifetime of the mice (Fraser 1983) (life span is shown in Fig. 2).

An aspect critically important to work in this area is the use of stringent "blind" coding for assessing the outcome of experiments. This applies at all levels of study: the assessment of the clinical status of live animals, the examination and evaluation of histological material as well as instances where more sophisticated analytical methods are adopted, such as special histological, histochemical, immunocytochemical, electron-microscopic and biochemical procedures. The design of appropriate controls for these more elaborate laboratory operations places an ever greater responsibility on investigators to establish stringency in coding. Another example is the obvious need to mix experimental subgroups of mice among several cages, rather than, for instance, grouping them in titrations, i.e. putting all mice from the same dilution group into the same cage. It is too easy for unconscious bias to influence objective analysis in scrapie research arising for example from the long time scale of the disease or the insidious way in which clinical signs develop. The literature abounds with examples of inadequate coding which have wasted much time and money.

Neuropathologic methods for routine work are relatively simple (Fig. 1), but a great deal of attention to detail is required to establish good quality standards in the preparation of specimens, as histologic artifacts can prevent the recognition or assessment of low-grade degenerative changes. It is important that scrapie experiments are monitored with histopathology to establish the status of so-called scrapie-affected mice. It cannot be assumed that all sick, even neurologically sick, animals are scrapie-positive; there are many reasons why animals become sick!

Survival studies are shown in Figs. 2, 3, and 8. Sampling procedures were carried out either on the basis of the entire experimental population (see caption to Fig. 2) or the survival of all animals in an experiment (see Figs. 3, 8).

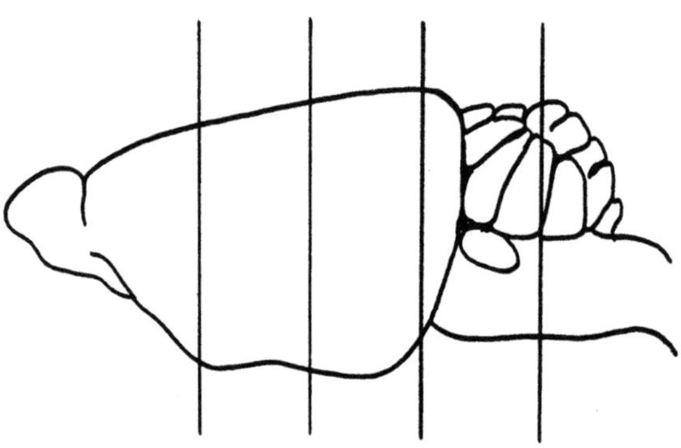

Fig. 1. The mouse brain is sectioned at four standard coronal levels. Histological staining is by haematoxylin and eosin and by Masson trichrome to highlight amyloid plaques (Bruce and Fraser 1975). For some purposes, serial sections are studied

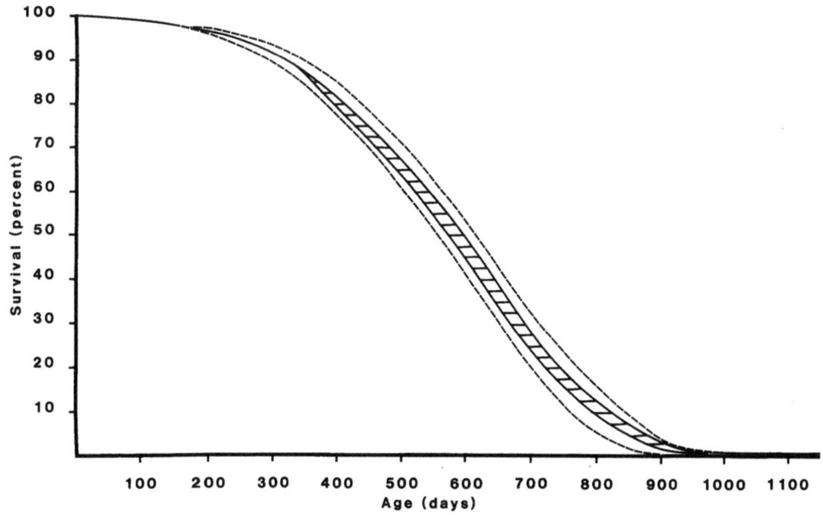

Fig. 2. Survival curve of mice of many inbred strains and crosses used in our scrapie programme over about 16 years. A total of 75,070 brains have been studied histologically; 60,250 were from mice killed as a result of experimentation; 14,820 from mice killed for nonexperimental, spontaneous intercurrent illness. This curve represents the losses of these 14,820 mice. One in ten of the total population was sampled for the survey. The *cross-hatched curve* represents the upper and lower estimate for mice of both sexes. The *upper dashed line* is the estimate for maximum female survival, and the *lower dashed line* is the estimate of the minimum male survival

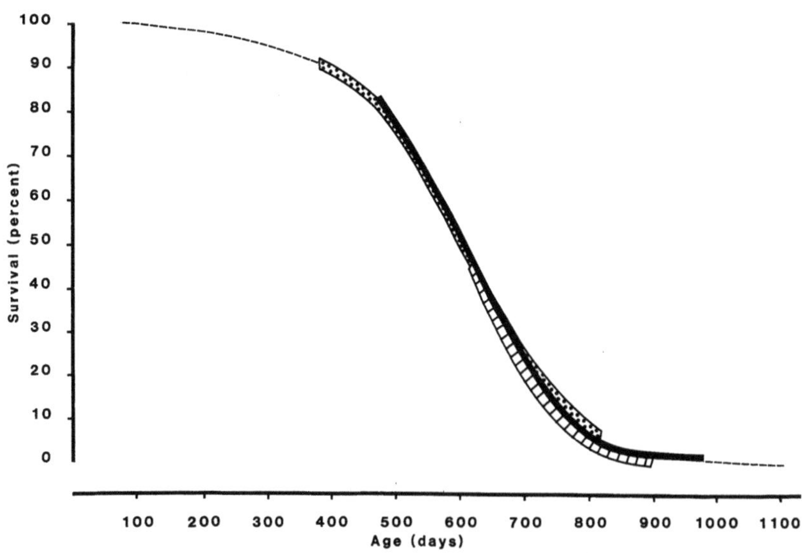

Fig. 3. Survival of mice infected with scrapie from five Icelandic sheep. All five had typical clinical signs and advanced brain pathology. Medulla and cerebral cortex of each were used separately for intracerebral injection (10% homogenates) into weaned mice (6–10 weeks old) of 12 inbred strains (including *Sinc*^{s7}, *Sinc*^{p7} strains and S7P7 crosses). The 700 injected mice were observed throughout their lifetimes. Scrapie-like or other neurologic signs were seen in 46 mice, but scrapie lesions (vacuolar spongiosis ⋯⋯, amyloid plaques ▬▬, both spongiosis and plaques ▭▭▭) were seen in only 15 of these mice. Histological confirmation that the majority of mice with neurologic signs had scrapie was thus not possible. Neuropathologic data were available on only 393 of the injected mice between 375 and 980 days after injection. Of the brains seen, 13% had positive evidence of transmission, but 32 of the 49 killed animals with scrapie lesions were killed for non-neurological reasons. Of the 49 mice with lesions, 15 had spongiosis alone, 15 had only amyloid plaques, and 19 showed both types of change (Fraser 1983)

Observations

There has been a consensus amongst histopathologists working on experimental scrapie in rodents that some pathologic changes occurring in brain sections can be confused with those of normal ageing. Our neuropathologic experience with 75,000 mice from many inbred strains over nearly 20 years, has resulted in a great deal of expertise in recognising and distinguishing the two processes. However, it has become clear that ageing changes and the degenerative pathology of scrapie may be difficult to distinguish when they coexist – as they inevitably must in some long-term experiments – and this can lead to difficulty in making a certain diagnosis of scrapie in a very aged individual.

Our studies have covered the entire life span (Fig. 2) utilizing different experimental systems and models with incubation periods ranging from around 150–1,000 days or even "beyond" an individual's life span by looking for infection rather than disease in very old, senile animals (Dickinson et al. 1975). Considerable experience has also been gained from attempted primary transmissions into mice from natural sheep scrapie. This has added not only to our knowledge of the diversity of the neuropathology of scrapie but also led to a recognition that the changes of ageing cause interpretative difficulties, especially in such types of experiments (Fraser 1983).

There are two categories of neuropathologic change in scrapie: spongiosis and argyrophilic amyloid plaques (which represent a close analogue of human senile plaques). Earlier work has already provided strong evidence first of all that plaques do not appear as an old age-associated lesion in mice and secondly that their occurrence in different scrapie models can be distinguished in important ways (Bruce and Fraser 1982; Bruce et al. 1976). Some scrapie strains do not cause recognisable plaques at all, others produce a few, while still other strains give rise to large numbers of plaques. The host genotype also exerts a major effect on their occurrence (Bruce et al. 1976). Spongiosis, on the other hand, is a lesion regarded as an almost pathognomonic feature of murine scrapie and, in our work, is treated as such.

There are some important unanswered questions about the origin and interdependence of each category of lesion, including the source and identity of amyloid precursors or possible cofactors and of the cells involved in their synthesis, the molecular and cellular basis of the spongy change and, lastly, the possible existence of a relationship between spongiosis and cerebral plaques. The wide discrepancies in the localisation of amyloid plaques and spongiosis in the CNS, especially in high-plaque models, as well as the absence or low numbers of plaques in other models remain unexplained. In some primary transmissions, large plaques can predominate, large numbers of which occur in the absence of spongiosis in some individuals, a phenomenon which is likewise not understood (see Figs. 3, 4) (Fraser 1979, 1983; Fraser and Bruce 1983).

An example of the wide pathological variety in primary transmission is illustrated in the survival curve of some 700 mice injected at around 6–10 weeks of age with inocula from five cases of natural scrapie in Icelandic sheep (Fig. 3) (Fraser 1983). Pathological evidence was obtained from 393 mice, but in only 49, killed between 360 and 980 days of age, were scrapie lesions found at all. The le-

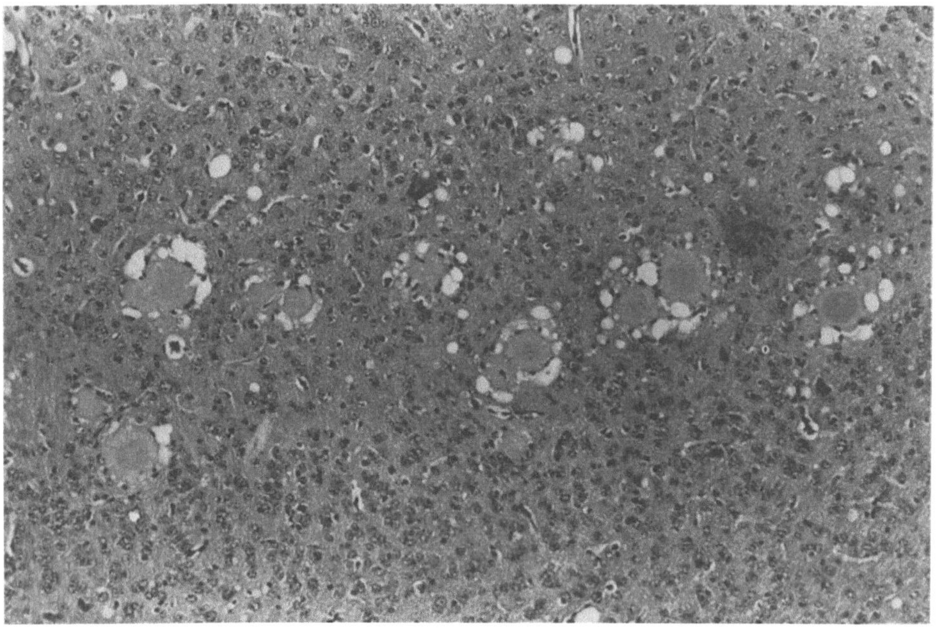

Fig. 4. Numerous unusually large amyloid plaques in an 850-day-old MB mouse showing an incoordinated gait killed 813 days following intracerebral infection of a 10% homogenate from the medulla of an Icelandic sheep with scrapie (rida). Spongiosis is conspicuously absent in some cases (Fraser 1983). Haematoxylin and eosin, × 100

sions consisted either of vacuolation alone (largely in s7s7, p7p7 and s7p7 mice) or of both types of lesions coinciding in the same brain (mostly in p7p7 mice) (Fig. 4). Clinical evidence of transmission was rarely convincing in individual mice. Half of those with clinically apparent neurologic deficits had no scrapie pathology, and most of the mice with positive scrapie lesions were killed for incidental reasons, usually systemic disease. Ageing changes such as vacuolation (see below), occurred in many and, in some animals, coexisted with scrapie lesions.

A model with a very low plaque occurrence is the ME7 scrapie strain in s7s7 genotype mice, especially following peripheral injection (Bruce et al. 1976). Spongiosis is widespread in this model, with generalised involvement of the cerebrum. Figure 5 illustrates the plaque distribution in coronal brain sections from VL mice (*Sinc*^{s7}) injected with the ME7 strain of scrapie, either intracerebrally ($n = 23$; incubation period, 170 ± 1 days, mean ± standard error) or intraperitoneally ($n = 18$; incubation period, 240 ± 4 days). The point to be made here is that, unlike some of the plaques produced by high-plaque strains and in primary transmission (Figs. 3, 4), plaques caused by ME7 are quite difficult to visualise and depend on trichrome staining for easier demonstration (Figs. 6, 7).

A major difference between natural scrapie and the experimental disease in mice concerns the question of maternal transmission of the infection. There are several reasons that suggest maternal transmission in sheep and point strongly to both prenatal and postnatal horizontal transmission from a ewe to her lamb

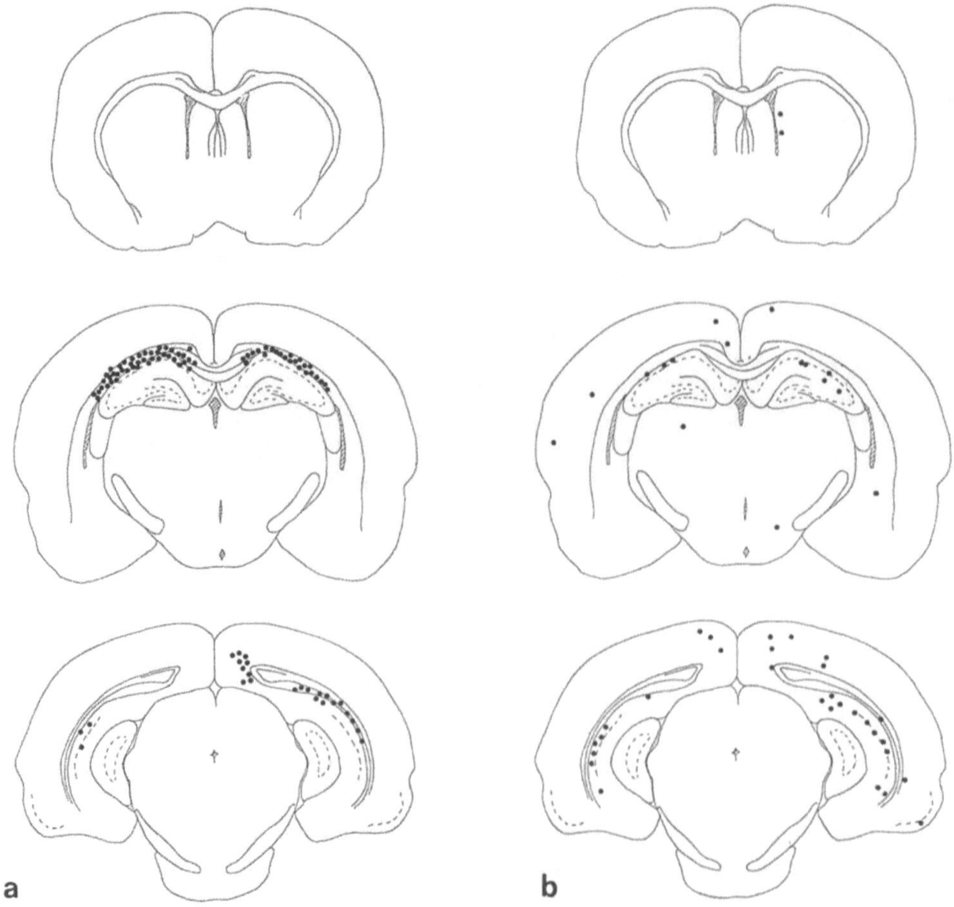

Fig. 5 a, b. Distribution maps of amyloid plaques in sections of VL mice injected with the ME7 scrapie agent. *Sinc*^{s7} injected **a** intracerebrally, $n=23$, or **b** intraperitoneally, $n=18$). Each *dot* represents one plaque revealed by Masson trichrome staining of serial sections at the level shown in Fig. 1

(Dickinson 1976; Hourrigan et al. 1979). However, all attempts to induce maternal transmission in mice with laboratory-passaged (mutant) strains have been unsuccessful. The reason for this failure is unknown; it could be due to the generally immature status of some unspecified organ systems in the perinatal mouse – for instance, immunological immaturity has been suggested (Dickinson 1976). However, an equally plausible explanation involves the differences between field strains of scrapie in sheep and the mutant strains used in laboratory experiments, the later having lost that part of their information system which might be the prerequisite for vertical transmission. This might also explain the absence of mutant strains (such as ME7) in natural epidemics in sheep.

In view of this possibility, it was decided to attempt maternal transmission in mice with 87A, a wild-type, high-plaque-producing agent. Young adult C57BL

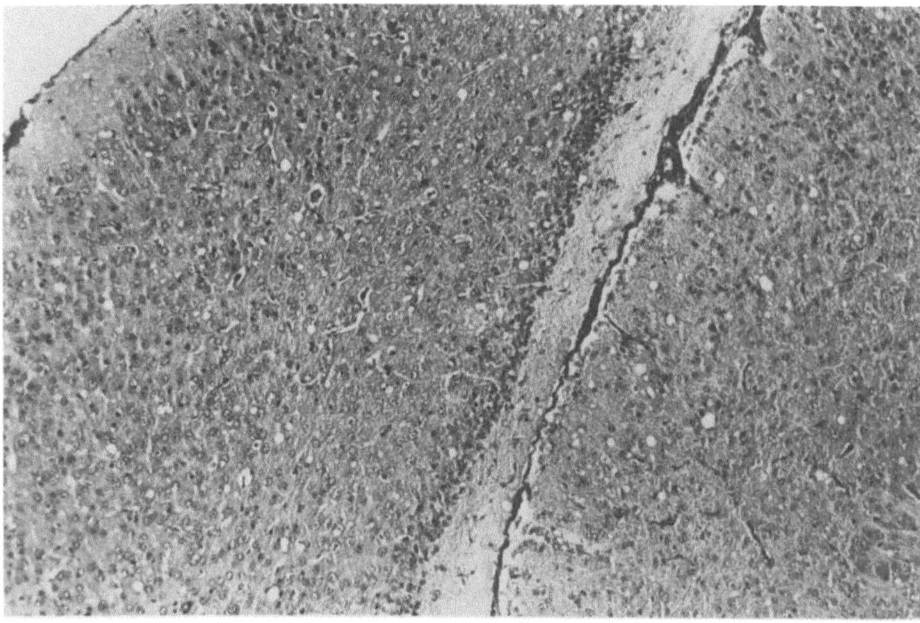

Fig. 6. Amyloid plaque in the retrosplenial cortex of a terminally scrapie-affected female VL mouse killed 266 days after intraperitoneal injection of ME7 scrapie agent. This section also shows scrapie-induced spongiosis in the cerebral cortex and superior colliculus. Masson trichrome, × 100

mice were injected by peripheral routes prior to breeding (see Table 1 and the caption to Fig. 8 for details). The survival of the 187 progeny of the 41 litters of these 87A-injected mothers is shown in Fig. 8. None developed scrapie, and the examination of serial, trichrome-stained brain sections failed to reveal amyloid plaques in any.

What is usually regarded as the pathognomonic lesion of scrapie, that most likely to be a significant reflection of neurologic dysfunction, consists of vacuolar degeneration of grey and sometimes white matter, which is conveniently described by the all-embracing term "spongiosis" (Fraser 1979). The distribution and regional intensity of spongiosis are controlled by a number of factors, of which the strain of agent and the host are the two most important (Dickinson and Fraser 1977; Fraser 1979). However, this lesion can bear a superficial similarity to a somewhat similar spongiosis accompanying old age, and some experience is needed to distinguish the two (Figs. 9, 10). The spongiosis of scrapie is associated with other indices of neuroparenchymal damage which the neuropathologist learns to recognise, whereas in old age, the vacuoles are clearly "punched out" from otherwise normal surrounding tissue. The scrapie lesion is a finer spongiosis compared with the characteristically large vacuoles observed in old mice (Figs. 11, 12). Moreover, changes in glia not seen in the old-age-associated vacuolation accompany the scrapie spongiosis. The most severe age-associated vacuolation seems to involve white matter (Fig. 12) and appears in very old females. It

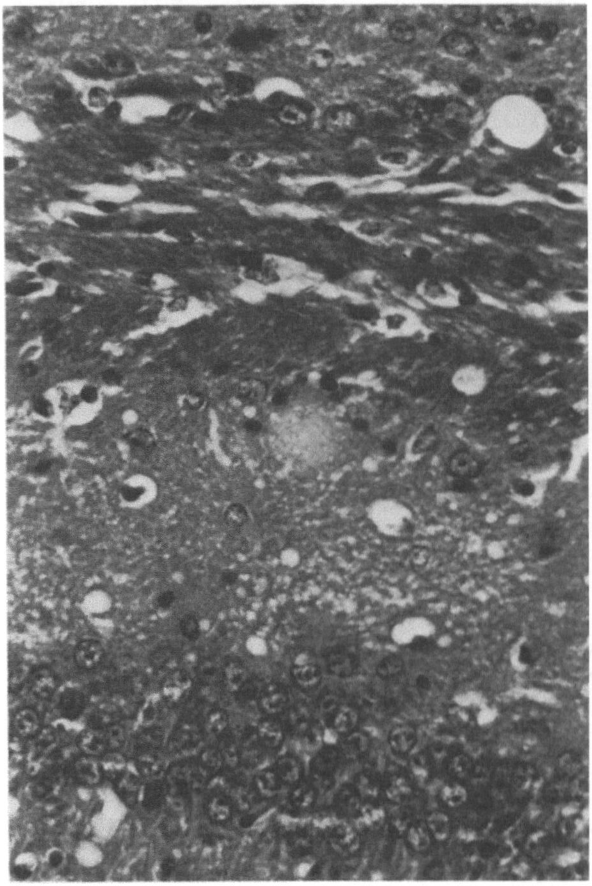

Fig. 7. Amyloid plaque in the hippocampus of a terminal scrapie-affected VL mouse killed 271 days after intraperitoneal injection of ME7 scrapie agent. Masson trichrome, × 400

Table 1. Attempted maternal transmission of 87A scrapie in C57BL mice

Mice injected (*n*)	Route	Incubation period (days ± SE)	Litters (*n*)
Breeding females			
5	IV	449 ± 8	17
4	SC	447[a]	13
3	SC and IP	359[b]	11
Controls			
4	IC	348 ± 13	
2	IV	372 ± 3	
1	SC	552	
4	SC and IP	404 ± 13	

[a] Based on two mice; the other two had not been identified as positive scrapie cases when killed at 230 and 391 days post injection

[b] Based on two mice; the other died at 241 days post injection, without brain histology having been carried out

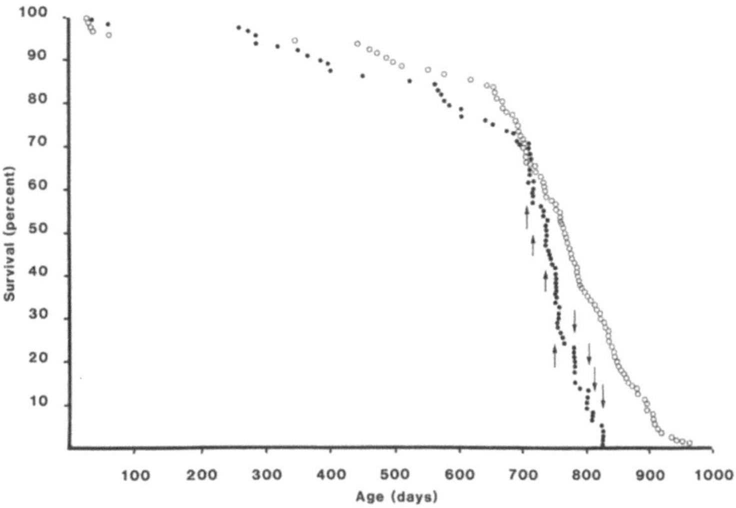

Fig. 8. Survival of 187 progeny of C57BL breeding females infected with 87A scrapie prior to breeding. No scrapie-type spongiosis or amyloid plaques were seen in serial, trichrome-stained sections taken at the levels shown in Fig. 1. o, mice left to survive to life span, of which some died and were not available for histology; •, mice sampled prior to being killed with intercurrent illness. *Arrows* indicate groups killed to avoid "in cage" deaths in older mice

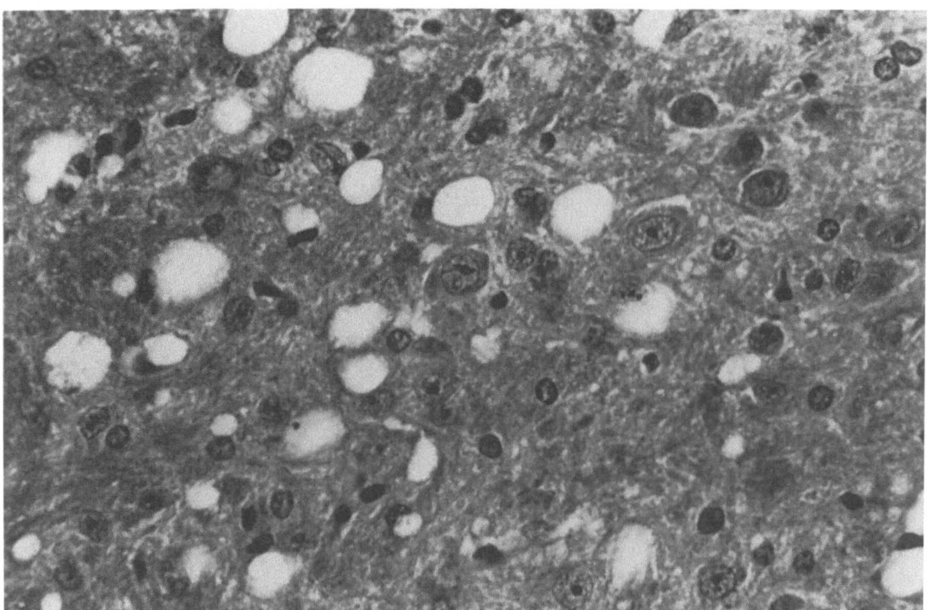

Fig. 9. Medulla of 920-day-old female C3H mouse killed when "senile", showing the vacuolation which is typically found in very old female mice. Haematoxylin and eosin, × 400

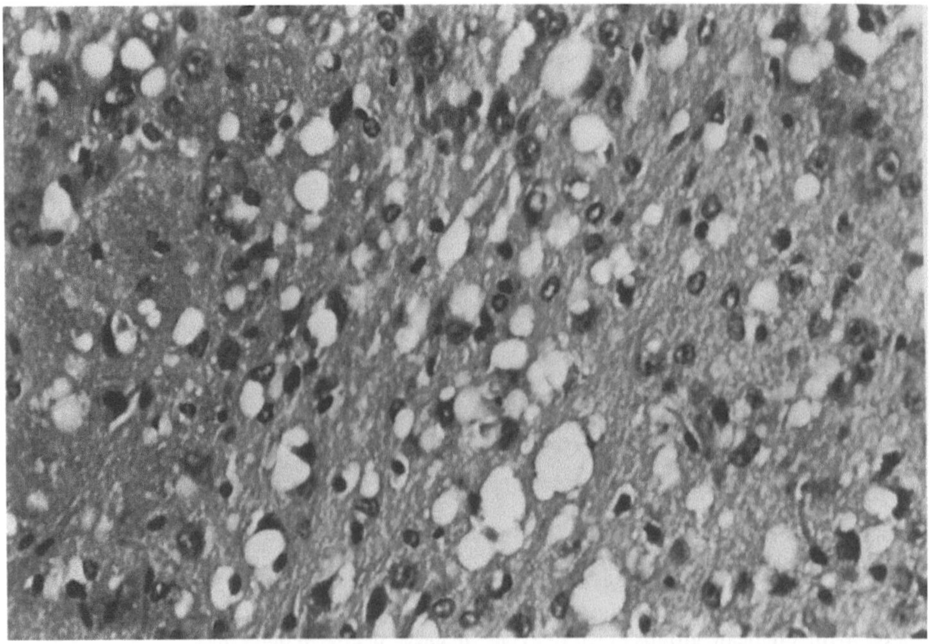

Fig. 10. Scrapie-type vacuolation in a VM mouse injected with ME7 scrapie. Haematoxylin and eosin, × 400

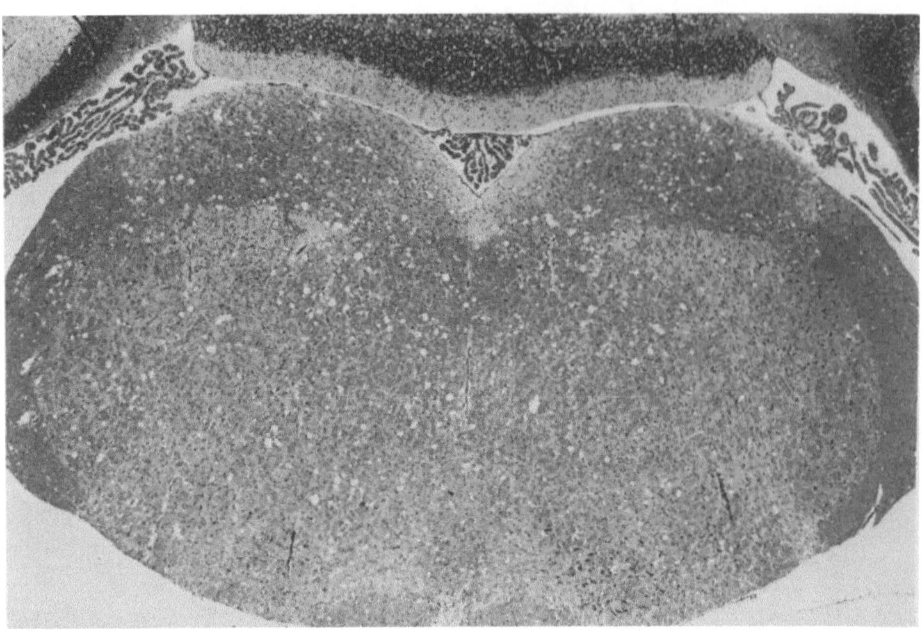

Fig. 11. Low-power view of ageing vacuolation in a very old female C3H mouse. Haematoxylin and eosin, × 20

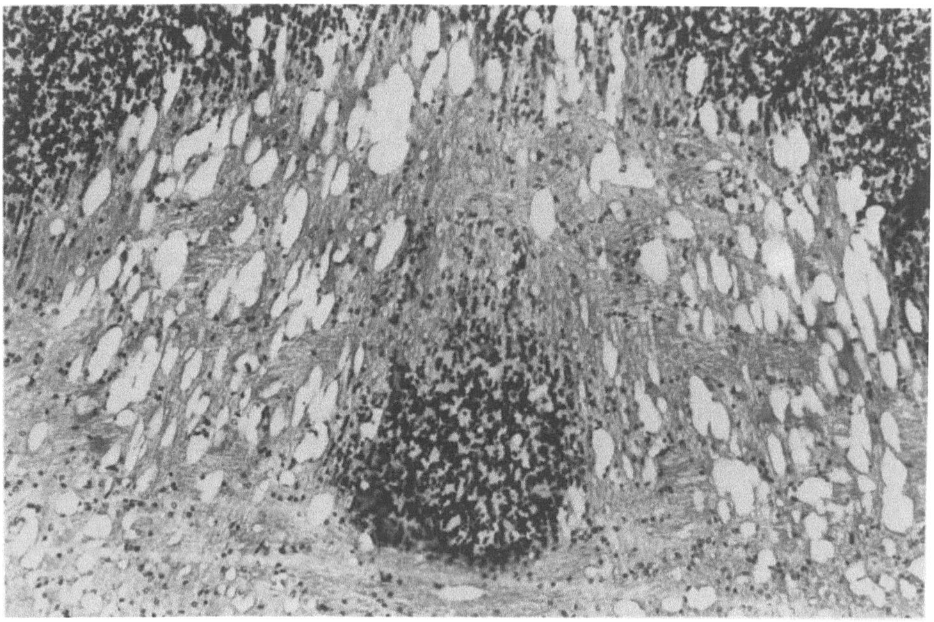

Fig. 12. Typical ageing-type vacuolation in 902-day-old female C57BL mouse in cerebellar white matter. Haematoxylin and eosin, × 100

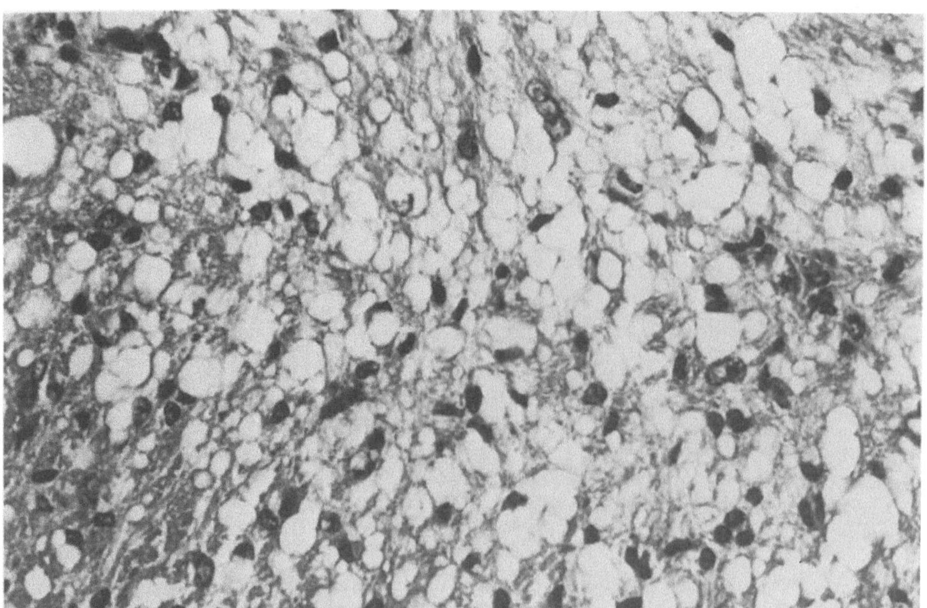

Fig. 13. Spongy leucoencephalopathy of the corpus callosum of a 967-day-old female RIII mouse, × 400

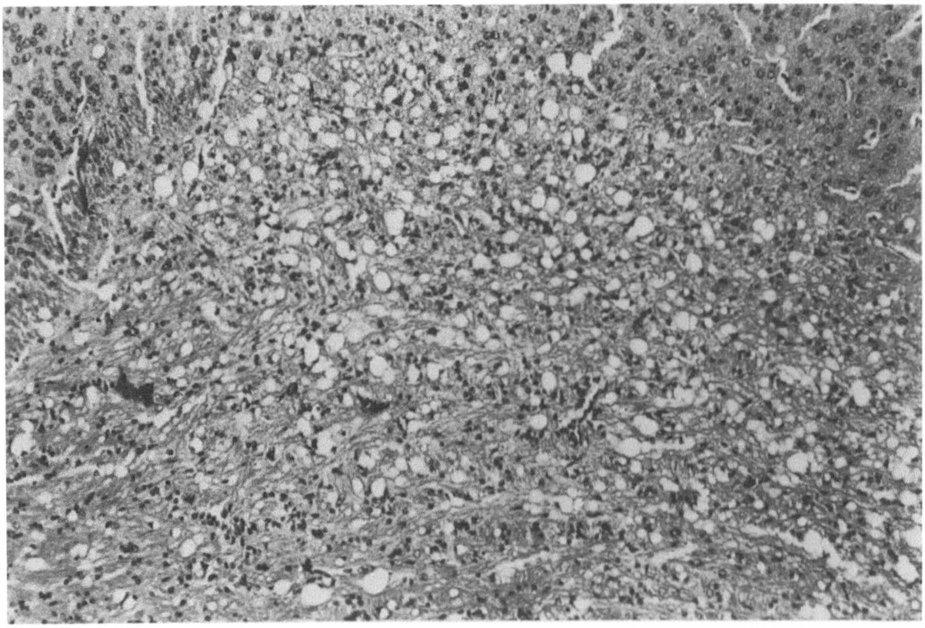

Fig. 14. Low-power view of spongy leucoencephalopathy in a 924-day-old female RIII mouse. × 100

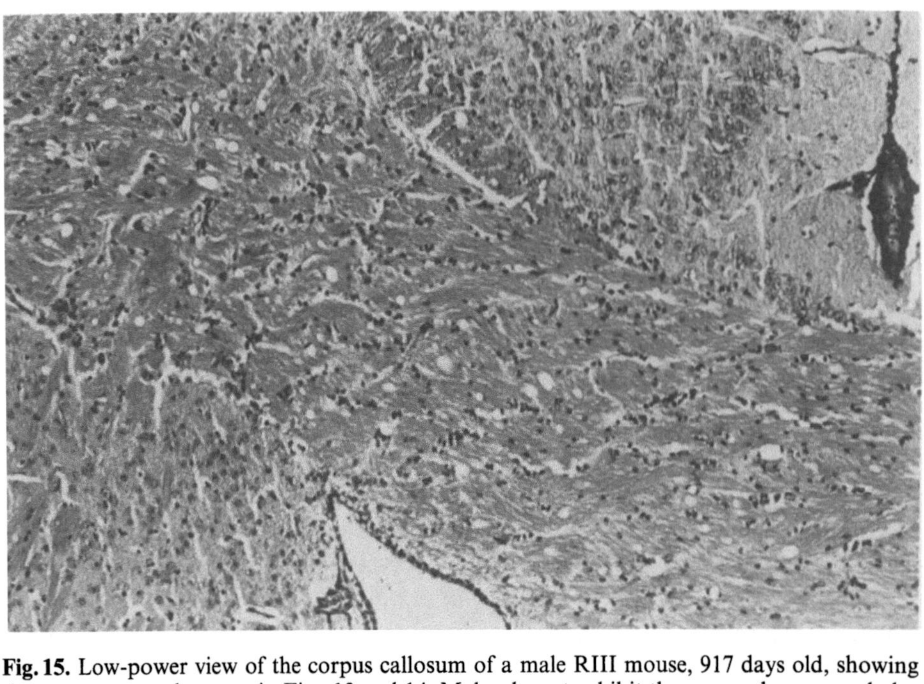

Fig. 15. Low-power view of the corpus callosum of a male RIII mouse, 917 days old, showing the same area as that seen in Figs. 13 and 14. Males do not exhibit the spongy leucoencephalopathy which affects the females. × 100

Table 2. Age incidence and sex ratios of the cases of nonscrapie-affected mice showing vacuolation in the brain

Age (days)	n (strains combined)	Corrected[a] sex ratio of cases with vacuolation (strains combined) F:M	Overall incidence %	Incidence in various mouse strains %					
				VM	MM	C57BL	RIII	C3H	All others
Overall	4,364	2.5:1	6	<1	14	7	8	67	4
>800	308	3.5:1	25	0		13	63	100	
−799	624	2:1	16	1	67	14	14	100	
−699	573	2:1	9	0	12	8	0	100	
−599	625	3:1	5	0	20	3	0	52	
−499	431	All F	3	0	38	4	6	0	
−399	402	All F	1	1	11	0	0	0	
−299	377		0	0	0	1	0	0	
<199	1,024		0	0	0	0	0	0	
n				737	129	1,282	210	81	1,925
Corrected[a] sex ratio of cases with vacuolation (ages combined)				All F	6.4:1	2.5:1	All F	0.8:1	2.7:1

[a] Adjusted to take account of the different numbers of each sex at different ages

Table 3. Estimation of overlap when cases of vacuolation associated with scrapie and with ageing appear to coexist, causing difficulty in scrapie diagnosis

Days	Cases (n) at age (days):									Corrected[a] sex ratio (M:F)
	<199	−299	−399	−499	−599	−699	−799	−899	<900	
Mouse strain										
VM	0	4	12	6	4	4	4	0	4	1:1
VL	0	4	1	7	2	3	4	0	0	1:1.4
C57BL	0	3	2	0	2	7	5	9	3	1:1.4
BALB/c	0	0	1	2	0	2	1	3	1	1:8.5
RIII	0	0	2	2	0	0	1	5	18	1:3.5
C3H	0	0	1	0	0	4	25	5	1	1:11
BRVR	0	0	0	0	2	3	2	3	2	1:5.4
Others	0	1	1	3	8	6	5	7	5	
% incidence (strains pooled)	0	0.1	0.5	0.8	1.1	2.8	0.8	14.7		1:2
% incidence (strains and ages pooled)					0.8					

[a] See Table 2 for definition of corrected sex ratio

can manifest itself as a spongy leucoencephalopathy affecting all the forebrain bundles and the corpus callosum (Figs. 13, 14), a phenomenon not seen in either age-matched or older males (Fig. 15). The leucoencephalopathy is particularly prominent in aged female RIII mice. Table 2 shows the incidence of old-age vacuolation in scrapie-free mice and illustrates the higher female incidence in most strains. Table 3 is a survey of cases where vacuolation developing in old age could have presented difficulties in diagnosing scrapie. These cases represent a selected series collected especially to illustrate examples where scrapie and old age might be confused by observers unfamiliar with their differences. It can be seen that, in most mouse strains, senile changes and scrapie are more likely to be confused in female than in male mice. There can be no doubt, however, that severe old-age-associated spongy change would obscure mild or low-grade scrapie spongiosis and that, because histologic distinctions cannot always be made, judgments may be arbitrary.

Conclusion

The foremost analogy between scrapie and AD has been based on the presence in some murine scrapie models of amyloid-containing, argyrophilic plaques which have essentially the same structure as the neuritic senile plaques of Alzheimer's disease (Bruce and Fraser 1975; Fraser and Bruce 1973; Wisniewski et al. 1975). Furthermore, the severe degeneration of the pyramidal neurons in some scrapie models is closely analogous to the cell-specific pathology of the hippocampus in AD (Bruce 1984; Bruce and Dickinson 1982; Hyman et al. 1984; Scott and Fraser 1984). However, another major feature of the human dementia, neurofibrillary tangles composed of paired helical filaments, have not been seen in any scrapie models (Table 4). On the other hand, the homology of scrapie and

Table 4. Contrasts between Alzheimer's disease and scrapie (Bruce 1984; Bruce and Dickinson 1982)

	Scrapie	Alzheimer's disease (AD)
Clinical circumstances	Natural and experimental	Natural disease only
	Infectious	Unknown
	(young adult →)[a] older	Adult to aged
Lesions	(→) amyloid plaques[a]	Argyrophilic plaques
	No tangles	Neurofibrillary tangles
	Degenerative pathology in grey matter (and white matter)	Grey matter
	(selective cell loss in hippocampus)	Selective cell loss in hippocampus
	Scrapie-associated fibrils, SAF	None found

[a] (→) indicates that there are a wide variety of scrapie models with characteristics extending beyond those of the AD models; characteristics in parentheses indicate inconstant features

Table 5. Network hypothesis for cerebral amyloid plaque occurrence

Status	Amyloid plaques	Spongiosis	Network
Nonscrapie	None	None	Intact
Wild-type scrapie	Many	Restricted	Partly intact
Mutant strain	Few or none	Widespread	Largely degenerate

Creutzfeld-Jakob disease (CJD), in which neurofibrillary tangles are not found, is now well-established. They clearly belong to a common group on the basis of their neuropathology and transmission characteristics. Any similarity between AD and scrapie can be of fundamental significance only when the aetiology of AD is discovered. There has been much speculation that AD may be a scrapie-like infectious process, and if this turns out to be the case, the two diseases will certainly be closely homologous – at least for those scrapie models, mostly associated with wild-type strains, in which a prominent pathological sign is the presence of plaques. Some sort of relation between AD and CJD is suggested based on the occurrence of both in some family studies, although this may simply reflect an unknown variety and overlap of the two diseases (Masters et al. 1979). AD is now recognised to be more variable than once thought, and the range of CJD neuropathology is still uncertain. It is therefore credible to draw a parallel between these human diseases if the CJD agent can be considered a derivative of a putative AD agent; this is the case with the known mutations of scrapie varieties, where wild-type, high-plaque scrapie strains can generate mutants producing rapid-onset disease and widespread spongiosis (Bruce and Dickinson 1984).

The origin of amyloid plaques is unknown, and a grasp of the differences in their occurrence between strains would therefore seem to be pivotal to an eventual understanding of much of the neuropathogenesis of scrapie. A sequence of occurrences between "normal" wild-type and mutant-strain types of pathology is shown in Table 5, showing the *network hypothesis* to help explain differences in amyloid plaque occurrence in four hypothetical steps of neuroparenchymal degeneration. If the amyloid precursors are products of normally functioning neuronal networks, normal turnover in the unaffected individual (synthesis and catabolism by different network components prevents accumulation of the locally generated products. With the partial loss of a network, as has been suggested for wild-type scrapie strains in which spongiosis is restricted to certain subcortical areas only, production of an amyloid precursor would be sustained by the functioning part of the network, but its removal could be prejudiced by the loss of the remaining components of the network. When the degeneration is more generalised, synthesis of precursor is stopped or reduced, meaning amyloid plaques would be absent or few: this is the case in such strains of scrapie as ME7, 7D, 22C and 79A, where spongiosis is widespread throughout the whole CNS. Figure 16 illustrates this network hypothesis.

An understanding of the changes normally accompanying old age becomes important when experimental observations over the whole period of an animal's life span are necessary. In experimental murine scrapie, the long incubation pe-

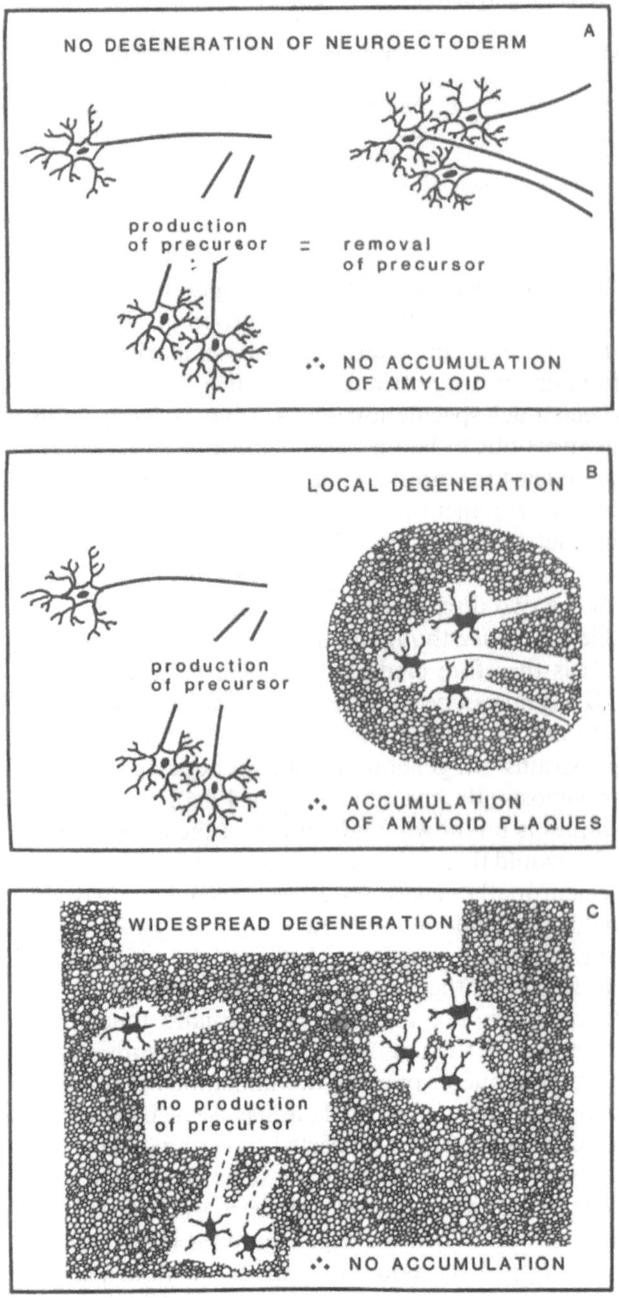

Fig. 16 A–C. Network hypothesis. **A** In a nonscrapie brain, putative amyloid precursors are produced, which are normally removed in an intact neuronal network. **B** scrapie caused by a high-plaque-producing, wild-type scrapie strain; the spongiosis occurs in restricted locations of the brain, leaving many cortical areas free of spongiosis. An amyloid precursor may be produced by neurons in the unaffected area, but its removal is compromised by degeneration of neurons elsewhere with which the normal neurons make connection. **C** widespread spongiosis in many CNS regions, leading to failure of precursor production

riods of some models can extend to life span or beyond (Dickinson et al. 1975). Clearly, ageing is accompanied by a wide range of homeostatic alterations which contribute to the survival of the individual. Some of these adaptations may be directly linked to the ageing process, while others are presumably initiated by environmental interactions (Sobel 1970). Some of the latter can constitute pathological alteration if they represent an atypical event in the existence of an individual. If, however, an environmental factor is ubiquitous, it may lead to a variety of responses, and a clear delineation between what constitutes a "disease" or a homeostatic response stopping short of disease becomes blurred. There are some cases where involving ageing processes to explain the aetiology of disease is justified (Sobel 1970). However, to conclude that ageing changes are identical to certain disease processes, as has been done, simply reflects ignorance of both. The fact that a disease occurs in old age does not justify confusing the two. If scrapie has any lessons for AD, it may be to suggest that the latter is an environmentally induced disorder independent of age or ageing (Bruce and Fraser 1982), in which homeostasis has "failed", bringing about a consequent pathological degeneration of the neuroectoderm. In other words, AD, like scrapie but unlike ageing, is a pathological and not a physiological process.

References

Bendheim PE, Barry RA, De Armond SJ, Stites DP, Prusiner SB (1984) Antibodies to a scrapie prion protein. Nature 310:418–421

Bruce ME (1984) Scrapie and Alzheimer's disease. Psychol Med 14:497–500

Bruce ME, Dickinson AG (1982) Dementia and unconventional slow infections. In: Wheatley D (ed) Psychopharmacology of old age, chapter 3. Oxford University Press, Oxford, pp 15–23

Bruce ME, Dickinson AG (1979) Biological stability of different classes of scrapie agent. In: Prusiner SB, Hadlow WJ (eds) Slow transmissible disease of the nervous system, vol 2. Academic, New York, pp 71–86

Bruce ME, Fraser H (1975) Amyloid plaques in the brain of mice infected with scrapie: morphological variation and staining properties. Neuropathol Appl Neurobiol 1:189–202

Bruce ME, Fraser H (1982) Effects of age on cerebral amyloid plaques in murine scrapie. Neuropathol Appl Neurobiol 8:71–74

Bruce ME, Dickinson AG, Fraser H (1976) Cerebral amyloidosis in scrapie in the mouse: effect of agent strain and mouse genotype. Neuropathol Appl Neurobiol 2:471–478

Collis SC, Kimberlin RH (1983) Further studies on the changes in immunoglobulin G in the sera and CSF of Herdwick sheep with natural and experimental scrapie. J Comp Pathol 93:331–338

Dickinson AG (1976) Scrapie in sheep and goats. In: Kimberlin RH (ed) Slow virus diseases of animals and man, chapter 10. Elsevier, Amsterdam, pp 209–241

Dickinson AG, Fraser H (1977) Scrapie: pathogenesis in inbred mice: an assessment of host control and response involving many strains of agent, chapter 1. In: Ter Meulen V, Katz M (eds) Springer, Berlin Heidelberg New York, pp 3–14

Dickinson AG, Fraser H, Outram GW (1975) Scrapie incubation period time can exceed natural lifespan. Nature 256:732–733

Diringer H, Gelderblom, Hilmert H, Ozel M, Edelbluth C, Kimberlin RH (1983) Scrapie infectivity, fibrils and low molecular weight protein. Nature 306:476–478

Diringer H, Ralm HC, Bode L (1984) Antibodies to proteins of scrapie-associated fibrils. Lancet II:345

Fraser H (1979) Neuropathology of scrapie: The precision of the lesions and their diversity. In: Prusiner SB, Hadlow WJ (eds) Slow transmissible diseases of the nervous system, vol 1. Academic, New York, pp 387–405
Fraser H (1983) A survey of primary transmission of Icelandic scrapie (rida) to mice. In: Court LA, Cathala F (eds) Virus non conventionnels et affections du système nerveux central, chapter 3. Masson, Paris, pp 34–46
Fraser H, Bruce ME (1973) Argyrophilic plaques in mice inoculated with scrapie from particular sources. Lancet I:617–618
Fraser H, Bruce ME (1983) Experimental control of cerebral amyloid in scrapie in mice. In: Behan PO, ter Meulen V, Clifford Rose F (eds) Immunology of nervous system infections; progress in brain research. Elsevier, Amsterdam, pp 281–289
Gardiner AC, Marucci AA (1969) Immunological responsiveness of scrapie-infected mice. J Comp Pathol 79:233–235
Hourrigan J, Klingspoorn A, Clark WW, de Camp M (1979) Epidemiology of scrapie in the United States. In: Prusiner SB, Hadlow WJ (eds) Slow transmissible diseases of the nervous system, vol 1. Academic, New York, pp 331–356
Hyman BT, Van Hoesen GW, Damasio AR, Barnes CL (1984) Alzheimer's disease: cell-specific pathology isolates the hippocampal formation. Science 225:1168–1170
Masters CL, Gajdusek DC, Gibbs CJ, Bernoulli C, Asher DM (1979) Familial Creutzfeldt-Jakob disease and other familial dementias: an inquiry into possible modes of transmission of virus-induced familial diseases. In: Prusiner SB, Hadlow WJ (eds) Slow transmissible diseases of the nervous system, vol 1. Academic, New York, pp 143–194
McKinley MP, Bolton DC, Prusiner SB (1983) A protease-resistant protein is a structural component of the scrapie prion. Cell 35:57–62
Merz PA, Somerville RA, Wisniewski HM, Iqbal K (1981) Abnormal fibrils from scrapie-infected brain. Acta Neuropathol 54:63–74
Merz PA, Somerville RA, Wisniewski HM (1983a) Abnormal fibrils in scrapie and senile dementia of Alzheimer type. In: Court LA, Cathala F (eds) Virus non conventionnels et affections du système nerveux central, chapter 21. Masson, Paris, pp 259–281
Merz PA, Somerville RA, Wisniewski HM, Manuelides L, Manuelides EE (1983b) Scrapie-associated fibrils in Creutzfeld-Jakob disease. Nature 306:474–476
Porter DD, Porter HG, Cox NA (1973) Failure to demonstrate a humoral immune response to scrapie in mice. J Immunol 111:1407–1410
Prusiner SB (1984) Some speculations about prions, amyloid, and Alzheimer's disease. N Engl J Med 310:661–663
Scott JR, Fraser H (1984) Degenerative hippocampal pathology in mice infected with scrapie. Acta Neuropathol 65:62–68
Sobel H (1970) Ageing and age-associated disease. Lancet II:1191–1192
Wisniewski HM, Bruce ME, Fraser H (1975) Infectious etiology of neuritic (senile) plaques in mice. Science 190:1108–1110

Animal Models of Geriatric Cognitive Dysfunction: Evidence for an Important Cholinergic Involvement

R. L. DEAN and R. T. BARTUS[1, 2]

Introduction

Cognitive impairments in the aged present an increasingly important health problem. More than 11% of the U.S. population is 65 years of age or older, and many of these people suffer some degree of intellectual dysfunction. In 1.5–3 million people, this cognitive decline is greatly exacerbated by the presence of senile dementia of the Alzheimer's type (SDAT). SDAT insidiously destroys the intellectual capacity of its victims (Reisberg et al. 1982), ultimately necessitating complete and perpetual institutional care. Annual costs for treatment and care are in excess of 20 billion dollars in the United States. At the same time, the devastating emotional burden and personal loss felt by family members, friends, and the patients themselves cannot be properly represented in financial terms. Improvement in other health care areas has been and is expected to continue to expand rapidly the aged sector of the population. The present magnitude of the health care problem posed by the elderly and clear projections for its increased incidence in the future demand a concerted efford to determine the nature, etiology, and treatment of cognitive impairments in the aged.

The number of clinical trials attempting to identify positive pharmacologic agents has likewise grown remarkably in recent years. Although a number of interesting and potentially promising approaches have emerged, no clearly effective drug has yet been discovered. Several reasons can be identified for the current lack of unqualified success, including the apparent complexity of the problem, ignorance of the underlying neurologic and neurochemical variables, and difficulty in controlling the clinical setting and/or accurately measuring subtle changes in clinical status. Clearly, the current situation suggests that much could be gained by the judicious use of information derived from valid and reliable animal models.

Although the task of developing meaningful animal models may seem quite difficult, recently published studies from our laboratory suggest that it is indeed possible to obtain information from animals that is reliable and has significant predictive value for problems of the aging human central nervous system. Over the past decade, our research has been oriented towards two primary objectives: (a) an understanding of the neurobiological changes that accompany age-related cognitive decline and (b) the development of animal models that reflect the neural and cognitive changes in aged and demented humans, with the ultimate goal of developing a treatment strategy.

1 Dept. of CNS Research, Lederle Laboratories, Medical Research Division, American Cyanamid Company, Pearl River, NY 10965, USA, and
2 New York University Medical Center, New York University, New York, NY 10016, USA

Senile Dementia of the Alzheimer Type
Ed. by J. Traber and W. H. Gispen

Our first published efforts in this area focused on the development of a nonhuman primate model of age-related changes in learning and memory performance (Bartus and Johnson 1976; Bartus et al. 1978). Nonhuman primates were selected for these studies for several reasons (Bartus 1979a). The similarity in the behavioral repertoire of humans and nonhuman primates makes it possible to achieve a high degree of correspondence between the two species in the experimental procedures used and the cognitive processes measured. Furthermore, the similarity in brain structure and organization simplifies the problem of identifying homologous brain regions. Finally, the close phylogenetic relationship between humans and nonhuman primates raises the possibility of studying age-related neurobiological changes that may not occur in subprimate species (e.g., senile plaques).

Automated General Experimental Device (AGED): The Behavioral Test Apparatus

For the nonhuman primate studies reviewed here, behavioral testing was conducted in the Automated General Experimental Device (AGED; Fig. 1). The AGED and its application to geriatric research has been discussed in detail previously (Bartus 1979a; Bartus and Johnson 1976; Bartus et al. 1978).

The AGED is a totally automated, computer-controlled testing system, which displays to the subject a 3- × -3 matrix of stimulus-response panels. Each stimulus-response panel is hinge-mounted in front of a reinforcement well. Both colored and patterned stimuli can be projected onto the stimulus-response panels. When the correct panel is pushed, a reed switch is magnetically activated, and the reinforcement well is exposed.

A plastic partition with a stimulus observation window and armholes separates the monkey from the stimulus-response matrix. The window is equipped

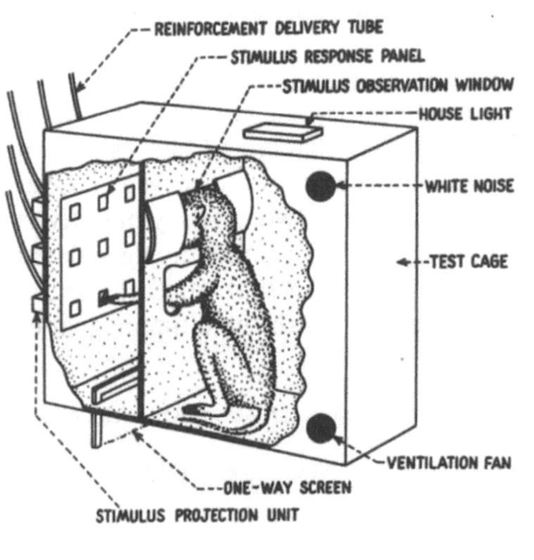

Fig. 1. Artist's conception of monkey making a choice response in the Automated General Experimental Device (AGED) used to collect the primate data reviewed in this paper. The most important features of the AGED are labeled, with the exception of the reinforcement feeder/router mechanism (not shown) and the photocell detecting unit located on either side of the stimulus observation window (not visible)

with a photocell and an infrared light source to detect when the monkey's head is oriented toward the stimuli. This allows the procedure to be subject-paced and increases the likelihood that the subject begins processing the stimuli at the start of each trial. A one-way viewing screen can separate the stimulus-response matrix from the monkey. When this screen is lit from the back, it is transparent, allowing the monkey to view, but not respond to, the panels. When it is not lit from the back, it is opaque, visually isolating the monkey from the stimulus-response matrix.

One of the AGED's main features is that it is totally automated and computer controlled. Thus, potential experimenter bias during the experimental procedure, problems of experimenter-subject interactions, and the need for extensive pre-experimental taming procedures required of manual procedures are eliminated or greatly minimized with an automated procedure. Furthermore, the degree of experimental control, accuracy, and specificity is substantially increased, as is the overall efficiency of the test.

Another important feature is that all trials are subject-paced, beginning each time the monkey's face enters the observation window. The self-pacing procedure is critical to an objective evaluation of performance in the aged, for many investigators have shown that experimenter-paced tasks produce spuriously low estimates of the aged subject's capacities (Canestrari 1963).

The final prominent feature of this apparatus is that the stimulus cue, response panel, and reinforcement well are spatially contiguous, thereby facilitating drug and gerontological testing. Because of this configuration, naive animals learn to operate the apparatus for food reinforcement very quickly, and relatively little effort is required on the part of a test-sophisticated monkey to perform in the apparatus for extended periods of time. This feature is important in evaluation and comparison of specific behavioral functions in aged subjects who may suffer from decreased motivation, attention, physical stamina, psychomotor coordination, and other noncognitive impairments.

Behavioral Profile of the Aged Monkey

In an early series of studies, we compared the ability of aged and young monkeys to perform a series of behavioral tasks. This was done to determine: (a) which behaviors in monkeys are most severely affected by the aging process, (b) how these changes compare with those occurring in humans and rodents, and therefore, (c) which behavioral measures would be most appropriate for future psychopharmacologic studies of age-related impairments.

Selective Behavioral Deficits

The results of this series of studies demonstrate clearly that aged monkeys indeed suffer dramatic behavioral deficits but that, just as importantly, other functions appear to remain relatively stable. The most impressive of these impairments is

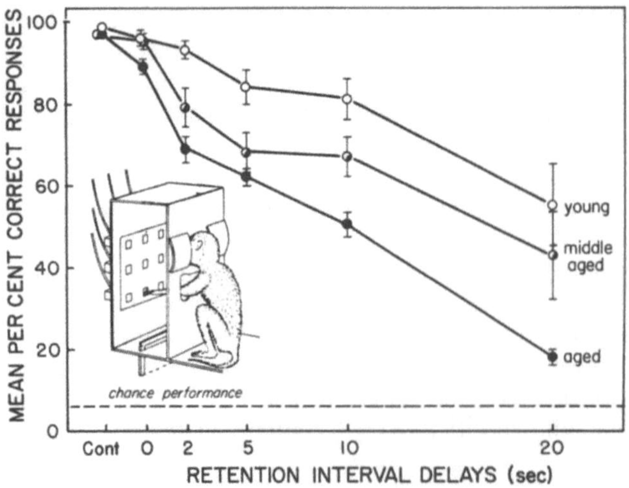

Fig. 2. Differences in ability of three age groups of *Cebus* monkeys to perform the delayed response task intended to measure accuracy of recent memory. Note progressively greater differences between age groups as duration of the retention interval increases, requiring monkeys to remember the stimulus location for increasingly longer periods. Young monkeys were 5–7 years, middle-aged ones were 10–15 years, and aged monkeys were over 18 years of age. (From Bartus et al., 1980; reprinted with permission)

the deficit in memory for recent stimulus events (Bartus et al. 1978, 1980). This deficit is best exemplified using an automated delayed response task which requires the monkey to locate visually and remember which of the nine panels has just been illuminated and to press that panel to obtain a food reward when the opportunity occurs. It was found that aged monkeys suffer severe deficits in their ability to remember the location of a stimulus. Further, this impairment was shown to be specific to memory mechanisms; the magnitude of this deficit is small at short retention intervals, but increases dramatically with retention interval duration (Fig. 2).

Subsequent experiments in our laboratory demonstrated that dysfunctions in motivation, sensory processing, or motor performance are not responsible for the age-related memory impairment. Further behavioral studies conducted with the same apparatus and general test procedure revealed that, in addition to the recent memory loss, significant deficits are observed on tasks requiring the attentional inhibition of irrelevant sensory stimulation (Bartus and Dean 1979) and the modification of previously formed stimulus reinforcement associations (Bartus et al. 1979). Once more, operationally and conceptually similar deficits have been reported in elderly and demented patients (Botwinick 1973; Reisberg et al. 1982). At the same time, however, not all behavioral functions were impaired in the aged monkeys, indicating that the deficits observed can not be explained on the basis of a general decline in behavioral function (Bartus 1979a).

In sum, this series of studies demonstrated that the changes observed in aged monkeys bear a strong resemblance to those seen in elderly humans (Craik 1977;

Kubanis and Zornetzer 1981) and, incidentally, to many deficits we and others have reported for aged rodents (Dean et al. 1981; Gold and McGaugh 1975; Lippa et al. 1980; Zornetzer et al. 1982). Further, the most severe deficit involves loss of memory for recent events, a deficit strikingly similar to the most severe and common behavioral impairment in elderly and demented humans. Thus, these behavioral data provide further justification for the use of aged monkeys as animal models for memory loss in elderly humans and help identify a reasonable behavioral deficit to use in evaluating the effects of experimental drugs intended to enhance geriatric memory.

Possible Relationship of Behavioral Deficits to Frontal Brain Lesions

We find it interesting that this preliminary behavior profile of the aged monkey closely parallels that observed in monkeys with destruciton or functional disturbances of the dorsolateral frontal cortex (Bartus 1979). A comparison of these two sets of observations appears in Table 1. On the basis of these striking similarities and the pharmacologic date we and others accumulated previously, we hypothesized that: (a) the cognitive decline associated with advanced age and dementia might be due in part to a functional deterioration of a cortical-subcortical system including the frontal cortex and (b) it is likely that at least some of the neurons involved are cholinergic in nature (Bartus 1979 a).

Concurrent collaborative studies demonstrating morphometric changes (e.g., cellular degeneration, sulcal size, neuronal/glial ratios) in the frontal cortex and hippocampus of aged monkeys in association with memory loss offered some independent support for this notion (Brizzee et al. 1980). At the time of these studies, the relationship between cholinergic cells in the basal forebrain and their termination in the cortex was not well-established. However, our observations now seem particularly intriguing in light of recent evidence indicating a large, topographically organized projection from areas of the nucleus basalis to the frontal cortex. It has been proposed that severe degeneration of the cortical cholinergic

Table 1. Similarities between behavior of aged rhesus monkeys and frontally ablated monkeys

Behavioral function	Aged monkeys	Frontally ablated monkeys
Recent or short-term memory	severely impaired	severely impaired
Sensitivity to interfering stimulation (intratrial)	increased	increased
Sensory processing ability (controlled for visual acuity problems)	no serious impairment	no obvious impairment
Visual discrimination learning	no consistent deficit	generally no deficit
Reversal learning (perseveration)	impaired	impaired
Long-term retention	no deficit	no deficit

projection from the basal forebrain plays a major role in the cognitive loss of SDAT (Coyle et al. 1983). By comparing normal aged and frontally lesioned monkeys, it is possible to extend this idea to suggest that less profound functional disturbances in this same system may contribute to the more subtle cognitive deficits seen with normal advanced age.

Similarities to Memory Loss in Aged and Demented Humans

Converging on these nonhuman primate studies are related investigations conducted on humans. In collaboration with Ferris and Flicker (New York University, New York), and Crook (National Institute of Mental Health, Bethesda, MD), we recently initiated a series of clinical studies aimed at the development of a test battery to assess the efficacy of pharmacologic treatments of the aged and demented. A fundamental objective of these studies is to devise human tests that are conceptually and operationally similar to available animal tests. Such tests would help bridge the gap between contemporary animal and human studies and would facilitate the evaluation of results obtained when a potential treatment is administered to both animals and humans.

The first study used a stimulus array and delayed response paradigm that is highly comparable to that of the AGED nonhuman primate apparatus. That is,

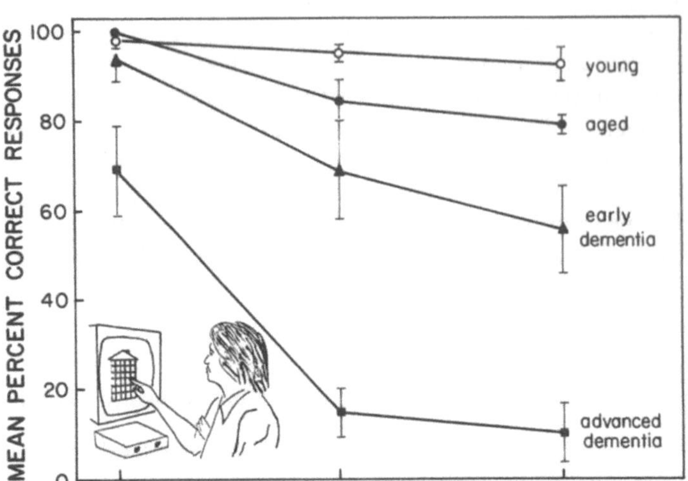

Fig. 3. Differences in performance between young humans (·····); normal aging (———); mild to moderate, clinically suspected Alzheimer's disease patients (– – –); and more severely demented patients (–·–·–·) on a delayed response task modeled after the nonhuman primate task in Fig. 2. *Insert* depicts subject responding to the window of a house which was illuminated prior to the retention interval. Note the clear differences between the various subject classifications and the similarity between these data and those obtained with the different age groups of monkeys in Fig. 2. (From Flicker et al. 1984, reprinted with permission)

subjects were required to remember, over periods of varying duration, which of several windows of a house had been illuminated, in a manner analogous to the monkey task. As shown in Fig. 3, a clear, time-related decay in performance occurred as the subjects were required to remember the location of the illuminated window over greater periods. More importantly, however, this task clearly differentiated young subjects from aged subjects, as well as normal healthy aged subjects from those with varying degrees of dementia (Flicker et al. 1984). Thus, the age-related deficits in nonhuman primates and in aged humans share certain common features. That is, some of the more pronounced and consistent deficits observed occur: (a) in situations where the event to be remembered is brief and discrete; (b) when little or no opportunity for rehearsal exists; and (c) over a relatively short time span, with retention often declining markedly within minutes. Taken together, the data suggest that a conceptually similar type of memory dysfunction may occur in aged members of the mammalian class.

The initial series of behavioral studies in aged monkeys described above is one of a few systematic investigations of the cognitive effects of aging in animals. However, more extensive studies involving a broader range of behaviors are needed as a prerequisite of: (a) developing a more complete understanding of the behavioral changes that occur with age, (b) establishing the role of basal forebrain cholinergic neurons in mediating these behaviors, and ultimately, (c) developing a valid and rational neurobehavioral model of the cognitive disturbances associated with aging and dementia.

Age-Related Cognitive Dysfunction: Role of the Cholinergic System

Because memory loss in nonhuman primates is similar to that of elderly and demented humans, it seems possible that aged monkeys can be used as models for studying memory disturbances and for evaluating experimental drugs intended to treat geriatric memory problems.

In addition to studying the effects of age on the cognitive behavior of nonhuman primates, considerable activity in our laboratory has been directed toward understanding the neurochemical variables involved in behavioral deficits. Guiding much of this research is the cholinergic hypothesis of age-related cognitive decline. The body of evidence supporting this hypothesis, which has been collectively generated by this laboratory and others, has been reviewed in detail elsewhere (Bartus et al. 1982b).

First, significant changes in cholinergic markers occur in the brains of aged humans and animals (reviewed in Bartus et al. 1982b). These changes are accompanied by electrophysiologic dysfunctions in cholinoceptive neurons (Lippa et al. 1981) and by a decline in memory/cognitive performance (Lippa et al. 1980; Perry et al. 1978; Strong et al. 1980). The cholinergic deficits and, in particular, the decline in choline acetyltransferase (ChAT) activity (reviewed in Bartus et al. 1982b) are exacerbated in SDAT patients. The magnitude of this decline in ChAT is correlated with both major neuropathologic markers and the degree of cognitive impairment produced bei the disease (Perry et al. 1978; Wilcock et al. 1982).

Although parallel neuropathologic changes have been reported for other neurotransmitter systems (Bondareff et al. 1981; Gottfries 1982; Kubanis and Zornetzer 1981), correlations between these changes and the cognitive deterioration in SDAT have yet to be established. Furthermore, it is unclear whether these changes exist in all SDAT patients (Rossor et al. 1984) or whether they may simply be due to confounding variables involving subject selection and diagnosis (Davies 1981). In contrast, the decrease in ChAT activity in SDAT and the correlation with cognitive deficits is remarkably consistent and has come to be regarded as a neurochemical hallmark of the disease.

It has been shown that the cholinergic blocker scopolamine produces behavioral effects in man similar to those arising in normal aging (Drachman and Leavitt 1974). In a similar series of tests in young monkeys, central anticholinergic agents like scopolamine (but not peripheral antagonists like methscopolamine) induced behavioral deficits strikingly similar to those occurring naturally in aged monkeys (Bartus and Johnson 1976).

Subsequent studies demonstrated that a deficit produced by scopolamine can be partially, but reliably, reduced by the anticholinesterase physostigmine in both humans (Drachman 1977) and monkeys in our laboratory (Bartus 1978). Similar beneficial effects were not observed with the CNS stimulants methylphenidate (Bartus 1978) or amphetamine (Drachman 1977). It is therefore unlikely that the retention deficit induced by scopolamine in either human or nonhuman primates can be related to its more general effects on arousal, attention, or similar, sedative-like properties. These findings suggest that the amnesia induced by scopolamine is due to a specific disruption of cholinergic mechanisms. That similar deficits are not observed with analogous pharmacologic blockade of dopaminergic, beta-adrenergic, or even nicotinic receptors further supports the notion of a specific role of the muscarinic cholinergic system in memory processes (Bartus 1980; Bartus et al. 1983 b). Taken together, these data suggest that an important functional relationship may exist between normal aging, cholinergic dysfunction, and loss of memory.

The consistent agreement of these results with predictions based on the cholinergic hypothesis encouraged us to pursue a e corrollary of the hypothesis, i.e., that the enhancement of cholinergic transmission would improve cognitive functioning in the elderly. We sought to determine whether this cholinergic manipulation would serve as a viable therapeutic approach to the problem of geriatric cognitive dysfunction.

Psychopharmacology of Cholinergic Enhancers in Aged Monkeys

Unless specified, all drugs were injected intramuscularly 30 min prior to the behavioral session. The doses for each drug were selected on the basis of published animal and clinical data (if available) and from previous dose range studies in our own laboratory. All doses were given in a quasi-random fashion, with a maximum of two doses per week given to each monkey and a minimum of 2 nondrug days separating each drug administration. Drug and saline control scores were compared directly by computing a "nondrug" statistical confidence limit for each monkey based on that monkey's own baseline control scores. In this way, it was possible to determine whether a change in performance under any single dose of drug reflected a significant and statistically reliable change from the particular monkey's normal baseline performance.

Using the automated delayed response task, we found improvements in the performance of aged monkeys after the facilitation of cholinergic transmission by administering two acetylcholinesterase inhibitors, physostigmine (Bartus 1979b; Bartus et al. 1980) and tetrahydroaminoacridine, and two direct-acting cholinergic agonists, arecoline (Bartus et al. 1980) and oxotremorine (Bartus et al. 1983a). The results obtained with physostigmine and arecoline have received subsequent confirmation in human subjects (Christie et al. 1981; Davis et al. 1979), thus providing strong support for the clinical relevance of the animal model. In contrast, we obtained negative effects in monkeys after acute administration of the cholinergic precursor choline (Bartus et al. 1980); these results received confirmation in human clinical trials (reviewed in Bartus et al. 1982b). It may also be noteworthy here that, of the many classes of drugs studied in the animal model (including CNS stimulants, neuropeptides, nootropics, and antidepressants), the cholinergic agents have thus far produced the most impressive improvement (Bartus and Dean 1981; Bartus et al. 1980, 1982a). Some further evidence of the specificity of ameliorative effects on the cholinergic system was obtained in the form of negative results after pharmacologic activation of other neurotransmitter receptor systems, via administration of apomorphine, muscimol, or clonidine (direct-acting dopaminergic, GABAergic, and alpha-adrenergic agonists respectively) (Bartus et al. 1983a).

These studies with aged monkeys are also a tentative guide for future studies in geriatric humans. The data reviewed here underscore the apparent importance of the cholinergic system in the memory loss observed in aged subjects. Although it seems most probable that other neurotransmitter systems playing equally important roles in this disturbance will be identified, to date, the cholinergic system is the only classic neurotransmitter system which, when stimulated, has produced a positive effect on memory performance in the aged monkey. Emerging from our investigations into manipulations of the cholinergic system, especially with centrally acting muscarinic agonists, is the hypothesis that the more closely one stimulates the muscarinic receptor, the more effective and consistent is the improvement in memory performance of aged subjects. If supported with additional data involving other drugs and replicated in human studies, this hypothesis may provide a clearer idea of where to look for neurochemical changes responsible for cognitive impairments and how to alleviate the dysfunction by the pharmacologic manipulation of the cholinergic system.

Nucleus Basalis of Meynert: Possible Model for SDAT

Another line of research closely related to our nonhuman primate program is our research on the aged rodent. This series of studies evolved in a manner comparable to the monkey experimentation. A wide array of behaviors was tested in the mouse (Dean et al. 1981) and rat (Bartus et al. 1983 b; Lippa et al. 1980) in order to identify those most sensitive to age-related change. Of these, passive avoidance retention was selected for further study because of its vulnerability to the effects of age and its operational and conceptual similarities to the impairment of recent memory observed in aged human and nonhuman primates. That is, as in other behavioral paradigms exhibiting robust, age-related deficits, the memory loss in the passive avoidance procedure is characterized by the facts that the event to be remembered is brief and discrete, there is little or nor practice or rehearsal, and retention of the events decays rapidly, usually within several hours.

Our rodent studies are relevant to the nonhuman primate studies in several respects. They have provided behavioral and pharmacologic evidence in support of the cholinergic hypothesis of age-related cognitive decline. For example, we have noted positive effects of physostigmine, arecoline, and oxotremorine on passive avoidance retention in aged rats (Bartus et al. 1983 b). Furthermore, our rodent studies have provided considerable evidence of a cholinergic neurochemical basis for age-related cognitive decline. These biochemical and electrophysiologic studies have demonstrated that, along with the deficit in passive avoidance retention the aged rodent exhibits decreased cortical and hippocampal muscarinic receptor binding (Lippa et al. 1980; Strong et al. 1980), decreased hippocampal choline uptake (Sherman et al. 1981), decreased cortical ChAT activity (Strong et al. 1980), and a large decrease in the responsiveness of hippocampal neurons to iontophoretically applied acetylcholine (Lippa et al. 1980). In many instances, parallel measures of other neurotransmitter markers revealed a much smaller effect or no deficit at all.

Thus, accumulated research from our own and other laboratories provides encouraging support for the cholinergic hypothesis of geriatric memory dysfunction. However, the majority of experiments have not specifically addressed the problem of memory dysfunction in SDAT. In part, this has been because a suitable animal model for SDAT has not been developed. Although aged humans and animals suffer from cognitive deficits and changes in cholinergic neurotransmission, these changes are typically not as severe as those seen in SDAT. In particular, there is a dramatic drop in cortical ChAT activity which seems to be specific to SDAT. Recent data (Whitehouse et al. 1982) suggest that degeneration of cholinergic cell bodies in the basal forebrain (medial septum, nucleus basalis) may account for this loss of ChAT. If it can be demonstrated that destruction of these cell bodies produces severe memory and cognitive deficits analogous to those of SDAT, it might be possible to use animals with basal forebrain lesions to study treatment alternatives for the major neurobehavioral symptoms of SDAT.

To investigate these possibilities, we have begun to examine the behavior of animals following basal forebrain lesions. For both ethical and practical reasons, rats were used as subjects in these preliminary experiments. In our initial study (Flicker et al. 1983), ibotenic acid was infused into the ventromedial globus pallidus, the basal forebrain area which provides the major cholinergic innervation to the cortex and is most homologous to the nucleus basalis of humans and monkeys. Histologic and biochemical evaluation of the rats' brains confirmed that the lesions destroyed the intended cell bodies and effectively reduced cortical ChAT activity. All rats were tested on a battery of behavioral tasks 2 weeks after surgery. Four different psychomotor tasks aimed at measuring muscle strength, stamina, and coordination revealed no effects of the lesion. Further, no differences were observed in shock sensitivity or initial latency to step from a bright to a dark compartment in a single-trial passive avoidance task. However, the nucleus-basalis–lesioned rats revealed severe impairment in the retention of the passive avoidance response.

Because these nucleus-basalis–lesioned animals exhibited deficits at both 1-h and 24-h retention intervals, it is unclear whether these deficits reflect problems in learning, memory, or both. Further, the passive avoidance procedure is recognized to be a relatively crude behavioral paradigm, and its results are often open to multiple alternative interpretations. For these reasons, we performed a second rodent experiment using a new group of rats which were first trained to obtain food reward by visiting each of 8 arms of a radial arm maze. Repeat visits to an arm were never reinforced and were scored as errors. Following several months of training and establishment of near-perfect performance, the rats received sham lesions or nucleus basalis lesions similar to those described above.

Two weeks after surgery, the rats were retested on the radial arm maze task. This retesting revealed normal postoperative retention of the learned task by the nucleus-basalis–lesioned animals. Thus, lesioned rats continued to perform the task as originally trained, going to each of the eight arms once without returning to any of the arms during the session. However, when a recent-memory variable was added to the task procedure, the nucleus-basalis–lesioned group revealed a profound deficit. Thus, when a retention interval was interposed between the selection of the first four arms and the remaining four arms, a time-related decrement in performance occurred (Fig. 4a).

Equally interesting, however, is the observation that, in the course of several months' training on the radial arm maze task, retention over the delay intervals gradually improved. By 6 months after surgery, the lesioned rats' performance was no different from that of the sham controls (Fig. 4b). Further, when trained and tested on the same passive avoidance task described earlier, these animals exhibited no retention deficit. These more recent findings raise questions concerning the adequacy of simply destroying neurons in the basal forebrain to model the major neuropathology of SDAT. Whether similar lesions in aged animals would have produced more lasting deficits is a question of definite import. Similarly, investigating the effects of multiple lesions involving the basal forebrain and other areas implicated in SDAT (i.e., hippocampus. locus ceruleus) would also be of great interest. Finally, the question of the functional significance of the classic neuropathology of SDAT (i.e., tangles and plaques) must be considered. For the time being, this study serves as a clear reminder of the limitations that exist with the brain lesion approach to animal models.

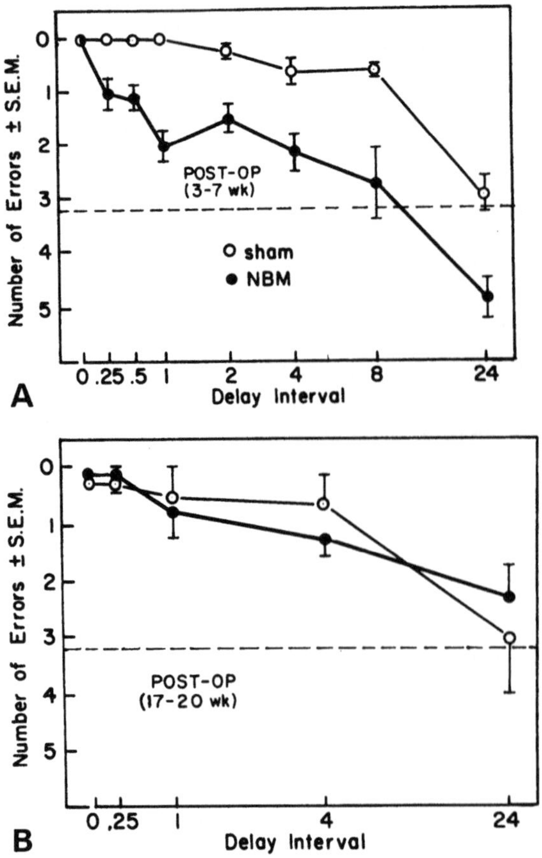

Fig. 4A, B. Retention of spatial location in the radial arm maze (8 arms) by nucleus-basalis- (*shaded circles*) and sham-lesioned (*open circles*) rats. The *dashed horizontal* line depicts chance performance was empirically determined by placing trained animals in the maze and arbitrarily designating four arms as correct and four as incorrect. It therefore approximates the performance that would be expected of animals with no memory for choices made prior to the retention interval. **A** Performance approximately 1 month after surgery. **B** Performance approximately 6 months after surgery. In contrast with performance 1 month after surgery, nucleus-basalis-lesioned animals no longer differed from sham controls in performance over the various delay intervals at 6 months after surgery

Additional studies, particularly in nonhuman primates, would seem to be warranted for several reasons. The basal forebrain nuclei (particularly the nucleus basalis) are poorly defined in many subprimate species; only the monkey has a well-defined cell population demonstrated to be clearly homologous to the nucleus basalis of Meynert in humans. The similarity of structure and organization of the basal forebrain nuclei in human and nonhuman primates, combined with the relative similarity of behavioral repertoire and cognitive test capabilities in these species, greatly reduces the number of assumptions needed to extrapolate from the effects of lesions in nonhuman primates to the functional consequences of degeneration in the basal forebrain nuclei in aged, demented humans. Furthermore, the availability of an extensive accumulation of data from our own and other laboratories concerning the effects of aging on cognitive performance by monkeys provides a strong foundation upon which to construct an optimal cognitive test battery. For these reasons, we are currently exploring this line of research in the development of a nonhuman primate model of the major cognitive problems associated with SDAT.

Acknowledgements. The autors would like to thank C. Flicker and M. Pontecorvo for technical assistance in certain phases of the research reported and for helpful comments on the manuscript and C. Nardella for her assistance in the preparation of this manuscript.

References

Bartus RT (1978) Evidence for a direct cholinergic involvement in the scopolamine-induced amnesia in monkeys: effects of concurrent administration of physostigmine and methylphenidate with scopolamine. Pharmacol Biochem Behav 9:833–836

Bartus RT (1979a) Effects of aging on visual memory, sensory processing and discrimination learning in the non-human primate. In: Ordy JM, Brizzee K (eds) Sensory systems and communication in the elderly. Raven, New York, pp 85–114 (Aging, vol 10)

Bartus RT (1976b) Physostigmine and recent memory: effects in young and aged non-human primates. Science 206:1087–1089

Bartus RT (1980) Cholinergic drug effects on memory and cognition in animals. In: Poon LW (ed) Aging in the 1980's: psychological issues. American Psychological Association, Washington DC, pp 163–180

Bartus RT, Dean RL (1979) Recent memory in aged non-human primates: hypersensitivity to visual interference during retention. Exp Aging Res 5:385–400

Bartus RT, Dean RL (1981) Age-related memory loss and drug therapy: possible directions based on animal models. In: Enna SJ, Samorajski T, Beer B (eds) Brain neurotransmitters and receptors in aging and age-related disorders. Raven, New York, pp 209–224 (Aging, vol 17)

Bartus RT, Johnson HR (1976) Short-term memory in the rhesus monkey: disruption from the anticholinergic scopolamine. Pharmacol Biochem Behav 5:39–46

Bartus RT, Fleming D, Johnson HR (1978) Aging in the rhesus monkey: debilitating effects on short-term memory. J Gerontol 33:858–871

Bartus RT, Dean RL, Fleming DL (1979) Aging in the rhesus monkey: effects on visual discrimination learning and reversal learning. J Gerontol 34:209–219

Bartus RT, Dean RL, Beer B (1980) Memory deficits in aged *Cebus* monkeys and facilitation with central cholinomimetics. Neurobiol Aging 1:145–152

Bartus RT, Dean RL, Beer B (1982a) Neuropeptide effects on memory in aged monkeys. Neurobiol Aging 3:61–68

Bartus RT, Dean RL, Beer B, Lippa AS (1982b) The cholinergic hypothesis of geriatric memory dysfunction. Science 217:408–417

Bartus RT, Dean RL, Beer B (1983a) An evaluation of drugs for improving memory in aged monkeys: Implications for clinical trials in humans. Psychopharmacol Bull 19:168–184

Bartus RT, Flicker C, Dean RL (1983b) Logical principles for the development of animal models of age-related memory impairments. In: Crook T, Ferris S, Bartus RT (eds) Assessment for geriatric psychopharmacology. Powley, New Canaan, CT, pp 263–299

Bondareff W, Mountjoy CO, Roth M (1981) Selective loss of neurons of origin of adrenergic projection to cerebral cortex (locus coeruleus) in senile dementia. Lancet I:783–784

Botwinick J (1973) Aging and behavior. Springer, New York

Brizzee KR, Ordy JM, Bartus RT (1980) Localization of cellular changes within multimodal sensory regions in aged monkey brain: possible implications for age-related cognitive loss. Neurobiol Aging 1:45–52

Canestrari RE (1963) Paced and self-paced learning in young and elderly adults. J Gerontol 18:165–168

Christie JE, Shering A, Ferguson J, Glen AIM (1981) Physostigmine and arecoline: effects of intravenous infusions in Alzheimer's presenile dementia. Br J Psychiatry 128:46–50

Coyle JT, Price DL, Delong MR (1983) Alzheimer's disease: A disorder of cortical cholinergic innervation. Science 219:1184–1190

Craik FIM (1977) Age-related differences in human memory. In: Birren JE, Schaie KW (eds) Handbook of the psychology of aging. Van Nostrand Reinhold, New York, pp 384–420

Davies P (1981) Theoretical treatment possibilities for dementia of the Alzheimer's type: the cholinergic hypothesis. In: Crook T, Gershon S (eds) Strategies for the development of an effective treatment for senile dementia. Powley, New Canaan, CT, pp 19–32

Davis KL, Mohs RC, Tinklenberg JR (1979) Enhancement of memory by physostigmine. N Eng J Med 301:946

Dean RL, Scozzafava J, Goas JA, Regan B, Beer B, Bartus RT (1981) Age-related differences in behavior across the life span of the C57Bl/6j mouse. Exp Aging Res 7:427–451

Drachman DA (1977) Memory and cognitive function in man: does the cholinergic system have a specific role? Neurology 27:783–790
Drachman DA, Leavitt J (1974) Human memory and the cholinergic system: a relationship to aging. Arch Neurology 30:113–121
Flicker C, Dean RL, Watkins DL, Fisher SK, Bartus RT (1983) Behavioral and neurochemical effects following neurotoxic lesions of a major cholinergic input to the cerebral cortex in the rat. Pharmacol Biochem Behav 18:973–981
Flicker C, Ferris SF, Bartus RT, Crook T (1984) Effects of aging and dementia upon recent visuospatial memory. Neurobiol Aging 5:75–83
Gold PE, McGaugh JL (1975) Changes in learning and memory during aging. In: Ordy JM, Brizzee KR (eds) Neurobiology of aging. Plenum, New York, pp 53–57
Gottfries CG (1982) The metabolism of some neurotransmitters in aging and dementia disorders. Gerontology 28(2):11–19
Kubanis P, Zornetzer SF (1981) Age-related behavioral and neurobiological changes: a review with emphasis on memory. Behav Neural Biol 31:115–172
Lippa AS, Pelham RW, Beer B, Critchett DJ, Dean RL, Bartus RT (1980) Brain cholinergic dysfunction and memory in aged rats. Neurobiol Aging 1:13–19
Lippa AS, Critchett DJ, Ehlert F, Yamamura HI, Enna SJ, Bartus RT (1981) Age-related alterations in neurotransmitter receptors: an electrophysiological and biochemical analysis. Neurobiol Aging 2:3–8
Perry EK, Tomlinson BE, Blessed G, Bergmann K, Gibson PH, Perry RH (1978) Correlation of cholinergic abnormalities with senile plaques and mental test scores in senile dementia. Br Med J 2:1457–1459
Reisberg B, Ferris SH, Crook T (1982) Signs, symptoms and course of age-associated cognitive decline. In: Corkin S, Davis KL, Growdon JH, Usdin E, Wurtman RJ (eds) Alzheimer's disease: a report of progress in research. Raven, New York, pp 177–182 (Aging, vol 19)
Rossor MN, Iversen LL, Reynolds GP, Mountjoy CQ, Roth M (1984) Neurochemical characteristics of early and late onset types of Alzheimer's disease. Br Med J 288:961–964
Sherman KA, Kuster JE, Dean RL, Bartus RT, Friedman E (1981) Presynaptic cholinergic mechanisms in brain of aged rats with memory impairments. Neurobiol Aging 2:99–104
Strong R, Hicks P, Hsu L, Bartus RT, Enna SJ (1980) Age-related alterations in the rodent brain cholinergic system and behavior. Neurobiol Aging 1:59–63
Whitehouse PJ, Price DL, Struble RG, Clark AW, Coyle JT, DeLong MR (1982) Alzheimer's disease and senile dementia: loss of neurons in the basal forebrain. Science 215:1237–1239
Wilcock GK, Esiri MM, Bowen DM, Smith CCT (1982) Alzheimer's disease: correlation of cortical choline acetyltransferase activity with severity of dementia and histological abnormalities. J Neurol Sci 57:407–417
Zornetzer SF, Thompson R, Rogers J (1982) Rapid forgetting in aged rats. Behav Neural Biol 36:49–60

Animal Models of Jacksonian Dissolution of Memory in the Aged

B. A. Campbell, C. B. Sananes, and J. R. Gaddy[1]

Introduction

The Jacksonian theory of dissolution of mental function due to injury, disease, or aging states that many infantile behaviors are eventually suppressed by continued growth of the central nervous system and that these functions often reappear following brain injury or dysfunction in adulthood (Jackson 1958). One classic example of this is the Babinski reflex, which is normally present only in infancy but which reappears following some types of brain injury (Willis and Grossman 1973). Senescent decline can also bring about a return of prenatal and infantile reflexes (Paulson 1977). Patients suffering from advanced senile dementia frequently show a return of infantile sucking and grasping reflexes (Paulson and Gottlieb 1968). Such signs do not represent a major part of the symptomatology during the initial phases of dementia, however. Early dementia and other forms of senescent decline are marked by more subtle losses, with the loss of memory seeming to be the commonest and most generally noted.

In keeping with the Jacksonian hypotheses, "organic" amnesias have been noted to resemble infantile amnesia (Schacter and Moscovitch 1984). Infantile amnesia, unlike senescent amnesia, is not a pathologic process. Rather, it is a period of early development marked by an inability to remember (Campbell and Spear 1972). Furthermore, the child's progress out of amnesia into mature memory is marked by the development of a hierarchy of memorial processes, with the recall of specific events emerging last. The different forms of senescent decline, in turn, are distinguished by the early loss of the ability to recall specific events, while memory of general principles remains relatively intact (Rozin 1976; Schacter and Moscovitch 1984). This is true both for the mild senescent amnesia known as benign senescent forgetfulness and for the severe and rapidly progressing senile dementias (Kral 1978).

Thus, in humans, the Jacksonian theory seems to hold quite well when applied to memory loss in old age. However, few direct inquiries into the accordance of this theory with memory function in aged animals have been made. Young rodents do show amnesic syndromes (infantile amnesia) when compared with adults (Campbell and Spear 1972), and long-term memory for some types of learning matures much earlier than for others. Although no animal model of senile dementia comparable to that available for infantile amnesia has yet been established, there is a rapidly increasing body of literature describing the changes in memory, or the absence thereof, that occur in the aged rat.

1 Department of Psychology, Princeton University, Princeton, New Jersey 08544, USA

Senile Dementia of the Alzheimer Type
Ed. by J. Traber and W. H. Gispen

At issue is the pertinence of the Jacksonian theory to these findings. Specifically, does loss of memorial function in the aged rat progress in an orderly fashion, with those capacities last gained in infancy being the first lost in senescence? A direct test of this theory would vary age from infancy through senescence and measure the emergence and decline of competence for different types of memory by means of tasks. As one might suspect, such experiments are not available. However, it is possible to identify several classes of learned behavior that develop sequentially in the rat which have also been studied in adult and aged rats. In short, there is an "infantile amnesia" literature and a "senescent deficit" literature which can provide a data base for an indirect test of the Jacksonian model.

Development of Memory in Rodents

A general search of these literatures has identified four representative tasks that measure the sequential emergence of long-term memory in the preweanling rat. The same tasks have also been used to study memory in senescent animals. The four types of learning include conditioned taste aversion, conditioned emotional response, passive avoidance, and spatial learning. Ontogenetically, the emergence of learning capability for these four tasks follows the sequential development of the sensory systems involved. As gustation is the first of these sensory modalities to mature, taste aversion learning is the first of the four behaviors to appear and the first to show the relatively slow rate of forgetting characteristic of adult rats. Audition is the next sensory system to mature, and auditorily conditioned emotional response is the next type of learning to emerge developmentally and reach adult retention levels. Passive avoidance and spatial memory both rely, at least to some extent, on the late-developing visual system and are the last to reach adult levels of learning and retention. In addition, both of these behaviors have been linked to the relatively late maturation of forebrain structures such as the hippocampus. With these different tasks as our bases of comparison, it appears that we have satisfied an initial requirement of constructing an animal model of senescent forgetting that mirrors infantile amnesia. That is, we have a hierarchy of abilities which immature rodents gain in successive order.

Analysis of Retention in Learning Studies

The next requirement for our effort was to develop a procedure for comparing these data on a common scale. To accomplish this, we first translated data given in the literature into percentages of retention, defining 100% retention as either the preset ceiling level or the terminal training score and 0% retention as either the score on the first training trial or the score of an untrained control group on a test trial. Omitted from this analysis for lack of a comparable data base is the spatial memory literature, which is discussed separately.

Our treatment of these data is presented in Figs. 1–3 which show the percentage of retention as a function of retention interval for the three tasks. The left-

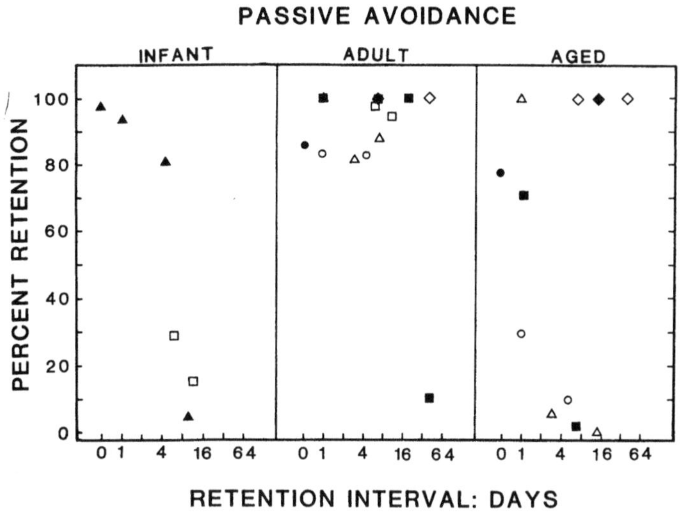

Fig. 1. Scatterplot of transformed, passive avoidance retention data (see text for procedure) for different-aged rodents. Data for the performances of infant, young adult, and aged adult rodents are presented in the *left, center,* and *right panels* respectively. *Solid triangles:* Stehouwer and Campbell (1980). *Open squares:* Schulenberg et al. (1981). *Open circles:* Bartus et al. (1983). *Solid squares:* Gold et al. (1981). *Open triangles:* Jensen et al. (1980). *Solid circles:* Dean et al. (1981). *Solid diamonds:* Bartus et al. (1983). *Open diamonds:* Campbell et al. (1980) (corrected for warm-up effects)

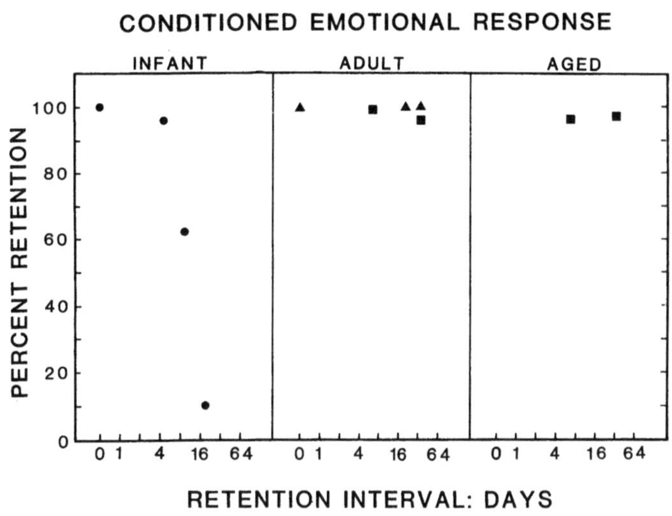

Fig. 2. Scatterplot of transformed, conditioned emotional response retention data (see text for procedure) for different-aged rodents. Data for the performances of infant, young adult, and aged adult rodents are presented in the *left, center,* and *right panels* respectively. *Solid circles:* Coulter et al. (1976). *Solid triangles:* Campbell and Campbell (1962). *Solid squares:* Campbell et al. (1980)

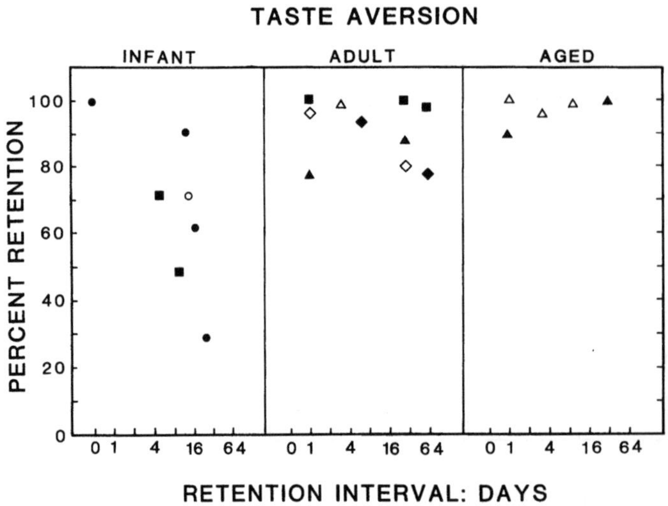

Fig. 3. Scatterplot of transformed, conditioned taste aversion retention data (see text for procedure) for different-aged rodents. Data for the performance of infant, young adult, and old adult rodents are presented in the *left, center,* and *right panels* respectively. *Open circle:* Gregg et al. (1978). *Solid square:* Campbell and Alberts (1979). *Solid circle:* Schweitzer and Green (1982). *Open triangle:* Cooper et al. (1980). *Solid triangle:* Guanowsky et al. (1983). *Open diamond:* Klein et al. (1977). *Solid diamond:* Steinert et al. (1980)

hand panels of the three figures reveal that we were indeed successful in finding three tasks that are forgotten rapidly during ontogenesis, confirming the general principle of infantile amnesia in animals.

Another requirement for our model, relatively low rates of forgetting in young adult animals, is more than adequately met by the data summarized in the center panels of Figs. 1–3. No appreciable retention loss is seen at any retention interval for any task except for one passive avoidance study that used a single-trial training procedure, a long retention interval, and a weak shock during training (Gold et al. 1981).

The final and most important requirement for an animal model of benign senescent forgetfulness and the relevance of the Jacksonian principle to describing the decline of memory in the aged is some evidence for a sequential loss of memory corresponding to the reverse of the order in which memorial functions are acquired during infancy. Examination of the right-hand panels of Figs. 1–3, which show retention of the three tasks reveals no overall tendency toward rapid forgetting in aged rats. The near perfect memory of aged rats for conditioned taste aversions is in no way comparable to the poor memory of infancy for that type of learning. Similarly, there is no indication that retention of the conditioned emotional response deteriorates with age to mimic the poor memory of infancy.

Only with the passive avoidance response, the last of the three types of learning to emerge during development, is there a return to the pattern of rapid forgetting characteristic of infancy. And even here, there is considerable ambiguity in the data presented. In some studies, retention of the passive avoidance response is nearly perfect over relatively long retention intervals, while in others, the retention loss in virtually complete in 2 or 3 days.

The preservation of function for two of the three tasks is not necessarily incompatible with the Jacksonian theory, since the theory does not demand that a deficit in a particular ability should develop in old age. It only requires that, when one appears, it should not precede the appearance of a deficit in a higher-order capacity. Thus, these data are in accord with the theory, since, of the three tasks reviewed, long-term retention of passive avoidance is among the last to develop in infancy and the first to diminish in senescence. However, the utility of the model is weakened by the failure to find age-related decrements in additional tasks.

Returning to the data presented in the right panel of Fig. 3, further examination indicates that there may be a theoretically consistent and reasonable explanation of the two types of findings. That is, those studies on aged animals in which rapid forgetting was obtained utilized a single-trial passive avoidance procedure (Bartus et al. 1970; Gold et al. 1981; Jensen et al. 1980), whereas those which employed multitrial procedures produced little or no evidence of loss of retention over the intervals studied (Rigter 1983; Campbell et al. 1980).

How does this pattern of single-trial passive avoidance results compare with the outcome of similar procedures in infancy? Unfortunately, there are no systematic studies comparing acquisition and long-term retention of multi- and single-trial passive avoidance learning in the developing rat. All of the infant data presented in the left-hand panel of Fig. 3 are based on multitrial training procedures. However, it is easy to infer from other studies that retention of single-trial passive avoidance would be poorer and later-maturing than retention of multitrial passive avoidance learning. An early study by Riccio et al. (1968) showed that 24-hour retention of a single-trial passive avoidance response did not reach adult levels until some time after 32 days of age, considerably later than for multitrial passive avoidance training (Schulenberg et al. 1981). Unfortunately, longer retention intervals were not included, making it impossible to trace the ontogenesis of long-term memory for single-trial passive avoidance in the rat. Although meager, the available data do allow us tentatively to conclude that single-trial passive avoidance retention deficits in aged rodents are the result of a loss of capacities which were gained relatively late in infancy.

Analyses of Spatial Memory

Another potential source of support for the Jacksonian principle of sequential development and dissolution of memory during the course of ontogeny and aging can be found in the spatial memory literature. In recent years, researchers have increasingly come to view the hippocampus as a repository of spatial information and to speculate that the deterioration of spatial memory that often occurs in the aged human (e.g., Barnes et al. 1983) is the result of hippocampal dysfunction. In support of this opinion, there is considerable evidence suggesting that the hippocampus is among those structures that reach functional maturity late in development (e.g., Nadel and Zola-Morgan, to be published; Altman et al. 1973) and that it shows an early decline with increasing age (e.g., Barnes et al. 1983). On the other hand, there is no clear-cut evidence showing that the hippocampus matures or declines significantly more rapidly than other forebrain structures, such as the cortex and striatum, in either rat or human (e.g., Bartus et al. 1982).

Behavioral analysis of spatial memory also provides some support for the Jacksonian principle. Spatial memory, as measured either in a radial maze with a food incentive (Rausch and Raskin 1984) or in a Morris water maze (Schenk et al. 1983), develops relatively late compared with other learning tasks. No evidence of learning was reported for either measure of spatial memory until the animals were at least 20 days of age. Conversely, performance on spatial tasks has been consistently poorer in aged than in young adult rats. Both Wallace et al. (1980) and Davis et al. (1983) reported that the asymptotic performance of aged rats in an 8-arm radial maze did not reach that of young adults even after extensive training. Similarly, Barnes and her co-workers (Barnes 1979, Barnes et al. 1980) have reported deficits in spatial memory using a hole-finding task, although the differences were primarily in retention rather than acquisition of the task. Research using the Morris water maze has produced similar results. Relatively minor differences in initial acquisition between young adult and aged animals were noted, but there was considerably greater disruption and lack of relearning when the goal (an invisible, submerged platform) was moved (Gage et al. 1984 b). Coupled with these findings are reports showing that cells in the dorsal hippocampus show declining "place sensitivity" in aged rats (Barnes et al. 1983) and that intracerebral implants of acetylcholine-containing cells reverse spatial deficits of aged rats in the Morris maze (Gage et al. 1984 a).

Although there are some difficulties in assessing the contribution of age-related sensory and motivational deficits to poorer spatial memory, these findings can be interpreted as supporting the Jacksonian principle of development and dissolution of function. There appears to be no question that spatial learning abilities emerge relatively late in ontogenesis and that they are more subject to age-related impairment than most other measures of learning and memory. Whether they are purely cognitive deficits or a combination of perceptual, motor, and motivational changes has yet to be determined.

Implications of Animal Models for Benign Senescent Forgetfulness in Humans

Since passive avoidance and spatial memory deficits occur in the absence of any invasive or pharmacologic manipulation, they may be taken as examples of the spontaneously occurring, progressive amnesia seen in old age. Can this amnesia in rodents be considered a model of human old-age amnesia? Both human and rodent populations should present increasing variability for memory tests with advancing age (Kral 1978; Rigter 1983). That is, many older people do not show any amnesia, some show the slight amnesia characteristic of benign senescent forgetting, while others show the deep amnesias of the senile dementias (Kral 1978). Although the same sort of divergence of memorial ability has been reported occasionally in rodent populations (Rigter 1983; Gage et al. 1984a), it has not yet been established that rodents show patterns of progressive amnesia which parallel or mimic those of humans.

The nature of the spatial memory and single-trial passive avoidance deficits in old rodents suggests that they might be examples of benign senescent forgetfulness. Rodents show spatial memory and passive avoidance impairment at ages where they do not exhibit losses of conditioned emotional response or conditioned taste aversion, demonstrating that their amnesic state is neither deep nor global. This finding is parallel to that observed in humans with benign senescent memory loss who show deficits in some types of memory but not others. On the other hand, scattergrams presented in the animal literature do not show a subpopulation of rodents resistant to single-trial passive avoidance retention deficits as would be predicted from the human literature (Bartus et al. 1983).

An even greater difficulty for the model arises in attempting to differentiate animals showing benign senescent forgetfulness from those manifesting signs of senile dementia. Indeed, it is not known if such a distinction exists. If human aging patterns apply to rodents, some rats should show deficits for a limited range of tasks, including spatial memory and single-trial passive avoidance, while others should show deficits for a much broader spectrum of learned behaviors. In addition, those developing more profound deficits should show a loss of spatial memory and single-trial passive avoidance at a younger age. One approach to evaluating this characteristic of the model would be to develop detailed forgetting curves for a large number of aged rodents. If the slopes of these curves show considerable diversity, it would suggest that the patterns of rodent senescent decline are, in some respects, similar to those of humans. However, it may be that the inbred rodent strains used for most laboratory research do not show the behavioral diversity during senescence that is characteristic of the varied human population.

In summary, the conformity of the Jacksonian theory to animal models of progressive senescent amnesias is by no means confirmed – but neither is it disproved. Much work remains to be done before a reasonable judgement can be made. The question more directly at hand is whether or not experiments designed to explore this issue will contribute toward our understanding of ontogenetic and senescent amnesias. Our evaluation of the data in the literature allows us to conclude that the Jacksonian theory is still viable and even vigorous enough to guide research into both normal and pathologic processes of development and aging.

Conclusion

The Jacksonian principle of hierarchical development and dissolution of function was applied to infantile amnesia and memory loss in senescence. When the Jacksonian model is generalized to include life span changes in memory, it predicts a last-in, first-out disappearance of memory processes. That is, those memory capacities that appear last in ontogeny should be the first to be compromised in aging. To evaluate this proposition in a specific context, the rodent literature on long-term memory in infant, adult, and aged animals was surveyed. Four types of memorial processes that emerge sequentially in development were identified and then examined in adult and aged rats. Moderate support of the Jacksonian principle emerged from this analysis; the theory is thus judged sufficiently viable to guide future research on both the normal and pathologic processes of development and aging.

References

Altman J, Brunner RL, Bayer SA (1973) The hippocampus and behavioral maturation. Behav Biol 8:557–596

Barnes CA (1979) Memory deficits associated with senescence: a neurophysiological and behavioral study in the rat. J Comp Physiol Psychol 93:74–104

Barnes CA, Nadel L, Honig WK (1980) Spatial memory deficits in senescent rats. Can J Psychol 34:29–39

Barnes CA, McNaughton BL, O'Keefe J (1983) Loss of place specificity in hippocampal complex spike cells of senescent rat. Neurobiol Aging 4:113–119

Bartus RT, Dean RL, Goas JA, Lippa AS (1980) Age-related changes in passive avoidance retention: Modulation with dietary choline. Science 209:301–303

Bartus RT, Dean RL, Beer B, Lippa AS (1982) The cholinergic hypothesis of geriatric memory dysfunction. Science 217:408–417

Bartus RT, Flicker C, Dean RL (1983) Logical principles for the development of animal models of age-related memory impairments. In: Crook T, Ferris S, Bartus R (eds) Assessment in geriatric psychopharmacology. Powley, New Canaan, pp 263–299

Campbell BA, Alberts JR (1979) Ontogeny of long-term memory for learned taste aversions. Behav Neurol Biol 25:139–156

Campbell BA, Campbell EH (1962) Retention and extinction of learned fear in infant and adult rats. J Comp Physiol Psychol 55:1–8

Campbell BA, Spear NE (1972) Ontogeny of memory. Psychol Rev 79:215–236

Campbell BA, Krauter EE, Wallace JE (1980) Animal models of aging: Sensory-motor and cognitive function in the aged rat. In: Stein DG (ed) Psychobiology of aging: problems and perspectives. Elsevier, Amsterdam, pp 201–226

Cooper RL, McNamara MC, Thompson WC, Marsh GR (1980) Vasopressin modulation of learning and memory in the rat. In: Poon L (ed) Aging in the 1980's, psychological issues. American Psychological Association, Washington DC, pp 201–211

Coulter X, Collier AC, Campbell BA (1976) Long-term retention of early Pavlovian fear conditioning in infant rats. J Exp Psychol [Anim Behav] 2:48–56

Davis HP, Idowu A, Gibson GE (1983) Improvement of 8-arm maze performance in aged Fischer 344 rats with 3,4-diaminopyridine. Exp Aging Res 9:211–214

Dean RL III, Scozzafava J, Goas JA, Regan R, Beer B, Bartus RT (1981) Age-related differences in behavior across the lifespan of the C57BL/6J mouse. Exp Aging Res 78:427–451

Gage FH, Bjorklund A, Stenevi U (1984a) Intrahippocampal septal grafts ameliorate learning impairments in aged rats. Science 225:533–535

Gage FH, Dunnett SB, Bjorklund A (1984b) Spatial learning and motor deficits in aged rats. Neurobiol Aging 5:43–48

Gold PE, McGaugh JL, Hankins LL, Rose RP, Vasquez BJ (1981) Age-dependent changes in retention in rats. Exp Aging Res 8:53–58

Gregg BE, Kittrell MW, Domjan M, Amsel A (1978) Ingestional aversion learning in preweanling rats. J Comp Physiol Psychol 92:785–795

Guanowsky V, Misanin JR, Riccio DC (1983) Retention of conditioned taste aversion in weanling, adult and old-age rats. Behav Neural Biol 37:173–178

Jackson JH (1958) Croonian lectures on evolution and dissolution of the nervous system. Br Med J 1:591 (Reprinted in: Taylor J (ed) Selected writings of John Hughlings Jackson, vol 2. Staples, London, pp 285–405)

Jensen RA, Martinez JL, McGaugh JL, Messing RB, Vasquez BJ (1980) The psychobiology of aging. In: Meletta GJ, Pirozzolo FJ (eds) The aging nervous system. Praeger, New York, pp 110–125
Klein SB, Mikulka PJ, Domato GC, Halstead C (1977) Retention of internal experiences in juvenile and young rats. Physiol Psychol 5:63–66
Kral VA (1978) Benign senescent forgetfulness. In: Katzman R, Terry RD, Bick KL (eds) Alzheimer's disease: senile dementia and related disorders. Raven, New York, pp 47–51 (Aging, vol 7)
Nadel L, Zola-Morgan S (to be published). Infantile amnesia: a neurobiological perspective
Paulson GW (1977) The neurological examination in dementia. In: Wells CE (ed) Dementia. Davis, Philadelphia, pp 169–188
Paulson G, Gottlieb G (1968) Development reflexes: the reappearance of foetal and neonatal reflexes in aged patients. Brain 91:37–52
Rauch SL, Raskin LA (1984) Cholinergic mediation of spatial memory in the preweanling rat: application of the radial arm maze paradigm. Behav Neurosci 98:35–43
Riccio DC, Rohrbaugh W, Hodges LA (1968) Developmental aspects of passive and active avoidance learning in rats. Dev Psychobiol 1:108–111
Rigter H (1983) Pitfalls in behavioural ageing research in animals. In: Gispen WH, Traber J (eds) Aging of the brain. Elsevier, New York, pp 197–208
Rozin P (1976) The psychobiological approach to human memory. In: Rosenzweig MR, Bennett EL (eds) Neural mechanisms of learning and memory. MIT Press, Cambridge, pp 3–48
Schacter DL, Moscovitch M (1984) Infants, amnesics, and dissociable memory systems. In: Moscovitch M (ed) Infant memory. Plenum, New York
Schenk F, Inglin F, Morris RGM (1983) Place navigation in rats as a function of age. Soc Neurosci 9:332 (abstract)
Schulenberg CJ, Riccio DC, Stikes ES (1981) Acquisition and retention of a passive-avoidance response as a function of age in rats. J Comp Physiol Psychol 74:75–83
Schweitzer L, Green L (1982) Acquisition and extended retention of a conditioned taste aversion in preweanling rats. J Comp Physiol Psychol 96:791–806
Stehouwer DJ, Campbell BA (1980) Ontogeny of passive avoidance: Role of task demands and development of species-typical behaviors. Dev Psychobiol 13:385–398
Steinert PA, Infurna RN, Spear NE (1980) Long-term retention of a conditioned taste aversion in preweanling and adult rats. Anim Learn Behav 8:375–181
Wallace JE, Krauter EE, Campbell BA (1980) Animal models of declining memory in the aged: short-term and spatial memory in the aged rat. J Gerontol 35:355–363
Willis WD, Grossman RG (1973) Medical neurobiology. Mosby, St. Louis

Mechanisms Underlying Pharmacologic Modifications of the Hippocampal Lesion Syndrome

R. L. ISAACSON and J. P. RYAN[1]

Introduction

In the volume arising from the first Tropon Conference 2 years ago, Hannigan and I noted that many people interpret the unfortunate mental and behavioral effects of aging as reflecting alterations in the functions of the hippocampal system (Isaacson and Hannigan 1983). In fact, there are many similarities between animals with hippocampal damage and symptoms of senility. The view that the animal with hippocampal damage is a reasonable model for Alzheimer's disease would find even greater endorsement if the interface between the hippocampal systems and the ascending dopaminergic systems at the basal ganglia level that, in turn, modulate the forebrain cholinergic systems were included. Indeed, reductions of dopamine and the enzymes necessary for its synthesis are correlated with advancing age (Adolfsson et al. 1979; McGeer and McGeer 1976). It has been proposed that aging is correlated with a reduction in a particular type of dopamine receptor (D1) at least in animals (Memo et al. 1980). Moreover, recent evidence indicates that Alzheimer's disease may not be entirely due to cell loss in the nucleus basalis, at least for patients with Parkinson's disease (Nakano and Hirano 1984). It is possible that losses of these cholinergic cells must be coupled with other structural and functional alterations before senile dementia of the Alzheimer type (SDAT) occurs.

Earlier Studies

Based on studies carried out in my laboratory over the past several years (Isaacson and Hannigan 1983; Isaacson 1984), the destruction of the hippocampus initiates a series of changes in the basal ganglia that can be demonstrated biochemically, pharmacologically, and behaviorally (Reinstein et al. 1982; Bär et al. 1981). Perhaps most important has been our demonstration that appropriate, direct dopaminergic intervention in the basal ganglia of animals with hippocampal damage can restore normal ranges of basal ganglia activities and, at least temporarily, of behavior.

However, direct intervention with basal ganglia systems through the injection of pharmacologic agents is an awkward process, one unlikely to be of use to human patients for whom such intervention might be desirable. Therefore, we have sought other ways of returning more or less to normal events in the basal ganglia of animals suffering from hippocampal damage.

1 University Center at Binghamton, Binghamton, NY 13901, USA

Senile Dementia of the Alzheimer Type
Ed. by J. Traber and W. H. Gispen

Cholinergic Interventions

A very useful hint or how to do this has come from the work of Lynn Wecker and her associates at Tulane University (e.g., Wecker et al. 1978; Wecker and Dettbarn 1979; Wecker and Schmidt 1979). They have found that the acute administration of choline, given peripherally, can produce alterations in both "free choline" levels and in acetylcholine levels in the brain that vary over time and show regional differences; that is, not every region changes in the same way at the same time. Alterations in cholinergic activities, for example, occur much earlier in the striatum than in the hippocampus. However, Wecker's results differ from the many, largely negative reports of central changes induced by peripheral choline administration in that she finds that the biochemical effects of choline administration occur only after a partial diminution of cholinergic activities. No effect is observed in the intact, normal animal. The effects of choline depend on the prior "stressing", or activation of the cholinergic systems, usually by the administration of a drug like atropine that increases cholinergic activities. The resultant decreases in acetylcholine levels can be offset by the systemic administration of choline.

Behavioral Studies

The work of Wecker and her associates has largely been devoted to understanding the biochemical changes produced by choline after interventions that increase cholinergic activities. We, on the other hand, have recently studied the behavioral effects of choline by stressing the cholinergic system directly through the administration of antimuscarinic drugs and, beyond this, by studying the effects of choline on animals with bilateral hippocampal destruction. Furthermore, to make our work more comparable to hers, we studied the animals at two time intervals (10 and 60 min) after choline administration, times at which regional biochemical differences following choline administration have been documented.

Choline and Scopolamine Interactions

Some of our results (Springer et al. 1985) indicating the effects of choline treatment on the hyperactivity induced by scopolamine are shown in Fig. 1. As can be observed, the usual effects of scopolamine on activity levels were obtained. In large open fields, anticholinergics produce enhanced locomotion, an effect similar to that produced by hippocampal destruction. Hyperactivity was not observed 10 min after choline treatment, but 60 min afterwards, the usual scopolamine effect was again observed, and the prior choline treatment had no effect. Not only was locomotor activity affected by the drug, but the *duration* of behaviors directed toward investigating the environment, for example, the animals' poking their heads into small holes and rearing, had decreased by about 50%. *It is the duration of such acts that changes, not their frequency*. Similar changes are found after both administration of antimucarinic drugs and hippocampal lesions. In the

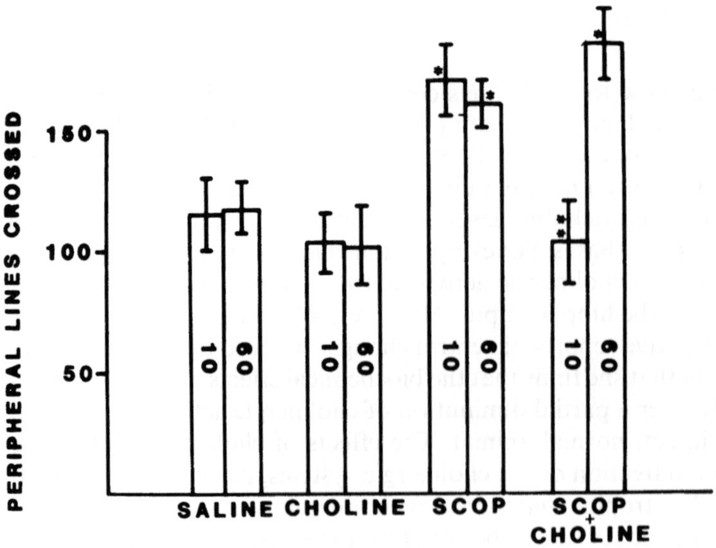

Fig. 1. Mean peripheral locomotion scores (±SEM) of animals receiving saline, choline, scopolamine (*SCOP*), or scopolamine and choline (*SCOP + CHOLINE*) tested 10 or 60 min after choline administration. (From Springer et al. 1985)

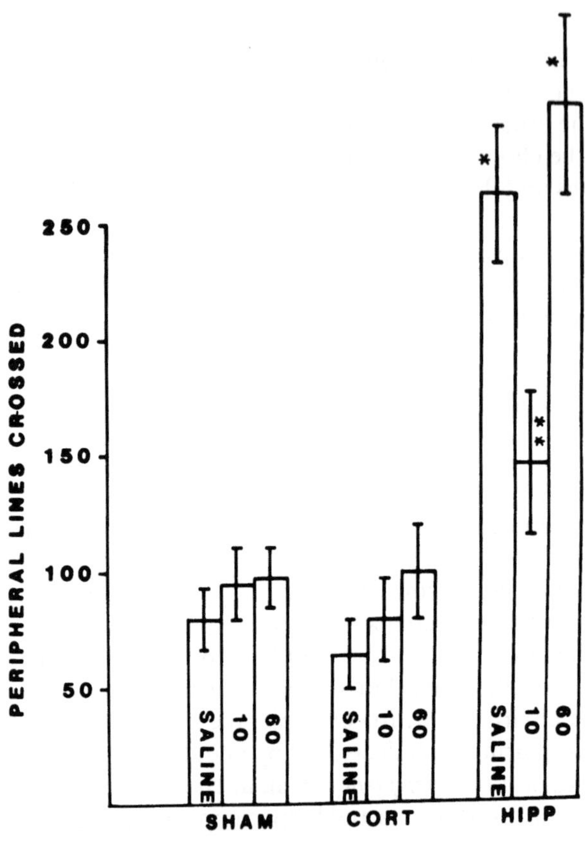

Fig. 2. Mean peripheral locomotion scores (±SEM) with sham operations (*SHAM*) or lesions restricted to posterior neocortex (*CORT*) or hippocampal damage (*HIPP*), tested after saline or at 10 or 60 min after systemic choline administration. Testing was conducted approximately 1 week after surgery. (From Springer et al. 1985)

rest of this report, we concentrate on the lesion-induced changes in locomotion, but in all cases, other aspects of the lesion-induced changes also show a tendency towards levels of normal animals.

Choline and Hippocampal Lesions

The effects of 100 mg/kg (free base) peripheral choline on the hippocampally lesioned animals are shown in Fig. 2 (Springer 1985a). Once again, a beneficial effect (i.e., reduction in hyperactivity) is seen 10 min after choline, but not 60 min afterwards. It is after an interval of 10 min that free choline levels reach their maximal levels in the striatum and hippocampus. By about 30 min after choline injection, the free choline levels have returned to normal levels. Resistance to atropine-induced reductions in striatal acetylcholine is found immediately after choline administration but takes 45 min to become noticeable in the hippocampus (Schmidt and Wecker 1981). Thus, the changes in acetylcholine levels induced in the hippocampal formation by choline begin later, but last longer, than those in the striatum. Since the behavioral effects we observed begin early but fade rapidly, they seem to be correlated with striatal changes in either free choline or acetylcholine.

Limited Duration of Choline Effects

The effects of peripheral choline administration are short-lived, lasting but 15–20 min. Furthermore, they are only effective directly after the brain damage occurs. By 28 days after the damage, and perhaps as early as 10–14 days after surgery, peripheral choline is without effect. This alteration in the effectiveness of choline should provide some insight into the series of changes initiated by hippocampal and neocortical destruction.

Relation of Effects of Choline to Interpretations of Brain Damage

Brain damage should not be thought of as producing a fixed alteration of the nervous system. Brain damage initiates a series of changes in at least some of the remaining brain systems. The greatest changes, or at least the most rapid, are probably those occurring immediately after damage, but others continue over a long period of time. Indeed, they may continue to evolve throughout the life of the animal or the person and suggest that the brain may be attempting in this way to compensate for the disruptions produced by the damage. Obviously, such compensatory mechanisms are more successful in some ways than in others. Progressive changes such as these can be documented both biochemically (Bär et al. 1981) and behaviorally (Reinstein et al. 1982), implying that interventions successful in restoring essentially normal behaviors at one postoperative period may not do so at another. As mentioned, this has proved to be the case with the peripheral administration of choline, the beneficial effect of which is found in hippocampally lesioned animals when given the drug a week after surgery but not in animals tested a month after surgery.

Peripheral Choline and Central Hemicholinium

Naturally, we were interesed in determining whether the effects obtained with choline are attributable to peripheral or central changes. In the Springer et al. (1985a) study, choline was given systemically (100 mg/kg), as had been done in other studies, and hemicholinium-3 then injected into the ventricular system to groups of sham-operated, cortically lesioned, and hippocampally lesioned animals 7 days after surgery. The rationale was that the hemicholinium would prevent the choline from being taken up into neurons, thus aborting the beneficial effects of choline – if it must be converted into acetylcholine to be effective. However, an unexpected result made it impossible to derive a decisive conclusion from the experiment. The hemicholinium, when given to animals with lesions restricted to the neocortex, produced substantial changes in behavior which made the cortically lesioned animals resemble those with hippocampal damage (see Fig. 3). Since the animals with hippocampal damage had also undergone neocortical destruction through the tissue removed to visualize the hippocampus, they, too, were subject to the same cortical-lesion–hemicholinium effect. The behavioral changes produced by this drug are similar to those found earlier by Clark (1968, 1970) using scopolamine. She found that the anticholinergic enhanced the activity of the animals with neocortical damage to a degree that made them indistinguish-

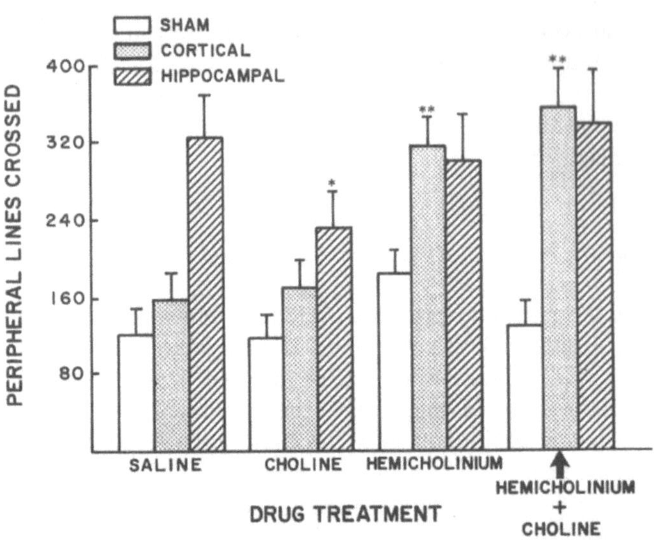

Fig. 3. Mean peripheral locomotion scores (±SEM). The three surgical groups are those shown in Fig. 2. All animals were tested 10 min after choline or saline injections. The 15-μg dose of hemicholinium-3 was given intracerebroventricularly 45 min before saline or choline. The *arrow* beneath the three groups on the right side of the figure indicates only that these were the three groups that received hemicholinium and choline. Significant reductions or increases in activity are represented by *single* ($P < 0.05$) or *double* ($P < 0.01$) *asterisks*. (From Springer et al. 1985)

able from animals with hippocampal damage. Hemicholinium also has antimuscarinic properties, which might account for the effects observed in the cortically lesioned subjects (Speth and Yamamura 1979). Unfortunately, these effects precluded any conclusion about whether the choline had produced its effects on animals with hippocampal damage through central or peripheral mechanisms.

Intracerebral Administration of Choline

Therefore, a series of studies was undertaken in which choline was directly injected into the cerebroventricular system (icv) or into the nucleus accumbens. We chose the nucleus accumbens because it is one location in which dopaminergic intervention can induce beneficial changes in the behavior of animals with hippocampal damage, an effect not shared by injection into the neostriatum (for a review, see Isaacson 1984). The results were surprising. First, on the negative side: icv injections of choline in doses of 0.01, 0.1, or 1.0 μg failed to influence the behavior of animals (Springer 1984). In contrast, choline injections into the nucleus accumbens produced a beneficial effect 7 days after the lesion, which was however lost by 28 days after the lesion.

Possible Interpretation

Collectively, these results suggest that the changes induced in the dopaminergic system after hippocampal lesions may in turn produce alterations that can be overcome by enhanced cholinergic activity in the nucleus accumbens, possibly on the basis of free choline acting as a direct cholinergic agonist when administered directly to selected central nervous system areas. It is conceivable that alterations induced by hippocampal damage in dopaminergic activities in the nucleus accumbens (and possibly in other basal ganglia structures as well) directly affect events in the cholinergic cells of the striatal complex and, secondarily, influence the cholinergic cells of the ventral pallidum via the direct (GABA) projections to it from the nucleus accumbens.

Because of the transitory nature of the choline-induced changes, we undertook to find other intervention procedures with longer-lasting effects and decided to replicate some potentially exciting results obtained earlier by Iuvone and Van Hartesveldt (1977).

Corticosteroid Influences

Effects of Chemical Reductions in Corticosteroids on Brain-Damaged Rats

Iuvone and Van Hartesveldt found that adrenalectomy resulted in the elimination of many features of the hippocampal lesion syndrome, an effect also found after adrenalectomy in animals with lesions induced by kainic acid (Nyakas et al.

1983). It was possible to restore this lesion effect by corticosterone replacement. This effect was ascribed to the loss of the corticosteroids, but many other changes are also produced by adrenalectomy, including alterations in the central and peripheral catecholaminergic activities (Dunn and Kramarcy 1985). Even though the complete nature of the effects of adrenalectomy in living animals is not known, we undertook to replicate the Iuvone and Van Hartesveldt (1976) experiment by carrying out a "chemical adrenalectomy" with the drug metyrapone (Ryan et al. 1985). This drug interferes with the synthesis of corticosterone at the 11-β-hydroxylation step and reduces corticosteroids by 90% or more within 10 min after administration (Jenkins et al. 1958; Chart and Sheppard 1959). The great advantage of this method over surgical adrenalectomy is that the precursor of the corticosteroids, normally present only in trace amounts, itself acts as as a mineralocorticoid. After corticosteroid suppression, it becomes abundant. It should also be noted that our study differed from most in the literature in that we used tartaric acid as the drug vehicle rather than propylene glycol. While the latter induces greatly aberrant behavior patterns of its own, making for very difficult interpretations of drug effects, tartaric acid does not alter the baseline behaviors of normal animals.

Metyrapone Effects on Animals with Hippocampal Damage

Following metyrapone treatment in animals with bilateral hippocampal damage returned to essentially normal levels. The behavior of animals with sham operations or lesions restricted to the neocortex was not altered, as shown in Fig. 4. Corticosterone replacement, also shown in this figure, produces a partial restoration of the deficit when given 2 h prior to the metyrapone. This was the optimal pretreatment interval, whereas corticosterone given 1 h before metyrapone was without effect. It should be emphasized that, when corticosterone was given at various times and dosages before testing in pilot studies, the lesion-induced normalities of behavior were never completely eliminated. This incomplete effect of corticosterone treatment suggests that metyrapone has multiple actions: a clear effect on the corticosteroid systems and another type of effect on other peripheral and/or central systems. The multiple actions of metyrapone are not surprising, since central effects of the drug on electrical activities of the brain can be found after it is administered to adrenalectomized animals (Helmy et al. 1970). Certainly, the reduction of corticosteroid production, like the peripheral administration of choline, alters the autonomic nervous system at several levels: at the adrenal medulla and the sympathetic ganglia and centrally. Since the effects produced by choline and metyrapone may exert their effects via peripheral rather than central actions, Ryan and I undertook to determine whether enhancement of catecholaminergic activities, by methods that are likely to have their greatest effects in the periphery, are capable of altering behavioral anomalies observed following hippocampal destruction.

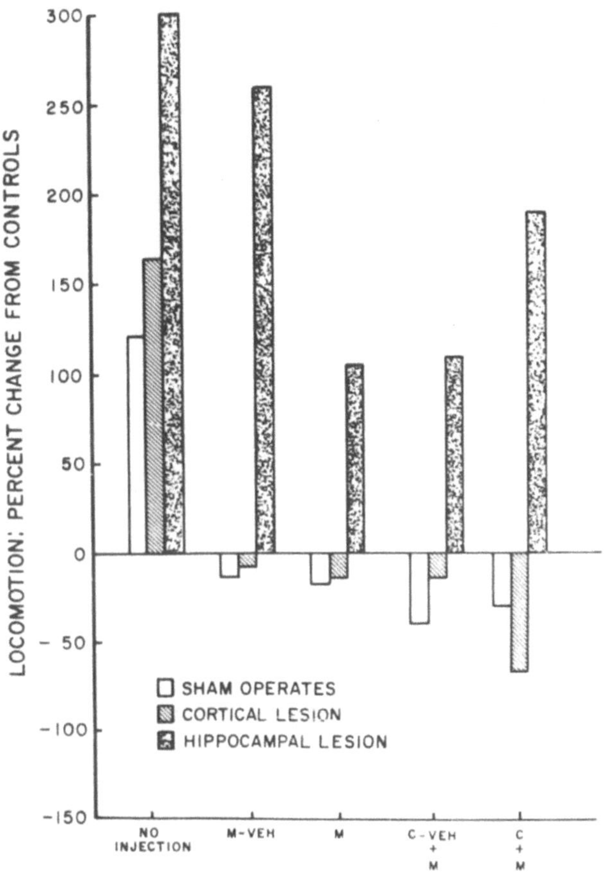

Fig. 4. Changes in locomotion (peripheral) of the sham-operated, neocortically lesioned, and hippocampally lesioned Long-Evans Hooded rats after various drug and vehicle treatments. The histogram depicts the percentage difference of the groups after the specified treatments relative to the mean of the locomotion scores of untreated (no injection), sham-operated animals and the locomotion scores after saline injections (ip). The *leftmost set of three bars* indicates that the activity of the sham-operated animals on the first day of testing (no injection) was higher than the average of this no-injection day and the reduced scores obtained after saline treatment. The *subsequent sets of three bars* on the graph indicate for each group of animals the effects of metyrapone vehicle (*M-VEH*), metyrapone (25 mg/kg), corticosterone vehicle 2 hours prior to metyrapone (*C-VEH+M*), and corticosterone treatment (0.006 mg/kg) 2 hours prior to metyrapone (*C+M*). Metyrapone significantly reduces the hyperactivity of the hippocampally lesioned animals whenever given. The M-VEH is ineffective in altering locomotor activity. Pretreatment with C-VEH+M results in a normalization of activity similar to metyrapone alone. Corticosterone pretreatment significantly restores the locomotor activity relative to that observed following C-VEH and M; however, this is only a "partial restoration" and differs significantly from baseline locomotor activity

Interaction of Metyrapone and Levodopa in Brain-Lesioned Animals

In one experiment (Ryan and Isaacson 1985), the results of which are illustrated in Fig. 5, levodopa was given peripherally with the simultaneous administration of metyrapone. As can be seen, levodopa at doses of 4 or 40 mg/kg produced a partial elimination of the hippocampal lesion-induced hyperactivity equivalent to that produced by metyrapone alone. Moreover, the levodopa effect did not summate with that of metyrapone; at these two dosages the effect is the same with

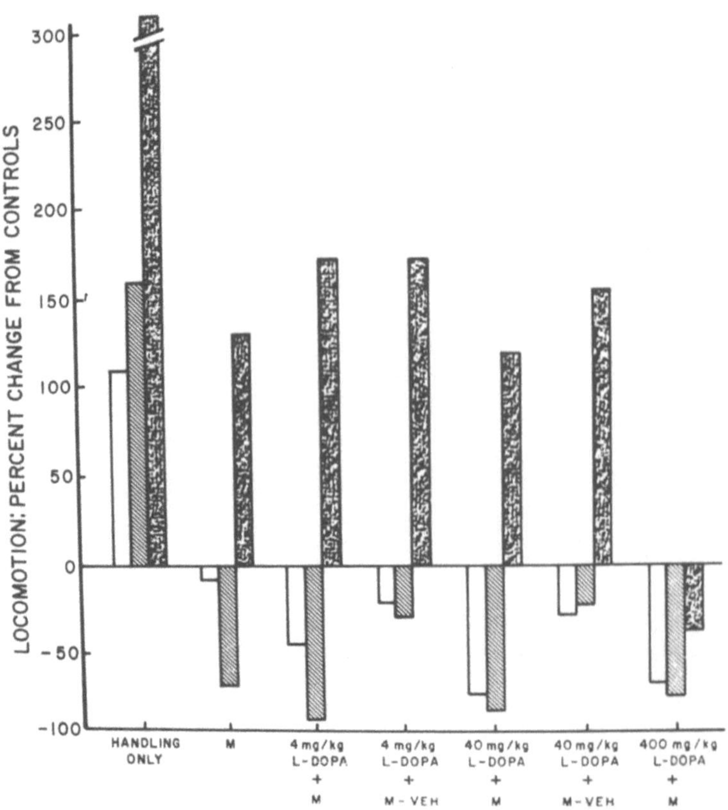

Fig. 5. Locomotion (peripheral) scores of sham and cortically and hippocampally lesioned groups. The histogram depicts the percentage difference of the various treatments based on the mean peripheral locomotion scores of untreated (handling only – no injection) and saline-treated, sham-operated rats. The treatments to the right of the handling-only *bars* (*leftmost*) show the effects of 25 mg/kg metyrapone (*M*), pretreatment with 4 mg/kg levodopa 30 min prior to the administration of M or metyrapone vehicle (*M-Veh*), the administration of 40 mg/kg levodopa 30 min prior to the administration of M or its vehicle. At the *right* are *bars* indicating the effects of 400 mg/kg levodopa and M. This levodopa dose in animals given M-Veh was virtually identical to that of the M-treated groups and is therefore not portrayed. Levodopa pretreatment (4 mg/kg or 40 mg/kg), whether followed by M or M-Veh, decreased locomotor activity of animals with hippocampal damage to an amount comparable to that of M treatment only. In contrast, 40 mg/kg of levodopa followed by M significantly decreased the locomotion of control animals in comparison to the same dose of levodopa followed by M-Veh. (□, sham-operated group; ▨, cortically lesioned group; ■, hippocampally lesioned group)

or without metyrapone. At a 400-mg/kg dose of levodopa, behavior is greatly suppressed in all groups, indicating a nonspecific, depressant effect.

A surprising and unexpected finding is that the lower doses of levodopa produced drastic reductions in the activity of animals with cortical damage. To a large extent, these levodopa effects were additive with respect to the metyrapone-induced alterations in behavior, an effect not found in animals with hippocampal lesions.

Since levodopa was given without the simultaneous administration of a peripheral decarboxylase inhibitor, it is possible that the drug's actions are at the peripheral level, although both with and without peripheral decarboxylase inhibition, levodopa, at the 400 mg/kg dose reaches the brain readily. If the beneficial effects were primarily at the peripheral level, a beneficial effect on the hyperactivity of the lesioned animals might also be obtained with the peripheral administration of epinephrine.

Epinephrine and Metyrapone Effects on Brain-Damaged Animals

To determine whether this is the case, rats were pretreated with 0.005 mg/kg epinephrine 30 min prior to the ip injection of metyrapone or its vehicle. This amount of epinephrine given in conjunction with metyrapone produced a beneficial effect equivalent to that achieved with metyrapone or levodopa. Extending the study to a dose-response study of epinephrine itself, the latter alone was insufficient to produce a remediation of the animals with hippocampal damage, except at the highest dose, which also produced a general depressant effect on all groups of animals. This global effect has been reported previously by others (Rothballer 1959). The effects of peripheral epinephrine administration (Fig. 6) are remarkable in several respects. A curvilinear effect characterizes the activity in the sham-operated animals: reductions were found at the lowest and highest doses, but an enhancement was observed at the middle dose (0.05 mg/kg). At the low and middle doses, the hippocampally lesioned animals were unaffected. Only at doses at which a general sedation became apparent were the locomotion scores of the hippocampally lesioned animals affected. However, at all doses, the animals with lesions restricted to the neocortex had greatly suppressed levels of activity (reductions of greater than 60% of control levels). Since this is not found in the hippocampally lesioned animals, this diminished activity may indicate that the secondary effects of hippocampal damage override those induced by neocortical damage alone in the systems affected by epinephrine. Such a result would be anticipated if the hippocampal effects were further along the "final common pathway" for behavior than those of the neocortex. In addition, considering the effects of hemicholinium-3 described earlier, it is apparent that posterior neocortical lesioning leads to pronounced hyperactivity in animals whose central cholinergic activities are interrupted and greatly depressed activity in animals subjected even to minimal adrenergic stimulation. It should be noted that none of the levodopa or epinephrine doses, with or without metyrapone, produced signs of autonomic changes (piloerection, urination, or changes in respiration rate).

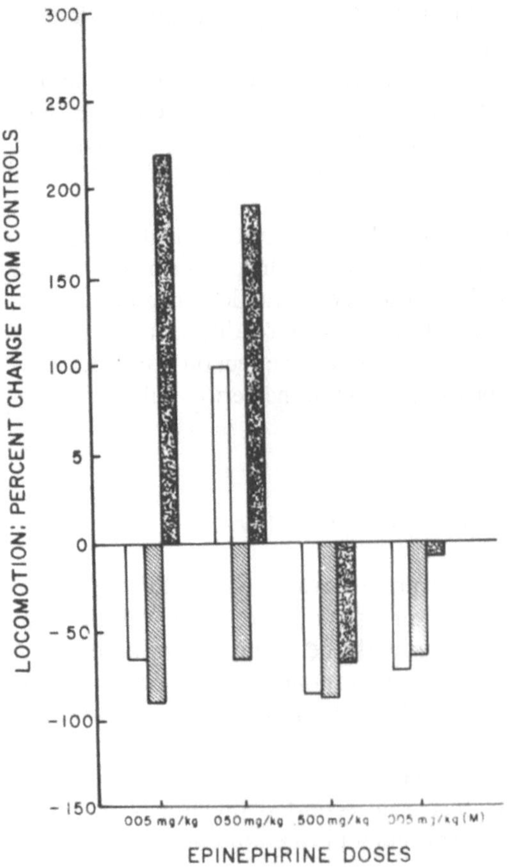

Fig. 6. Changes in locomotion (peripheral) in sham-operated group and in groups with cortical and hippocampal lesions. The histogram depicts the percentage difference of the various epinephrine doses relative to the mean locomotion scores of handled-only and saline-treated, sham-operated controls. The highest dose of epinephrine (0.5 mg/kg) reduced the locomotor activity of all groups to the same degree as the lowest dose of epinephrine (0.005 mg/kg) when given in conjunction with metyrapone (M). This low dose of epinephrine without M was ineffective in altering the locomotor activity of the hippocampal group. All doses of epinephrine reduce the locomotion of the cortical lesion group whereas a curvilinear effect is observed with the sham operates. (□, sham-operated group; ▧, cortically lesioned group; ■, hippocampally lesioned group)

Conclusion

At this stage of our research, it is clear that adrenalectomy, whether physical or chemical, can selectively reduce at least some of the impairments usually found after hippocampal destruction. The adrenalectomy seems to produce two different types of changes: one related to corticosteroid levels and a second involving the catecholamine systems. At this time, however, direct intervention with the peripheral catecholamine system produces an extensive reduction in the activity of both sham-operated and cortically lesioned animals. Furthermore, it is not clear whether the primary catecholamine effects are peripheral or central. On the other hand, it is possible that the changes involved are not only simple distinctions between central and peripheral effects of hormones or drugs – perhaps both types of effects are synergistic and cooperative, as our own data suggest. In any case, much more research is required to sort out the importance of each of these factors.

The important feature, however, is that it *is* possible to change in a very radical fashion lesion-induced behavioral changes by hormonal and pharmacologic interventions. Such interventions offer great hope for improving the abilities of impaired individuals, as well as understanding the physiologic effects produced by the lesions. The ways in which these intervention procedures may be applied to the human problems associated with aging depend on the degree to which the hippocampal lesion model approximates aspects of human dementia and is able to provide new diagnostic approaches to identifiying the neural systems most affected by brain damage.

References

Adolfsson R, Gottfries CG, Ross BE (1979) Postmortem distribution of dopamine and homovanillic acid in human brain, variations related to age and a review of the literature. J Neural Trans 45:81–106

Bär PR, Gispen WH, Isaacson RL (1981) Behavioral and regional neurochemical sequelae of hippocampal destruction in the rat. Pharm Biochem Behav 14:305–312

Chart JJ, Sheppard H (1959) Amphenone analogues as adrenal cortical inhibitors. J Med Pharm Chem 1:407–441

Clark CVH (1968) Ph.D. Dissertation, University of Rochester

Clark CVH (1970) Effect of hippocampal and neocortical ablation on scopolamine-induced activity in the rat. Psychopharm 17:289–301

Dunn AJ, Kramarcy NR (1985) Neurochemical responses in stress: relationships between the hypothalamic-pituitary-adrenal and catecholamine systems. In: Iversen LL, Iversen SD, Synder SH (eds) Handbook of psychopharmacology, vol 18. Plenum, New York

Helmy L, Bohus B, Frey ZS, Endröczi E (1970) Direct metyrapone effect on the central nervous system. Endokrinologie 57:139–141

Isaacson RL (1984) Hippocampal damage: effect on dopaminergic systems of the basal ganglia. Int Rev Neurobiol 25:339–359

Isaacson RL, Hannigan JH Jr (1983) The hippocampus and age-related disorders. In: Gispen WH, Traber J (eds) Aging of the brain. Elsevier, Amsterdam, p 139

Iuvone PM, Van Hartesveldt C (1976) Locomotor activity and plasma corticosterone in rats with hippocampal lesions. Behav Biol 16:515–520

Iuvone PM, Van Hartesveldt C (1977) Diurnal locomotor activity in rats: effects of hippocampal ablation and adrenalectomy. Behav Biol 19:228–237

Jenkins JJ, Meakin JW, Nelson DH, Thorn GW (1958) Inhibition of adrenal steroid 11-oxygenation in the dog. Science 128:478–479

McGeer EG, McGeer PL (1976) Neurotransmitter metabolism in the aging brain. Neurotransmitter metabolism in the aging brain. In: Terry RD, Gerson S (eds) Neurobiology of aging, vol 3. Raven, New York, p 389

Memo M, Lucchi L, Spano PF, Trabucchi M (1980) Aging process affects a single class of dopamine receptors. Brain Res 202:488–492

Nakano I, Harano Y (1984) Parkinson's disease: neuron loss in nucleus basalis without concomitant Alzheimer's disease. Ann Neurol 15:415–418

Nyakas CS, De Kloet ER, Veldhuis HD, Bohus B (1983) Hippocampal corticosterone receptors and novelty-induced behavioral activity: effect of kainic acid lesion in the hippocampus. Brain Res 288:219–228

Reinstein DK, Hannigan JH Jr, Isaacson RL (1982) The time course of certain behavioral changes after hippocampal damage and their alteration by dopaminergic intervention into nucleus accumbens. Pharm Biochem Behav 17:193–202

Rothballer AB (1959) The effects of catecholamines on the central nervous system. Pharmacol Rev 11:494–547

Ryan JP, Isaacson RL (to be published) The effects of catecholaminergic enhancement on the behavior of animals with hippocampal lesions

Ryan JP, Springer JE, Hannigan JH Jr, Isaacson RL (1985) Suppression of corticosterone synthesis alters the behavior of hippocampally lesioned rats. Behav Neural Biol 44:47–59
Schmidt EI, Wecker L (1981) CNS effects of choline administration: evidence for temporal dependence. Neuropharmacology 20:535–539
Speth RC, Yamamura H (1979) On the ability of choline and its analogues to interact with muscarinic receptors in the rat brain. Eur J Phharmacol 58:197–201
Springer JE, Ryan JP, Isaacson RL (1985) Acute choline administration produces transient reductions in the effects of hippocampal destruction. (to be published)
Springer JE (1984) Ph. D. Dissertation, State University of New York at Binghamton
Wecker L, Dettbarn W-D (1979) Relationship between choline availability and acetylcholine synthesis in discrete regions of rat brain. J Neurochem 32:961–967
Wecker L, Schmidt DE (1979) Central cholinergic function: Relationship to choline administration. Life Sci 25, 375–3844
Wecker L, Dettbarn W-D, Schmidt DT (1978) Choline administration: modification of the central actions of atropine. Science 199:86–87

Lesions of the Nucleus Basalis in the Rat: Functional Changes*

G. Pepeu[1], F. Casamenti[1], L. Bracco[2], H. Ladinsky[3], and S. Consolo[3]

Anatomical Definition

Kelly and Moore (1978) demonstrated in the rat that an electrolytic lesion of the globus pallidus results in a 50% decrease in choline acetyltransferase (ChAT) activity in the ipsilateral frontal and parietal cerebral cortex. Further evidence for an important cholinergic projection to the neocortex from neurons in the basal forebrain accumulated rapidly thanks to the work of Johnston et al. (1979), Wenk et al. (1979), and Lehman et al. (1980).

In the rat, the cholinergic neurons of the basal forebrain are divided into six major sectors (Mesulam et al. 1983b). The Ch_4 sector includes the cholinergic neurons of the nucleus basalis of Meynert (NB). These neurons are localized ventrally and medially to the globus pallidus. Some neurons intensely stained for acetylcholinesterase (AChE) are occasionally found within the pallidum proper (Bigl et al. 1982). The Ch_4 sector also contains the cholinergic neurons of the substantia innominata of Reichert (Wainer et al. 1984), which, in primates, according to Mesulam et al. (1983a), is located in the NB. Bigl et al. (1982) consider the substantia innominata in the rat to be part of the ventral pallidum.

The organization of the cholinergic neurons of the NB is similar in the rat and monkey (Wainer et al. 1984), in the cat (Irle and Markowitsch 1984), and in man (Davies and Feisullin 1982). The large neurons of the NB, intensely stained for AChE and with strong ChAT immunoreactivity, provide the major cholinergic innervation of the cortical mantle. In the cat, these neurons project to all neocortical fields. However, they give rise to a surprisingly strong projection to the medial prefrontal cortex, whereas lateral prefrontal areas receive the same low number of afferents as do all other neocortical regions (Irle and Markowitsch 1984).

Similarly, the caudal substantia innominata and NB are the source of afferent fibers innervating the rat neocortical regions (Bigl et al. 1982). Lamour et al. (1982a) also demonstrated in the rat that the injection of horseradish peroxidase into the frontal cortex labeled for the most part neurons in the substantia innominata while injections into the temporal and parietal cortices labeled neurons in the medial and ventral boundaries of the globus pallidus. These locations can also be considered within the limits of the NB.

* This study was supported by CNR grants CT 81.00137.04, 82.02043.04, and 83.02411.04

1 Department of Pharmacology, University of Florence, Viale Morgagni 65, 50134 Florence, Italy
2 Department of Neurology, University of Florence, Careggi, 50134 Florence, Italy
3 Istituto di Ricerche Farmacologiche "Mario Negri", Via Eritrea 62, 20127 Milan, Italy

Senile Dementia of the Alzheimer Type
Ed. by J. Traber and W.H. Gispen

ChAT and AChE distribution in the various layers of the lateral neocortex is uneven, with the lowest degree of activity associated with layers II and III. Lesions of the NB resulted in a 43% decrease in ChAT and a 53% decrease in AChE for all layers of the cortex, as well as the equalization of the uneven distribution of these markers within the cortex (Johnston et al. 1981).

Lesioning Procedures

The anatomical information reviewed above demonstrates that the destruction of the NB offers a unique possibility for investigating the functional role of cortical cholinergic fibers originating in this location.

Unilateral lesions were used initially, since the survival rate after bilateral lesions was low. In our work (Lo Conte et al. 1982a, 1982b; Pedata et al. 1982), unilateral electrolytic lesions were made according to the following coordinates taken from the Koenig and Klippel (1963) atlas of the rat brain: 0.2 mm anterior to the bregma, 2.5 mm lateral to the bregma, 7 mm below the dura. Male rats of 140–150 g body weight were anesthetized with ketamine, and a current of 1.0 mA was passed through a unipolar electrode for 30 s. An example of the lesion obtained using this procedure is shown in Fig. 1.

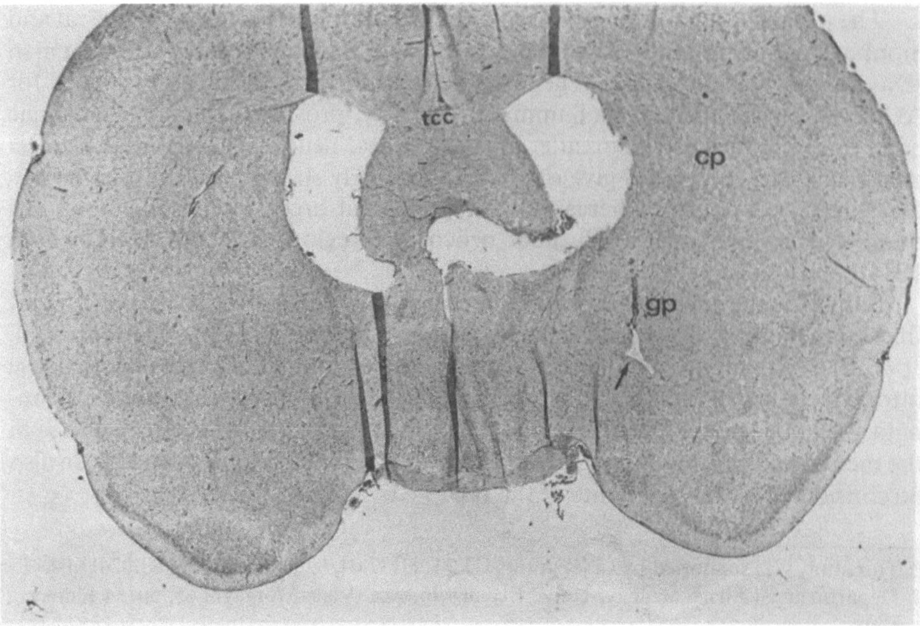

Fig. 1. Unilateral electrolytic lesion of the nucleus basalis. Coronal section of rat brain, Nissl staining. Magnification: × 35. The *arrow* indicates the lesion. The trace left by the electrode can be also seen. (*cp*, caudate putamen; *gp*, globus pallidus; *tcc*, truncus corporis callosi)

Unilateral excitotoxic lesions were made by Johnston et al. (1978) and Lehman et al. (1980) through local injection of kainic acid or ibotenic acid with the intent of selectively destroying the neurons while preserving other kinds of fibers.

Recently, several authors were able to obtain a high survival rate in rats with bilateral excitotoxic lesions (Flicker et al. 1983; Friedman et al. 1983). A careful description of the placement and size of the lesions as well as of the postoperative care making it possible to obtain both a large decrease in cortical ChAT and a high survival rate can be found in the work of Wenk et al. (1984).

Even if the NB and the substantia innominata are considered separate areas, they are anatomically so close that the cholinergic neurons of both areas are usually affected by lesions placed in the ventromedial pallidum.

Biochemical Changes

Choline Acetyltransferase (ChAT)

As first shown by Kelly and Moore (1978) and repeatedly confirmed, lesions of the NB bring about a diminution in ChAT activity in the cerebral cortex. In most studies, the decrease was measurable 7–20 days after the lesion. It has however been detected as early as 72 h following the lesion (McKinney and Coyle 1982).

Table 1 lists some of the changes reported in the literature. In the frontal cortex, the decrease varies from 24% to 58% depending upon the size and position of the lesion. Although according to Mesulam et al. (1983 a) and Bigl et al. (1982) the neurons of the NB do not project extensively to the posterior cortex, a reduction in ChAT activity has been found in this region. However, in these cases, there is the possibility that the lesion might involve cholinergic neurons of the diagonal

Table 1. Percentage decrease in ChAT activity in the cerebral cortex of rats with lesions of the nucleus basalis

Days after lesion	Cortical areas investigated	% Decrease	Reference
14	Frontoparietal	45	Johnston et al. (1979)
7–14	Lateral frontoparietal	43	Johnston et al. (1981)
7	Frontal	44	Wenk et al. (1980)
7–14	Frontal	24	Lehman et al. (1980)
20	Frontal	41	Pedata et al. (1982)
20	Parietal	38	Pedata et al. (1982)
20	Occipital	35	Pedata et al. (1982)
7	Frontal	58	Hartgraves et al. (1982)
7	Parietal	42	Hartgraves et al. (1982)
7	Posterior	33	Hartgraves et al. (1982)
14–16	Frontal	47	Friedman et al. (1983)
14–16	Parietal	35	Friedman et al. (1983)
14–16	Posterior	17	Friedman et al. (1983)

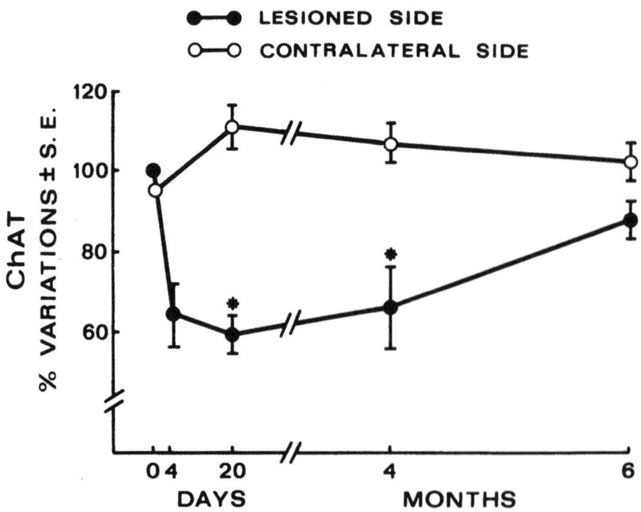

Fig. 2. Spontaneous recovery of ChAT activity in the frontal cortex following a unilateral electrolytic lesion of the NB, placed as described by Lo Conte et al. (1982a). Radiometric determination of ChAT as described by Pedata et al. (1982). Each *point* is the mean of 4–6 rats. *, Statistically significant difference between the two hemispheres, $P < 0.01$

band which project to the occipital cortex (Henderson 1981) and are part of the Ch_3 sector in the classification proposed by Mesulam et al. (1983b).

Lehman et al. (1980) demonstrated that an electrolytic lesion or a kainic acid infusion placed at the same coordinates bring about a decrease of similar magnitude in cortical ChAT activity.

A small but consistent increase in ChAT activity in the controlateral cortex was observed in rats with unilateral electrolytic lesions of the NB (Pedata et al. 1982). On the other hand, Wenk et al. (1984) found a 58% decrease in ChAT activity in the frontolateral cortex of both hemispheres 1 week after the bilateral infusion of ibotenic acid in the NB.

As shown by Wenk and Olton (1984), ChAT activity gradually returned to normal within 3 months after a unilateral infusion of ibotenic acid in the NB that caused a 60% decrease in the frontolateral cortex. We also observed spontaneous recovery in rats with a unilateral electrolytic lesion of the NB, as illustrated in Fig. 2. The recovery was almost complete 6 months after the lesion. In this regard, it may be mentioned that Flicker et al. (1983) found only a 16%–23% decrease in ChAT activity in the frontal cortex of rats sacrificed 2.5 months after receiving an infusion of ibotenic acid in the NB.

Acetylcholinesterase (AChE)

NB lesions also induce a marked decrease in AChE activity in the cerebral cortex, as demonstrated by histochemical and neurochemical methods. Wenk et al. (1980) produced a decrease in AChE levels of up to 82% in the frontal cortex, depending on the position of the lesion. Lehman et al. (1980) reported a 21%–26% decrease in AChE in the frontal cortex of rats killed 2 weeks after receiving a kainic acid infusion or electrolytic NB lesions respectively.

High-Affinity Choline Uptake (HACU)

ACh synthesis is regulated by choline availability through the sodium-dependent HACU system. HACU is therefore considered a biochemical marker for the localization of cholinergic terminals (Kuhar 1976), but it is also an indicator of the activity of cholinergic neurons (Atweh et al. 1975).

Johnston et al. (1979) found a 45% decrease in cortical HACU, together with a 50% decrease in ChAT activity 7–10 days after unilateral kainic acid injections in the NB. Pedata et al. (1982) reported 33% and 38% decreases in HACU activity in the frontal and parietal cortices respectively 4 days following the infliction of a unilateral electrolytic lesion. Decreases of 42% and 39% respectively were found 10 days after lesioning, but a remarkable recovery in HACU activity occurred within 20 days in the ipsilateral cortical areas, accompanied by a significant increase in HACU activity in the corresponding cortical areas of the opposite hemisphere. The rapid recovery and the increase in activity in the controlateral hemisphere may be interpreted as a compensatory increase in HACU activity in surviving neurons, which is presumably coupled with an increase in impulse flow.

Levels, Release, and Turnover of Acetylcholine (ACh)

We have seen that extensive degeneration resulting from lesions of the NB of cholinergic fibers ascending to the cortex causes a reduction in ChAT activity. A decrease in neurotransmitter content should be expected as a direct consequence. Table 2 demonstrates that decreases in ACh levels of 30% and 39% in rat frontal and parietal cortices respectively were found 8 days after unilateral electrolytic lesioning of the NB. After an interval of 20 days, the decreases measured only 18% and 15% respectively. The difference between ACh levels 7 and 20 days after lesioning suggests that the recovery in HACU activity occurring in these animals [see section on "High-Affinity Choline Uptake (HACU)"] is associated with an increase in ACh formation.

Johnston et al. (1978) reported a 45% decrease in cortical ACh level 7–10 days after unilateral kainic acid injections in the NB.

As a consequence of the reduced ACh level in the cerebral cortex of the lesioned hemisphere, less ACh is spontaneously released from the cortical surface in unanesthetized, freely moving rats. For example, 20 days after the lesion, spontaneous ACh output from the cerebral cortex, as measured by the cortical cup technique, showed a 40% decrease in one group of rats (Lo Conte et al. 1982 b) and a 18% decrease in a second group (Lo Conte et al. 1982 a), depending on the size of the lesion.

A further demonstration of the functional impairment of the cortical cholinergic network after a NB lesion is derived from ACh turnover studies. In fact, 20

Table 2. ACh content (nmol/g, mean ± SE) in the cerebral cortex of rats with unilateral electrolytic lesions of the nucleus basalis

Conditions	Cortical areas			
	Frontal		Parietal	
Days after lesions	8	20	8	20
Sham operated ($n=12$)				
Both hemispheres	16.0 ± 0.5	16.2 ± 0.5	14.9 ± 0.7	14.8 ± 0.4
Lesioned ($n=11$)				
Ipsilateral	11.2 ± 0.4*	13.2 ± 0.4*	9.1 ± 0.5*	12.5 ± 0.5*
(% decrease from normal ACh levels)	−30	−18	−39	−15.4
Controlateral	17.0 ± 0.8	15.4 ± 0.5	13.8 ± 1.2	13.9 ± 0.5

Rats killed by microwave radiation. ACh levels measured by a radioenzymatic method (Ladinsky et al. 1983). Electrolytic lesions placed as described by Lo Conte et al. (1982a).
* Statistically significant difference, $p<0.01$ Student's t test

Table 3. Turnover rates (TR) of ACh (pmol/min/mg tissue) in the cerebral cortex of rats 20 days after a unilateral electrolytic lesion of the nucleus basalis

Conditions	Frontal areas		Parietal areas	
	TR_{ACh}	decrease (%)	TR_{ACh}	decrease (%)
Sham operated ($n=5$)				
Both hemispheres	3.63 ± 0.4		2.85 ± 0.31	
Lesioned ($n=5$)				
Ipsilateral	1.65 ± 0.11*	54.4	1.39 ± 0.18*	51.2
Controlateral	3.18 ± 0.52		3.07 ± 0.20	

The rats were killed by microwave radiation 4–6 min after the i.v. infusion of (methyl ^{3}H)choline. ACh turnover was measured according to the method of Ladinsky et al. (1983).Electrolytic lesions according to Lo Conte et al. (1982)
* Statistically significant difference between lesioned and sham-operated rats, $p<0.01$ with Student's t-test

days after lesion, when only a 15%–18% decrease in cortical ACh level was detectable, a 55% decrease in ACh turnover in the frontal cortex and a 52% decrease in the parietal cortex were found, as shown in Table 3.

Muscarinic Receptors

McKinney and Coyle (1982) demonstrated that 72 h after ibotenic acid injections in the NB that caused a 66% decrease in ChAT activity, there was a small but significant decrease in the total number of muscarinic binding sites, with no change in affinity. Carbachol agonist displacement curves indicate a loss of low-affinity sites. These results are compatible with a partial localization of low-affinity agonist receptors on cortical cholinergic terminals arising from the NB. The number of muscarinic antagonist binding sites did not significantly differ from that of controls 5 weeks after the lesion, whereas the number of receptors was elevated in comparison with the number observed 3 days after lesioning. The carbachol agonist displacement curves revealed a significant increase in the number of high-affinity sites, with no alteration in the number of low-affinity sites.

Lamour et al. (1982b) found a dramatic increase in the percentage of cortical neurons excited by ACh and an increase in their sensitivity 2 weeks after electrolytic lesions of the NB. The proportion of neurons excited by carbachol and nicotine was also increased. Both changes occurred in layers II, III, and IV and were not accompanied by changes in glutamate sensitivity. Since the effect tended to disappear by the 3rd week after the lesion, the authors interpret their findings as an indication of the transient supersensitivity of cortical cholinoceptive neurons.

The disappearance of muscarinic presynaptic autoreceptors located on the cholinergic nerve endings regulating ACh release is also supported by the finding that the increase in ACh output from the cerebral cortex induced by scopolamine is strongly reduced in NB-lesioned rats (Lo Conte et al. 1982a).

Other Neurotransmitters

According to Johnston et al. (1981), unilateral kainic acid lesions of the NB decreased only cortical cholinergic markers, leaving unmodified the activity of the enzymes glutamate decarboxylase, tyrosine hydroxylase, and histidine decarboxylase and levels of gamma-aminobutyric acid (GABA), noradrenaline, and 5-hydroxytryptamine (5HT). Cortical glutamate decarboxylase was also unaffected by kainic acid lesions of the NB in experiments by Lehman et al. (1980).

Electrolytic lesions of the NB causing a 39% decrease in ChAT activity in the frontoparietal cortex did not affect noradrenaline levels in the same area (Casa-

Table 4. Effects of unilateral electrolytic lesions of the nucleus basalis on 5HT and HVA levels (pmol/mg, mean ± SE) in the rat cerebral cortex ($n = 5$)

Hemisphere	Frontoparietal area	
	5HT	HVA
Intact	2.06 ± 0.05	0.19 ± 0.05
Lesioned	1.56 ± 0.16*	0.16 ± 0.01
% decrease from normal levels	−25	−16

Rats killed by decapitation 14 days after lesion. 5HT and HVA levels measured by the HPLC method of Kilts et al. (1981). Electrolytic lesions according to Lo Conte et al. (1982a).
* Statistically significant difference, $p < 0.01$ Student's t test

menti et al. 1985). However, similar lesions induced a 25% decrease in 5HT and a 16% reduction in homovanillic acid (HVA) levels in the ipsilateral frontoparietal cortex, as shown in Table 4.

Changes in Electrocortical Activity

Electrocorticograms recording electrical activity in rats 20 days after unilateral electrolytic lesions of the NB showed an asymmetry of the two hemispheres, with a diminuton of total electrical activity on the lesioned side. Spectrum analysis showed that the reduction in electrical activity involved all frequencies, but was more evident for high-frequency bands (Lo Conte et al. 1982b).

The amplitude of conditioned cortical slow potential was significantly decreased in rats with a unilateral electrolytic lesion of the NB or after inactivation of the NB by a local injection of procaine (Pirch et al. 1984). However, recordings of the spontaneous activity of cortical neurons in the somatosensory cortex of urethane-anesthetized rats 2 weeks after an electrolytic NB lesion were no different than for controls (Lamour et al. 1982b). The possibility that anesthesia alone depresses the effect of cholinergic input, thereby masking the effect of the NB lesion, should be considered.

Behavioral Changes

Lo Conte et al. (1982a, 1982b) demonstrated that unilateral electrolytic lesions of the NB are associated with changes in behavior, indicating an impairment of cognitive functions. The lesioned rats showed both impairment in the acquisition of a two-way active avoidance response (shuttle box) and suppression of the facilitating effect of scopolamine on shuttle box performance. In the same rats, impairment of passive avoidance response was noted. In this test, the effect of lesioning was potentiated by scopolamine. Furthermore, when placed in a Y maze 20 days after being lesioned the rats showed an increase in spontaneous motility, since the number of entries in both arms of the maze over a 3-min period was significantly greater for these rats than for controls.

Unilateral electrolytic lesions also impaired the acquisition of a one-way active avoidance (pole jumping) and a water maze task (Banfi 1984, personal communication).

Bilateral excitotoxic lesions of the NB were followed by an impairment of cognitive function similar to that described after unilateral lesions, without affecting the rats' performance on a battery of psychomotor tasks (Flicker et al. 1983). These authors reported that 3–5 weeks after lesioning, the rats were mildly impaired in the acquisition of a one-way active avoidance and exhibited a severe deficit in the retention of a passive avoidance response 1 h and 24 h after the training trial. The latter deficit was also observed by Friedman et al. (1983). On the other hand, no changes in the extinction of the task were observed.

Memory deterioration following bilateral lesions of the NB was also detected in T maze and radial maze tasks (Hepler et al. 1984), but none was observed for choice accuracy in a complex maze task involving trial-independent memory (Knowlton et al. 1984). These results demonstrate that NB lesions impair working memory (recall of recent events of transient importance) but not reference memory (information stored over the long term). This conclusion is also supported by the work of Beninger et al. (1984) using a delayed alternation task in a T maze.

It is, however, relevant to mention that Hepler et al. (1983) demonstrated on three behavioral tasks that bilateral lesions of both the NB and the medial septal area produce similar impairments. The medial septal area is the main source of the major cholinergic projection to the hippocampus (Mesulam et al. 1983b).

Conclusion

From the data reported in this review, it appears that lesions of the NB cause a marked impairment of the cortical cholinergic system, which is in turn associated with a loss of cognitive functions. These findings demonstrate the importance of the cortical cholinergic network in information acquisition and in working memory, thus confirming previous observations arrived at through the administration of anticholinergic drugs in animals or man (Warburton and Wesnes 1984).

It is interesting to note that unilateral and bilateral lesions of the NB causing a less than 40% decrease in cortical ChAT activity in one or both hemispheres produce similar cognitive deficits. This and the observation of Hepler et al. (1983) that medial septal and NB lesions also cause similar impairments suggest that a number of cognitive functions require the integrity of the cortical and hippocampal network.

Electrolytic lesions of the NB also affect serotoninergic and dopaminergic fibers slightly, as shown by the decrease in cortical levels of 5HT and HVA. However, it appears both from this review and from the direct comparison made by Hepler et al. (1983) of the effects of electrolytic and excitotoxic lesions that there are no differences between the behavioral deficits induced by the two types of lesions. This finding further emphasizes the crucial role of the cortical cholinergic system in the behaviors investigated.

A remarkable recovery seems to take place in the rat cholinergic system after NB lesions. An initial, partial functional recovery is demonstrated by the almost complete normalization within 20 days of cortical HACU activity. ChAT activity returns to normal levels within 3–6 months. Whether these recovery processes depend on the increased activity of surviving cholinergic neurons or on processes of sprouting and regeneration still needs to be defined. It is important to point out, however, that recovery can be stimulated by repeated administrations of gangliosides (Casamenti et al. 1985; Pedata et al. 1984).

Finally, a decrease in cortical and hippocampal ChAT activity related to a degeneration of the cholinergic neurons of the NB is the main neurochemical and neuropathologic change detected so far in senile dementia of the Alzheimer type (Price et al. 1982). This disorder is clinically characterized by severe impairment of cognitive functions. Animals with lesions of the NB therefore offer a useful experimental model of senile dementia.

References

Atweh SF, Simon JR, Kuhar MJ (1975) Utilization of sodium-dependent high-affinity choline uptake as a measure of the activity of cholinergic neurons in vivo. Life Sci 17:1535–1544

Beninger RJ, Jhamandas K, Boegman RJ, El-Defrawy SR (1984) Effects of scopolamine and nucleus basalis lesions on working and reference memory in the rat. Abstracts Soc Neurosci 10:1188

Bigl V, Woolf NJ, Butcher LL (1982) Cholinergic projections from the basal forebrain to frontal, parietal, temporal, occipital and cingulate cortices: a combined fluorescent tracer and acetylcholinesterase analysis. Brain Res Bull 8:727–749

Casamenti F, Bracco L, Bartolini L, Pepeu G (1985) Effects of ganglioside treatment in rats with a lesion of the cholinergic forebrain nuclei. Brain Res (338:45–57)

Davies P, Feisullin S (1982) A search for discrete cholinergic nuclei in the human ventral forebrain. J Neurochem 39:1743–1747

Flicker C, Dean RL, Watkins DL, Fisher SK, Bartus RT (1983) Behavioral and neurochemical effects following neurotoxic lesions of a major cholinergic input to the cerebral cortex in the rat. Pharmacol Biochem Behav 18:973–981

Friedman E, Lerer B, Kuster J (1983) Loss of cholinergic neurons in the rat neocortex produces deficits in passive avoidance learning. Pharmacol Biochem Behav 19:309–312

Hartgraves SL, Mensah PL, Kelly PH (1982) Regional decrease of cortical choline acetyltransferase after lesions of the septal area and in the area of the nucleus basalis magnocellularis. Neuroscience 7:2369–2376

Henderson Z (1981) A projection from acetylcholinesterase-containing neurones in the diagonal band to the occipital cortex of the rat. Neuroscience 6:1081–1088

Hepler D, Wenk G, Olton D, Lehman J, Coyle J (1983) Lesions in the nucleus basalis of Meynert and medial septal area of rats produce similar memory impairments in three behavioral tasks. Abstract Soc Neurosci 9:639

Hepler DJ, Wenk GL, Cribbs BL, Olton DS, Coyle JT (1984) Memory impairment following basal forebrain lesions. Brain Res (to be published)

Irle E, Markowitsch HJ 81984) Basal forebrain efferents reach the whole cerebral cortex of the cat. Brain Res Bull 12:493–512

Johnston MV, McKinney M, Coyle JT (1979) Evidence for a cholinergic projection to neocortex from neurons in the basal forebrain. Proc Natl Acad Sci USA 76:5392–5396

Johnston MV, Young AC, Coyle JT (1981) Laminar distribution of cholinergic markers in neocortex: effects of lesions. J Neurosci Res 6:597–607

Kelly PH, Moore KE (1978) Decrease of neocortical choline acetyltransferase after lesion of the globus pallidus in the rat. Exp Neurol 61:479–484

Kilts CD, Breese GR, Mailman RB (1981) Simultaneous quantification of dopamine, 5-hydroxytryptamine and four metabolically related compounds by means of reversed-phase high-performance liquid chromatography with electrochemical detection. J Chromatogr 225:347–357

Knowlton BJ, Wenk GL, Olton DS, Coyle JT (1984) Basal forebrain lesions produce a dissociation of trial-dependent and trial-independent memory performace. Brain Res (to be published)

Koenig JF, Klippel R (1963) The rat brain, a sterotaxis atlas. Williams and Wilkins, Baltimore

Kuhar MJ (1976) The anatomy of cholinergic neurons. In: Goldberg AM, Hanin I (eds) Biology of cholinergic function. Raven, New York, pp 3–27

Ladinsky H, Consolo S, Zatta A, Vezzani A (1983) Mode of action of gamma-butyrolactone on the central cholinergic system. Naunyn-Schmiedebergs Arch Pharmacol 322:42–48

Lamour Y, Dutar P, Jobert A (1982 a) Topographic organization of basal forebrain neurons projecting to the rat cerebral cortex. Neurosci Lett 34:117–122

Lamour Y, Dutar P, Jobert A (1982b) Spread of acetylcholine sensitivity in the neocortex following lesion of the nucleus basalis. Brain Res 252:377–381

Lehman J, Nagy JI, Atmodja S, Fibiger HC (1980) The nucleus basalis magnocellularis: the origin of a cholinergic projection to the neocortex of rat. Neuroscience 5:1161–1174

Lo Conte G, Bartolini L, Casamenti F, Marconcini Pepeu I, Pepeu G (1982a) Lesions of cholinergic forebrain nuclei: changes in avoidance behavior and scopolamine actions. Pharmacol Biochem Behav 17:933–937

Lo Conte G, Casamenti F, Bigl V, Milaneschi E, Pepeu G (1982b) Effect of magnocellular forebrain lesions on acetylcholine output from the cerebral cortex, electrocorticogram and behaviour. Arch Ital Biol 120:176–188

McKinney M, Coyle JT (1982) Regulation of neocortical muscarinic receptors: effects of drug treatment and lesions. J Neurosci 2:97–105

Mesulam MM, Mufson EJ, Levey AI, Wainer BH (1983a) Cholinergic innervation of the cortex by the basal forebrain: cytochemistry and cortical connections of the septal area, diagonal band nuclei, nucleus basalis (substantia innominata) and hypothalamus in the Rhesus monkey. J Comp Neurol 214:170–197

Mesulam MM, Mufson EJ, Wainer BH, Levey AI (1983b) Central cholinergic pathway in the rat: an overview based on an alternative nomenclature (Ch1–Ch6). Neuroscience 10:1185–1201

Pedata F, Lo Conte G, Sorbi S, Marconcini Pepeu I, Pepeu G (1982) Changes in high-affinity choline uptake in rat cortex following lesions of the magnocellular forebrain nuclei. Brain Res 233:359–367

Pedata F, Giovannelli L, Pepeu G (1984) GM_1 ganglioside facilitates the recovery of high-affinity choline uptake in the cerebral cortex of rats with a lesion of the nucleus basalis magnocellularis. J Neurosci Res 12:421–427

Pirch JH, Corbus MJ, Rigdon GC, Lyness WH (1984) Role of the nucleus basalis in generation of conditioned cortical slow potentials in the rat. Abstract Soc Neurosci 10:128

Price DL, Whitehouse PJ, Struble RG, Clark AW, Coyle JT, DeLong MR, Hedreen JC (1982) Basal forebrain cholinergic systems in Alzheimer's disease and related dementias. Neurosci Comm 1:84–92

Warburton DM, Wesnes K (1984) Drugs as research tools in psychology: cholinergic drugs and information processing. Neuropsychobiology 11:121–132

Wainer BH, Levey AI, Mufson EJ, Mesulam MM (1984) Cholinergic systems in mammalian brain identified with antibodies against choline acetyltransferase. Neurochem Int 6:163–182

Wenk GL, Olton DS (1984) Recovery of neocortical choline acetyltransferase activity following ibotenic acid injection into the nucleus basalis of Meynert in rats. Brain Res 293:184–186

Wenk H, Bigl V, Meyer U (1980) Cholinergic projections from magnocellular nuclei of the basal forebrain to cortical areas in rats. Brain Res Rev 2:295–316

AF64A Cholinotoxicity: Functional Aspects*

S. M. Leventer and I. Hanin[1]

Neurotoxins: An Overview

Over the past 20 years, neurotoxins have played an increasingly important role in the elucidation of neural mechanisms in the CNS. Neurotoxins have been utilized not only for the study of particular neurotransmitter systems, but also for the study of interactions between such systems. In addition, neurotoxins have been used to *simulate* neuronal, biochemical, and behavioral observations. This particular use of neurotoxins as tools for the production of *animal models* of human disease states has recently generated a great deal of enthusiasm.

Perhaps the best known of the neurotoxins is 6-hydroxydopamine (6-OHDA), a structural analog of the catecholamines. In 1967, Thoenen and Tranzer observed that systemic administration of this drug leads to selective destruction of peripheral adrenergic nerve terminals (Thoenen and Tranzer 1968). Subsequent studies in which 6-OHDA was injected either directly into brain or intracerebroventricularly clearly demonstrated both loss of nigrostriatal neurons and behavioral abnormalities (Ungerstedt 1968, 1971; Zigmond and Stricker 1972). This chemically induced dopaminergic hypofunction closely parallels the human disease state of Parkinsonism.

It is widely felt that this selective toxic effect of 6-OHDA results from its accumulation by the high-affinity uptake system present on catecholaminergic terminals. Once concentrated, 6-OHDA, a highly unstable compound, apparently forms several toxic compounds, including hydrogen peroxide and free radicals, leading to cell death (for review, see Rotman 1977). Another neurotransmitter-specific neurotoxin is 5,7-dihydroxytryptamine. This compound has been shown to produce a long-lasting reduction in brain tryptophan hydroxylase, a marker for serotonergic neurons (Victor et al. 1973).

A second group of neurotoxins consists of a family of compounds which have been collectively termed "excitotoxins." Included in this group are the three amino acids: kainic acid, ibotenic acid, and quinolinic acid. Each of these substances is capable of producing axon-sparing lesions in specific brain areas (Schwarcz et al. 1978 a). Interestingly, these compounds differ from one another in several important aspects.

First, the lesions produced by the injection of ibotenic acid tend to be more localized than those caused by kainic acid (Aldinio et al. 1981). The distant neuro-

* This study was supported by NIMH grant no. MH 34893 and by a grant from UCB, S. A., Brussels, Belgium

1 University of Pittsburgh School of Medicine Western Psychiatric Institute and Clinic 3811 O'Hara Street Pittsburgh, PA 15213, USA

Senile Dementia of the Alzheimer Type
Ed. by J. Traber and W. H. Gispen

nal degeneration caused by kainic acid injection, possibly due to its sustained convulsant activity (Ben-Ari et al. 1979), limits its use in the production of lesions. In contrast, the more discrete effect of ibotenic acid may make it more attractive than kainic acid for the production of localized striatal lesions intended to mimic the neural degeneration seen in Huntington's chorea (Kohler and Schwarcz 1983). On the other hand, kainic acid produces a better animal model of seizure disorders, in that intraventricular injection of this substance produces a pattern of seizures and pyramidal cell destruction similar to that seen in severe temporal lobe epilepsy (Schwarcz et al. 1978 b; Nadler et al. 1978).

It is also important to note that marked variations in susceptibility to the effects of each of these compounds exist, both between different regions of the brain and within individual brain areas. For example, cell groups in the medial septum and locus ceruleus are much more resistant to kainic acid administration than ibotenic acid (Kohler and Schwarcz 1983). Also, a wide range of vulnerability to kainic acid is seen in various regions of the hippocampus; such differences are not observed with ibotenic acid (Kohler and Schwarcz 1983). Similarly, quinolinic acid, a neuroexcitatory metabolite of tryptophan, exerts a neurodegenerative action which varies widely in different cell groups (Schwarcz and Kohler 1983).

Although the mechanism(s) of action of each of these compounds is still under debate, recent evidence indicates that prolonged depolarization induced by the excitatory amino acids may lead to unregulated chloride influx down its electrochemical gradient. This chloride influx is balanced ionically by increased cation influx and osmotically by water influx, leading finally to cell lysis (Samson et al. 1984; Rothman 1984).

Cholinotoxins: Rationale and Need

The availability of a neurotoxin capable of producing a specific and persistent central *cholinergic* deficit would be of great research value for several reasons. First, the central cholinergic system is important in the regulation of memory and learning processes (Glick et al. 1973; Beatty and Carbone 1980; Bartus 1979); additionally, there is an impressive body of evidence indicating that a central cholinergic deficit may be the important biochemical manifestation of Alzheimer type senile dementia (Wilcock et al. 1983; Rossor 1982; Coyle et al. 1983; Bird et al. 1983; Davies and Maloney 1976). A "cholinotoxin" might be expected to affect high-affinity choline transport (HAChT), choline acetyltransferase (ChAT) activity, acetylcholine (ACh) synthesis, storage or release, all of which are biological indicators of cholinergic neuronal function. Until recently, drugs known to affect central cholinergic function have been either short-lasting (for example, the HAChT inhibitor hemicholinium-3) or not cholinospecific [for example, venoms such as β-bungarotoxin (Mebs 1983; Smith et al. 1980)]. However, a relatively new group of compounds, the choline mustard analogs, has recently emerged. These compounds show a great deal of promise as potential cholinotoxins. In particular, ethylcholine mustard aziridinium (AF64A) has been proposed as a compound capable of producing long-lasting central cholinergic hypofunction (Mantione et al. 1981; Fisher et al. 1982).

AF64A: A Brief Summary of Findings

This section reviews some recent findings concerning AF64A, and provides a rationale for the role of this compound in the study of cholinergic function. Early experiments demonstrated that various choline mustard analogs inhibit both HAChT into synaptosomes (Rylett and Colhoun 1976, 1980a) and ChAT activity in vitro (Rylett and Colhoun 1979, 1980b). These interesting properties of the choline mustard analogs led to the suggestion that these compounds might be cholinotoxic, and could be used in animals to model disease states characterized by cholinergic dys- or hypofunction (Fisher and Hanin 1980).

Three days after injecting 65 nmol of AF64A intracerebroventricularly (i.c.v.) into mice, there was a large reduction in HAChT in both the hippocampus and the cortex (Mantione et al. 1981). This was the first indication that AF64A can be used in vivo to produce a persistent central cholinergic deficit. Further work in mice demonstrated that, in addition to decreased HAChT, i.c.v. injection of AF64A also leads to a depletion of ACh levels and to greatly reduced ChAT activity in several brain areas 7 days after injection (Fisher et al. 1982). In the same tissues, AF64A had no effect on the number of muscarinic receptors, as measured by ^{3}H-QNB binding, indicating that the site of action is probably presynaptic as well as persistent.

These initial demonstrations in the mouse of the ability of i.c.v. administered AF64A to produce deficits in a wide variety of cholinergic parameters led to the study of the cholinotoxic effects of AF64A in other species. Consistent with the earlier findings, Walsh et al. (1984) found that the bilateral injection of 7.5 or 15 nmol of AF64A (i.c.v.) in the rat causes a reduction in ACh levels in both the cortex and the hippocampus for as long as 120 days after AF64A treatment. No concurrent changes were seen in catecholamine or indoleamine levels in any brain area studied, thus supporting the "cholinospecificity" of the administered neurotoxin. In the same study, this group noted marked impairment of radial-arm maze performance 60–80 days after treatment. Similarly, Jarrard et al. (1984), using lower doses of AF64A (3–6 nmol, i.c.v.), found a reduction in hippocampal and striatal ACh levels 1 week after treatment, while reporting no changes in striatal dopamine (DA) or hippocampal norepinephrine (NE) levels. Like Walsh et al., this group also noted behavioral deficits in the form of impaired performance on complex place and cue tasks as a result of AF64A administration.

Other groups have investigated the effects of injection of AF64A directly into specific rat brain areas. Mantione et al. (1983) injected 2 nmol of AF64A into the hippocampus and found a significant reduction in ACh levels, HAChT, and ChAT activity 5 days later. As in the i.c.v. studies, the cholinospecificity of AF64A was supported, in that NE levels and 5-HT uptake in the same tissue were not affected by AF64A treatment. Similarly, Sandberg et al. (1984) found that 8 nmol of AF64A injected directly into rat striatum led to a large decrease in ChAT activity which persisted for at least 9 weeks. Importantly, striatal tyrosine hydroxylase and glutamate decarboxylase activity in the same tissue were unaffected by the AF64A treatment.

These and other studies, then, have firmly established the efficacy of using AF64A to produce long-lasting cholinergic hypofunction at both the neurochemical and behavioral level.

Recently, our group carried out a comprehensive study of the *functional* effects of a low dose of AF64A on rat central cholinergic function. In addition to analyzing cortical, hippocampal, and striatal ChAT activity, HAChT, [^{3}H]QNB binding, and acetylcholinesterase (AChE) activity, we also examined the functional state of the hippocampal cholinergic system after in vivo treatment with AF64A. This was accomplished through the determination of K^+-stimulated ACh release from superfused hippocampal slices. As the methods and results of this study are currently in press (Leventer et al., to be published), they are only briefly summarized here. Essentially, rats were infused bilaterally with AF64A (3 nmol/3 μl/side) or vehicle solution, and were killed 7 or 21 days posttreatment. In experiments measuring accumulation of [^{3}H]Ch and synthesis of [^{3}H]ACh, tissues were homogenized in 1.7 *N* HCl, and the levels of these substances in the supernatants were measured by means of thin layer chromatography (TLC) following centrifugation. In experiments involving K^+-stimulated ACh release, hippocampal slices (0.5 mm) were incubated with [^{3}H]Ch for 30 min, washed, mounted in small chambers, and superfused with buffer. This superfusion buffer was switched to one containing high (40 m*M*) K^+ for two periods (5 min each; S1 and S2 in Table 1) during the superfusion. These stimulations led to a large tritium efflux, as determined by TLC analysis, consisting almost entirely of [^{3}H]ACh. K^+-stimulated ACh release was then calculated as the sum of the two stimulations.

As shown in Table 1, AF64A caused a very large decrease in K^+-stimulated ACh release, both 7(−76%) and 21(−65%) days posttreatment. In contrast, the

Table 1. Effect of AF64A on K^+-stimulated ACh release, [^{3}H]choline accumulation, and [^{3}H]ACh synthesis 7 or 21 days posttreatment

	ACh release (S1+S2)[a]	[^{3}H]Choline accumulation (dpm × 10^6/ hippocampus)	% ACh	% Ch
7 Days				
Vehicle	18.8±1.3 (*n*=6)	2.6±0.1 (*n*=5)	17.5±0.7 (*n*=5)	77.3±1.3 (*n*=5)
AF64A	4.5±1.1 (*n*=6)***	2.4±0.2 (*n*=6)	12.4±1.7 (*n*=6)*	78.5±1.9 (*n*=6)
21 Days				
Vehicle	19.1±1.4 (*n*=6)	2.4±0.3 (*n*=6)	19.5±1.2 (*n*=6)	73.4±1.8 (*n*=6)
AF64A	6.7±0.9 (*n*=6)***	1.9±0.2 (*n*=5)	9.9±2.6 (*n*=5)**	77.8±3.2 (*n*=5)

Values shown represent the mean ±S.E. of (*n*) animals

[a] For each depolarization period, stimulated release was calculated by subtracting the basal release from the total release. The sum of the stimulated release from the two depolarization periods (S1+S2) represents ACh release. Values shown represent fractional release ×100. Fractional release was calculated as a percentage of the total amount of radioactivity available in the slices at the time of fraction collection

* $P<0.05$ as compared with vehicle

** $P<0.01$ as compared with vehicle

*** $P<0.001$ as compared with vehicle

accumulation of [^{3}H] after incubation with [^{3}H]Ch was comparable in hippocampal slices taken from either the AF64A-treated or the control animals (Table 1). However, the percentage of the accumulated label present in the form of [^{3}H]ACh was much lower in the animals treated with AF64A, both 7(−29%) and 21(−49%) days posttreatment (Table 1).

Hippocampal ChAT activity (Table 2) was also significantly reduced by treatment with AF64A, both 7 and 21 days posttreatment (−42% in both groups). Striatal and cortical ChAT, on the other hand, were not affected by AF64A treatment.

The effect of AF64A on AChE activity, HAChT, and [^{3}H]QNB binding is shown in Table 3. Both AChE activity and HAChT were decreased in the hippocampus by treatment with AF64A. Striatal and cortical AChE activity, HAChT, and [^{3}H]QNB binding were not affected by AF64A treatment (data not shown). Hippocampal [^{3}H]QNB binding was not affected 7 days after AF64A treatment, and was only slightly decreased (−11%) 21 days posttreatment.

Table 2. Effect of AF64A on ChAT activity in hippocampus, cortex, and striatum 7 or 21 days posttreatment

	% of control
7 Days	
Striatum ($n=12$)	98.5±2.5
Hippocampus ($n=7$)	58.0±7.3*
Cortex ($n=12$)	97.1±2.4
21 Days	
Striatum ($n=13$)	110.1±3.6
Hippocampus ($n=8$)	58.2±5.5*
Cortex ($n=13$)	97.0±3.4

Values shown represent the mean ±S.E. of (n) animals
* $P<0.001$ as compared with vehicle

Table 3. Effect of AF64A on AChE activity, HAChT, and [^{3}H]QNB binding in hippocampus 7 or 21 days posttreatment

	AChE activity (μmol/mg prot/h)	*HAChT* (pmol/mg prot/8 min)	*[^{3}H]QNB binding* (pmol/mg prot/40 min)
7 Days			
Vehicle	7.4±0.4 ($n=6$)	14.7±2.6 ($n=5$)	0.65±0.01 ($n=5$)
AF64A	2.9±0.6 ($n=5$)***	4.8±1.6 ($n=5$)*	0.60±0.03 ($n=5$)
21 Days			
Vehicle	8.7±0.4 ($n=7$)	12.4±0.6 ($n=6$)	0.65±0.01 ($n=6$)
AF64A	2.6±0.3 ($n=7$)***	6.0±1.2 ($n=6$)***	0.58±0.02 ($n=6$)**

Values shown represent the mean ±S.E. of (n) animals
* $P<0.02$ as compared with vehicle
** $P<0.01$ as compared with vehicle
*** $P<0.001$ as compared with vehicle

Taken as a whole, these data lend further support to the use of AF64A as a tool for the production of a persistent presynaptic cholinergic deficit in the rat. This deficit is not merely biochemical, but also functional in nature, in that both ACh synthesis and ACh release are reduced by treatment with AF64A in vivo. Interestingly, a similar functional deficit in ACh synthesis has also been noted in neocortical tissue from patients with Alzheimer's disease (Sims et al. 1982).

Cholinergic Specificity of AF64A: Special Considerations

While these findings are most encouraging from a developmental point of view, caution must be exercised in the interpretation of the effects of AF64A. Under conditions of excess, the action of AF64A may not be restricted to the cholinergic system; in fact, it can affect noncholinergic neurons as well. The question of the cholinergic specificity of AF64A may be approached neurochemically and/or morphologically.

Direct *neurochemical* evidence regarding the cholinospecificity of AF64A has been reviewed earlier (Walsh et al. 1984; Jarrad et al. 1984; Mantione et al. 1983; Sandberg et al. 1984). In each of these studies, AF64A affected only cholinergic values, while noncholinergic measures remained unchanged by various methods (i.c.v., intrastriatal, and intrahippocampal) of AF64A administration. Moreover, although we did not directly investigate noncholinergic factors in our study of the effects of i.c.v. AF64A treatment on K^+-stimulated ACh release, the findings provide additional, indirect neurochemical evidence for the cholinergic specificity of AF64A. As previously mentioned, while treatment with AF64A greatly reduced the capacity of hippocampal slices to synthesize [^{3}H]ACh, the accumulation of [^{3}H]Ch by hippocampal slices was unaffected by AF64A treatment. Had the AF64A acted nonspecifically, one would have expected some reduction in the transport of choline into the slices. This was not the case in our experiments. Although AF64A obviously affects HAChT both in vivo and in vitro, it had little or no effect, under the conditions of our study, on low-affinity choline transport. Our present study, then, also favors the concept of AF64A cholinospecificity.

One neurochemical study, however, has demonstrated that under certain conditions, AF64A may affect noncholinergic values. In this study, Levy et al. (1984) found that AF64A (3 nmol), injected directly into the substantia nigra of the rat, caused a large reduction in striatal DA levels. In addition, this group reported extensive damage at the injection site. The reason for this discrepancy has yet to be elucidated.

Morphological studies also indicate that, under certain conditions, AF64A is capable of affecting noncholinergic as well as cholinergic cells. Kozlowski and Arbogast (to be published) injected AF64A directly into the region of the nucleus basalis of Meynert in the rat, and noted that as low a dose as 0.02 nmol of AF64A produced nonspecific lesions at the injection site. Larger doses caused even greater nonspecific damage at the site of injection.

Other groups have also noted noncholinergic changes with high doses of AF64A, while, in contrast, lower doses caused changes specific to the cholinergic system. For example, Kasa et al. (1984) have found that, although i.c.v. injection of 8 nmol of AF64A produced degeneration of noncholinergic pyramidal cells in the CA2 and CA3 regions of the hippocampus 3 days after treatment, injection of 5 nmol selectively affected cholinergic terminals. Similarly, when Gaal et al. (1984) injected 40 nmol of AF64A i.c.v. in the rat, they noted pronounced nonspecific hippocampal degeneration; 10 nmol, in contrast, affected only cholinergic neurons in the hippocampus.

The above studies indicate that one must be careful to administer AF64A under the appropriate conditions when it is to be used as a cholinospecific neurotoxin. At low doses, ($\leqq$ 5 nmol, i.c.v.), the effects of AF64A appear to be limited to the cholinergic system. At higher doses (i.c.v.), noncholinergic effects become prominent.

Special caution must also be exercised when injecting AF64A directly into specific brain regions, since even very low doses may cause general damage to tissue surrounding the injection site. Also, as seen with the excitotoxins, individual brain areas may exhibit very different degrees of susceptibility to AF64A. One must, therefore, titrate the dose and concentration of the substance administered for each specific brain area to be studied. Finally, the preparation of AF64A must be performed carefully, as small variations in pH may have a deleterious effect on the compound.

Summary

AF64A is capable of producing a selective cholinergic deficit in the rat which is not merely neurochemical in nature. This deficit is, in fact, *functional,* as well as *biochemical.*

Not only does AF64A treatment lead to decreases in HAChT, ChAT activity and AChE activity, such treatment also produces a functional deficit in both *ACh synthesis* and in *ACh release.* In addition, functional deficits in learning and memory occur after AF64A treatment. These functional deficits are long-lasting; moreover, recent work in our laboratory has indicated that, like its behavioral effects, the neurochemical effects of AF64A treatment develop over a period of several days. This time course of the action of AF64A makes the compound extremely useful as a tool for the study of cholinergic function in general.

The AF64A-treated animal, then, continues to show promise as a model for human disease states, especially Alzheimer's disease, in which a cholinergic deficit is apparent.

Acknowledgements. The authors gratefully acknowledge the secretarial assistance of J. O'Leary in the preparation of this manuscript.

References

Aldinio C, French ED, Schwarcz R (1981) Seizures and neuronal degeneration: relationships investigated by intrahippocampal kainic and ibotenic acid. Neuroscience 7:589 (abstract)

Bartus RT (1979) Physostigmine and recent memory: effects in young and aged nonhuman primates. Science 206:1087–1089

Beatty WW, Carbone CP (1980) Septal lesions, intramaze cues and spatial behavior in rats. Physiol Behav 24:675–678

Ben-Ari Y, Tremblay E, Ottersen OP, Naquet R (1979) Evidence suggesting secondary epileptogenic lesions after kainic acid: pretreatment with diazepam reduces distant but not local brain damage. Brain Res 165:362–365

Bird TD, Stranahan S, Sumi SM, Raskind M (1983) Alzheimer's disease: choline acetyltransferase activity in brain tissue from clinical and pathological subgroups. Ann Neurol 14:284–293

Coyle JT, Price DL, DeLong M (1983) Alzheimer's Disease: a disorder of cortical cholinergic innervation. Science 219:1184–1190

Davies P, Maloney AJF (1976) Selective loss of central cholinergic neurons in Alzheimer's disease. Lancet 2:1403

Fisher A, Hanin I (1980) Minireview: choline analogs as potential tools in developing selective animal models of central cholinergic hypofunction. Life Sci 27:1615–1634

Fisher A, Mantione CR, Abraham DJ, Hanin I (1982) Long-term central cholinergic hypofunction induced in mice by ethylcholine aziridinium ion (AF64A) in vivo. J Pharmacol Exp Ther 222:140–145

Gaal G, Potter PE, Harsing LG Jr, Kakucska I, Fisher A, Hanin I, Vizi ES (1984) Histological changes caused by AF64A in rat hippocampus. Vizi ES, Magyar K (eds) Regulation of transmitter function: Basic and clinical aspects. Akademiai Kiado, Budapest, pp 295–300

Glick SD, Mittag TW, Green JP (1973) Central cholinergic correlates of impaired learning. Neuropharmacology 12:291–296

Jarrard LE, Kant GJ, Meyerhoff JL, Levy A (1984) Behavioral and neurochemical effects of intraventricular AF64A administration in rats. Pharmacol Biochem Behav 21:273–280

Kasa P, Farkas Z, Szerdahelyi P, Rakonczay Z, Fisher A, Hanin I (1984) Effects of cholinotoxin (AF64A) in the central nervous system: morphological and biochemical studies. In: Vizi ES, Magyar K (eds) Regulation of transmitter function: Basic and clinical aspects. Akademiai Kiado, Budapest, pp 289–293

Kohler C, Schwarcz R (1983) Comparison of ibotenate and kainate neurotoxicity in rat brain: a histological study. Neuroscience 8:819–835

Kozlowski MR, Arbogast RE (in press) Histochemical and biochemical effects of the injection of AF64A into the *nucleus basalis* of Meynert: relevance to animal models of senile dementia of the Alzheimer type. In: Hanin I (ed) Dynamics of cholinergic function. Plenum, New York

Leventer SM, McKeag D, Clancy M, Hanin I, Wulfert E (to be published) Intracerebroventricular AF64A reduces acetylcholine release from rat hippocampal slices. Neuropharmacology

Levy A, Kant GJ, Meyerhoff JL, Jarrard LE (1984) Non-cholinergic effects of AF64A in the *substantia nigra*. Brain Res 305:169–172

Mantione CR, Fisher A, Hanin I (1981) The AF64A-treated mouse: Possible model for central cholinergic hypofunction. Science 213:579–580

Mantione CR, Zigmond MJ, Fisher A, Hanin I (1983) Selective presynaptic cholinergic neurotoxicity following intrahippocampal AF64A injection in rats. J Neurochem 41:251–255

Mebs D (1983) Myotoxic and neurotoxic phospholipases A. In: Hucho F, Ovchinnikov YA (eds) Toxins as tools in neurochemistry. De Gruyter, Berlin

Nadler JV, Perry BW, Cotman C (1978) Intraventricular kainic acid preferentially destroys hippocampal pyramidal cells. Nature (Lond) 271:676–677

Rossor MN (1982) Neurotransmitters in CNS disease: dementia. Lancet 1:200–204

Rothman SM (1984) Excitatory amino acid neurotoxicity is produced by passive chloride influx. Neuroscience 10:24 (abstract)

Rotman A (1977) The mechanism of action of neurocytotoxic compounds: Life Sci 21:891–900

Rylett BJ, Colhoun EH (1976) Effects of acetylcholine mustard aziridinium ion and its choline analogue on choline transport into synaptosomes. Can J Physiol Pharmacol 55:769–772

Rylett BJ, Colhoun EH (1979) The interactions of choline mustard aziridinium ion with choline acetyltransferase. J Neurochem 32:553–558

Rylett BJ, Colhoun EH (1980a) Kinetic data on the inhibition of high-affinity choline transport into rat forebrain synaptosomes by choline-like compounds and nitrogen mustard analogues. J Neurochem 34:713–719

Rylett BJ, Colhoun EH (1980b) Carrier-mediated inhibition of choline acetyltransferase. Life Sci 26:909–914

Samson L, Olney JW, Price JT, Labruyere J (1984) Kyenurate protects against excitotoxin-induced neuronal necrosis in chick retina. Neuroscience 10:24 (abstract)

Sandberg K, Hanin I, Fisher A, Coyle JT (1984) Selective cholinergic neurotoxin: AF64A's effects in rat striatum. Behav Neurosci 98(1):162–166

Schwarcz R, Kohler C (1983) Differential vulnerability of central neurons of the rat to quinolinic acid. Neurosci Lett 38:85–90

Schwarcz R, Scholz D, Coyle JT (1978a) Structure-activity relations for the neurotoxicity of kainic acid derivatives and glutamate analogues. Neuropharmacology 17:145–151

Schwarcz R, Zaczek R, Coyle JT (1978b) Microinjection of kainic acid into the rat hippocampus. Eur J Pharmacol 50:209–220

Sims NR, Bowen DM, Davison AN (1982) Acetylcholine synthesis and glucose metabolism in aging and dementia. In: Giacobini E, Filogamo G, Giacobini G, Vernadakis A (eds) The aging brain: cellular and molecular mechanisms of aging in the nervous system. Raven, New York, pp 153–160

Smith CCT, Bradford HF, Thompson EJ, MacDermot J (1980) Actions of β-bungarotoxin in amino acid transmitter release. J Neurochem 34:487–494

Thoenen H, Tranzer JP (1968) Chemical sympathectomy by selective destruction of adrenergic nerve endings with 6-hydroxydopamine. Naunyn Schmiedebergs Arch Pharmacol Exp Pathol 261:171–288

Ungerstedt U (1968) 6-hydroxy-dopamine induced degeneration of central monoamine neurons. Eur J Pharmacol 5:107–110

Ungerstedt U (1971) Adipsia and aphagia after 6-hydroxydopamine induced degeneration of the nigro-striatal dopamine system. Acta Physiol Scand [Suppl] 367:95–122

Victor SJ, Baumgarten HG, Lovenberg W (1973) Effect of intraventricular administration of 5,6 and 5,7 dihydroxytryptamine on regional tryptophan hydroxylase activity in rat brain. Fed Proc 32:564 (abstract)

Walsh TJ, Tilson HA, DeHaven DL, Mailman RB, Fisher A, Hanin I (1984) AF64A, a cholinergic neurotoxin selectively depletes acetylcholine in hippocampus and cortex, and produces long-term passive avoidance and radial-arm maze deficits in the rat. Brain Res 321:91–102

Wilcock GK, Esiri MM, Bowen DM, Smith CCT (1983) The nucleus basalis in Alzheimer's disease: cell counts and cortical biochemistry. Neuropathol Appl Neurobiol 9:175–179

Zigmond MJ, Stricker EM (1972) Deficits in feeding behavior after intraventricular injection of 6-hydroxydopamine in rats. Science 177:1211–1214

Novel Approaches in the Study of Brain Acetylcholine Function: Neuropharmacology, Neuroanatomy, and Behavior

D. G. SPENCER, JR.,[1] E. HORVATH,[1] P. LUITEN,[2] T. SCHUURMAN,[1] and J. TRABER[1]

Introduction

Over the last 30 years, it has become well-recognized that drugs blocking the muscarinic subtype of acetylcholine (ACh) receptors in the brain have selective and reproducible effects on behaviors requiring learning, memory, and stimulus discrimination in both animals (Hearst 1958; Carlton 1963; Warburton and Heise 1972; Bartus and Johnson 1976; Heise et al. 1976; Moore et al. 1976; Milar 1981; Spencer and Lal 1983; Spencer et al. 1985) and humans (Ostfeld and Aruguete 1962; Hrbek et al. 1971; Crow and Grove-White 1973; Drachman 1978; Mewaldt and Ghoneim 1979; Wesnes and Warburton 1984). Behavioral effects that are in many ways similar to those observed after central muscarinic blockade are also seen after electrolytic lesions of brain structures that involve a major cholinergic pathway, such as the medial-septal–hippocampal system (Douglas 1967; Walker et al. 1972; Myhrer 1975; Jarrard 1975, 1976; Johnson et al. 1977; Sinnamon et al. 1978), and after local infusions of muscarinic antagonists into the hippocampus (Leaton and Rech 1972; Ross and Grossman 1974; Leith and Barrett 1975; Ross et al. 1975; Blozovski 1979; Solomon and Gottfried 1981). Another major cholinergic projection passes from the nucleus basalis magnocellularis (nBM) to the neocortex, and lesions in this nucleus also produce antimuscarinic-like behavioral deficits (Flicker et al. 1983; Friedman et al. 1983), which are further increased by concurrent administration of centrally active muscarinic antagonists (Lo Conte et al. 1982).

The development of histologic techniques for the demonstration of cholinergic cell markers, such as the cholinergic metabolic enzymes acetylcholinesterase (AChE) and choline acetyltransferase (ChAT), has permitted the correlation of behavioral lesion effects with changes in the appearance of these cholinergic markers in specific brain structures. The exact circuitry of cholinergic projections has also begun to be elucidated through the combination of AChE or ChAT staining with retrograde tracing techniques (Bigl et al. 1982; McKinney et al. 1983; Milner et al. 1983; Woolf et al. 1983; Wahle et al. 1984). The retrograde technique, often employing fluorescent dyes or horseradish peroxidase as the transported agent, allows identification of the sources of the projection pathways terminating in a specific area. In this way, the nBM has been identified as a major source of cholinergic innervation of the cerebral cortex. Despite this information, however, the inherent properties of the retrograde method hamper further eluci-

1 Neurobiology Department, Troponwerke, Neurather Ring 1, 5000 Cologne 80, FRG
2 Department of Animal Physiology, State University of Groningen, P.O. Box 14, 9750 AA Haren, The Netherlands

Senile Dementia of the Alzheimer Type
Ed. by J. Traber and W. H. Gispen

dation of this pathway. Typically, retrograde tracers have little spatial resolution in the projection terminus due to spread of the injected tracer and thus cannot reveal the manner in which the projections interact with the target cells. In addition, retrograde techniques cannot reveal all the projections of the source nucleus, but only those already suspected. To detect all projections, anterograde tracing techniques are required. Phaseolus vulgaris lectin (PHA-L) can be used as such a specifically anterogradely transported tracer, and it has several useful advantages over autoradiographic detection of anterogradely transported amino acids (Ter Horst et al. 1984). The results of PHA-L experiments are described below.

Another approach to the localization and quantification of cholinergic transmission is receptor ligand autoradiography. In this procedure, brain sections are incubated with radiolabelled receptor ligands. After washing, the slices are exposed to radioactivity-sensitive film. When developed, the film reveals relative degrees of ligand binding in the brain section.

Until recently, all muscarinic drugs seemed to have affinity for only one homogenous population of muscarinic receptors. This tendency hampered further understanding of central cholinergic function because no drug "tools" existed that were capable of selectively interacting with subsets of the cholinergic muscarinic system. However, in the last 5–7 years, three independent lines of evidence have been reported for muscarinic receptor heterogeneity.

First, Goyal and Rattan (1978) reported that two kinds of cholinergic muscarinic response exist in the opossum lower esophageal sphincter: stimulation of the vagus nerve causes relaxation, while administration of the muscarinic agonist bethanechol results in contraction. The receptors mediating relaxation were found on the inhibitory intraluminal neurons, were preferentially activated by the agonist McN A 343, and were termed M1 receptors. The contraction-inducing receptors were found on the sphincter muscle itself, were preferentially activated by bethanechol, and were called M2 receptors. Later studies confirmed this differentiation and showed that the muscarinic antagonist pirenzepine preferentially blocked the M1 response to McN A 343 (Gilbert et al. 1984).

Second, Birdsall et al. (1980) studied the pattern of displacement of radiolabelled antagonist binding produced by concurrent incubation with agonists such as carbachol. The displacement functions indicated three separate receptor affinities for carbachol, which were called superhigh- (SH), high- (H), and low- (L) affinity sites. Subsequent studies showed that while SH and H binding were strongly affected by divalent cation concentrations and were regulated by a guanine nucleotide-binding protein, the same was not the case for L binding (Hulme et al. 1983). In addition, the L sites were found to have a 20-fold higher affinity than the SH and H sites for pirenzepine (Birdsall and Hulme 1983).

Third, the binding characteristics of radiolabelled pirenzepine to membrane receptors have also been studied. Hammer et al. (1980) first reported that pirenzepine has affinities across brain structures, glands, heart, and smooth muscle that differ from those of nonselective antagonists such as *N*-methyl scopolamine (*N*MS). Pirenzepine and McN A 343 have pharmacologic activities that correlate well with these affinities (Hammer and Giachetti 1982), and more recent studies of pirenzepine binding have confirmed the regional variations in brain receptor affinity as well as the probable characterization of these receptors as M1 (Watson et al. 1982, 1983; Luthin and Wolfe 1984). Potter et al. (1983) have attempted to integrate the SH, H, and L receptor terminology with the M1 and M2 classification scheme. They provide evidence that M1 and M2 receptors are independent, but that each can exist in high- and low-affinity forms, the high-affinity forms being coupled and the low-affinity forms being uncoupled. Thus, SH is the same as high-affinity M2, L is the same as low-affinity M1, but H represents an overlap between low-affinity M2 and high-affinity M1. The issue is further complicated by the fact that in different brain areas, there are different relative proportions of M1 and M2 receptors.

Although autoradiographic localization of M1 receptors in the brain using labelled pirenzepine has been well described (Yamamura et al. 1983; Wamsley et al. 1984), no complete reports exist of direct M2 brain receptor autoradiography. Radiolabelled oxotremorine-M would seem to be a good candidate ligand for such studies, since its binding in brain (Hulme et al. 1983; Bevan 1984) and heart (Waelbroek et al. 1982; Harden et al. 1983; Martin et al. 1984) is highly specific and well-characterized. Therefore, oxotremorine-M was selected for our autoradiographic studies described below.

As the title of this paper implies, three main topics within the broad subject of central acetylcholinergic function are presented. The first consists of autoradiographic differentiation of M1 and M2 receptors in the rat brain, using tritiated *N*-methyl scopolamine (^{3}H-*N*MS), pirenzepine (^{3}H-PZ), and oxotremorine-M (^{3}H-OXO). The second deals with preliminary determination of the projection patterns of the rat nBM in the cerebral cortex, using the PHA-L anterograde tracing technique. The third involves the histologically determined pathologic and behavioral consequences of chemical lesions of two cholinergic brain nuclei: the nBM and the medial septum.

Methods and Materials

Muscarinic Cholinergic Receptor Autoradiography

Rapidly removed male rat brains were frozen in 2-methylbutane (−45 °C) and stored at −70 °C until use. 20-μm thick coronal sections were cut on a cryostat microtome and mounted on chrome alum/gelatine-coated slides. After 10 min preincubation in 20 m*M* Hepes-TRIS buffer (pH, 7.5) containing 10 m*M* Mg^{++}, slices were then incubated in the same buffer along with 1 n*M* ^{3}H-OXO, 1 n*M* ^{3}H-PZ, or 0.1 n*M* ^{3}H-*N*MS. Nonspecific binding was always determined through displacement by 1 μ*M* atropine sulfate. After 30 min incubation at 30 °C, slides were transferred through three 2-min successive changes of ice-cold buffer and then rinsed with cold, deionized water. After overnight air-drying at room temperature, brainsections were apposed to LKB Ultrafilm for a period of 4–5 weeks. For purposes of binding site localization, alternate brain sections were fixed and stained with cresyl violet.

Anterograde Tracing Using PHA-L

PHA-L (2.5% in TRIS-buffered saline) was iontophoretically injected into the anterior part of the nBM of male Wistar rats at the interaural coordinates AP 7.7, LR 3.5, and V 2.5 of Paxinos and Watson (1982). The rats were sacrificed, and their brains fixed 7 days after the PHA-L injection. The PHA-L was visualized by the PAP technique of Sternberger, as described by Ter Horst et al. (1984).

Morphological and Behavioral Consequences of Chemical Lesions of Cholinergic Nuclei

Male rats were given local pressure injections of ethylcholine mustard aziridinium ion (AF64A) over a 10-min period into either the nBM (bilaterally) or the medial septal nucleus (one injection on the midline). Behavioral evaluation took place 10–14 days after the lesion. Lesion pathology was evaluated on cresyl-violet–stained brain sections taken from rats 2 weeks after lesioning. The following behavioral tests were performed.

Response to a Novel Environment. Rats were inserted singly into small glass chambers and observed over a 50-min period. Behavior was sampled every 15 s, categorized, and entered into a computer. The behavioral categories were: locomotion, rearing, grooming, licking/sniffing (directed away from the animal itself), gnawing, hunched posture, sitting, and sleeping (Traber et al. 1982).

Passive Avoidance. Following control or lesion treatment, rats were individually trained in a step-through passive foot shock avoidance task, as described by Ader et al. (1972). Briefly, rats received a foot shock after entering a large dark compartment (shock trial), and the time required to enter was recorded. After a 27-h interval, latency to enter was again measured, but no shock was delivered (retention trial).

Active Avoidance. Training of lesioned and control rats took place in a two-compartment shuttlebox, as described by Bauer (1982). Subjects received 20 pairings of signal (combined tone and light) and foot shock in each daily session and the percentage of trials in which the rats successfully avoided to shock by running to the opposite compartment during the signal was taken as an index of acquisition. In order to measure lesion effects on retention of this behavior, a separate group of untreated rats were trained as above, lesioned, and then tested again after the lesion.

Water Maze. Lesioned and control rats were individually placed at one end of a water-filled tank. In order to escape from the tank, rats were required to swim around a series of barriers until the ladder at the opposite end was reached. Sessions were conducted daily and the number of errors (turning the wrong direction) was measured on each trial. Simple learning was studied in water maze type 1 (Fig. 1, top), whereas reversal learning was examined in water maze type 2 (Fig. 1, bottom).

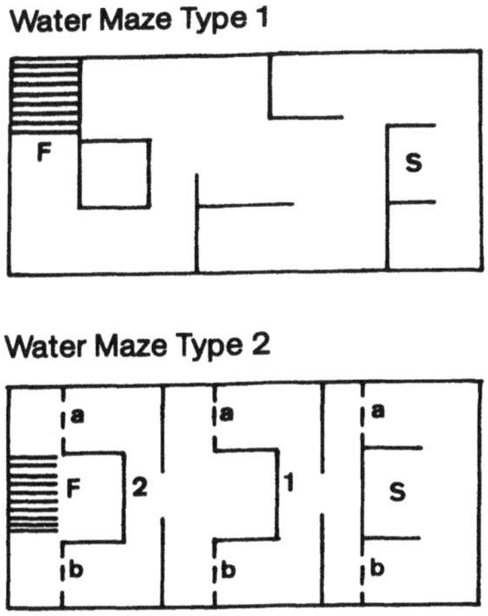

Fig. 1. Schematic drawing of water mazes used in behavioral evaluation of AF64A lesion effects. In both mazes, rats were placed at the locations marked *"S"* and were required to swim to the areas marked *"F"* in order to find the escape ladder. For reversal learning (water maze type 2), barriers were placed at either locations marked *"a"* or at those marked *"b."* Training on this maze began on the 1st day with subjects placed at location 2, proceeded to location 1 on the 2nd day, and finished at location *"S"* on the next 2 days. On the final (reversal) day, barricades were shifted from *"a"* to *"b,"* or vice versa

Student's *t*-test was used for statistical evaluation of all lesion effects on behavior, except in the case of water maze acquisition, where the Mann-Whitney *U*-test was performed.

Results and Discussion

Muscarinic Cholinergic Receptor Autoradiography

The results of autoradiographic experiments with ^{3}H-*N*MS, ^{3}H-PZ, and ^{3}H-OXO are presented in Fig. 2. With each of the three ligands, nonspecific binding after incubation with atropine was not visually apparent. In order to quantitatively determine the degree of specific binding of each ligand, the slices were transferred to scintillation vials containing 3 ml Quickszint 402 (Zinsser Analytic, Frankfurt, FRG), shaken for 30 min, allowed to sit at 4 °C overnight, after which radioactivity was measured, Analysis revealed that the percentage of specific binding of ^{3}H-*N*MS, ^{3}H-PZ, and ^{3}H-OXO was 95%, 94%, and 90% respectively. At the most rostral coronal level (Fig. 2, tow row), ^{3}H-*N*MS binding was strong in the cortex, caudate putamen, septal nuclei, and olfactory tubercle, but was relatively undifferentiated, ^{3}H-PZ was also localized in the cerebral cortex (mostly in the superficial layers), primary olfactory cortex, caudate putamen, and olfactory tubercle, but was not detectable in the septal nuclei. ^{3}H-OXO bound in a pattern similar to that of the other two ligands in the caudate putamen, but displayed a marked lamination in the cerebral cortex that continued into the cingulate cortex. Although intense binding was found in the medial septum and the vertical limb of the diagonal band of Broca, the olfactory tubercle and primary olfactory cortex were much less strongly labelled. The second row of Fig. 2 shows binding patterns for the three ligands at a more caudal coronal level. In the cerebral and cingulate cortices, the ^{3}H-*N*MS distribution was again rather homogenous. ^{3}H-PZ was detected in superficial cerebral cortical layers and the primary olfactory

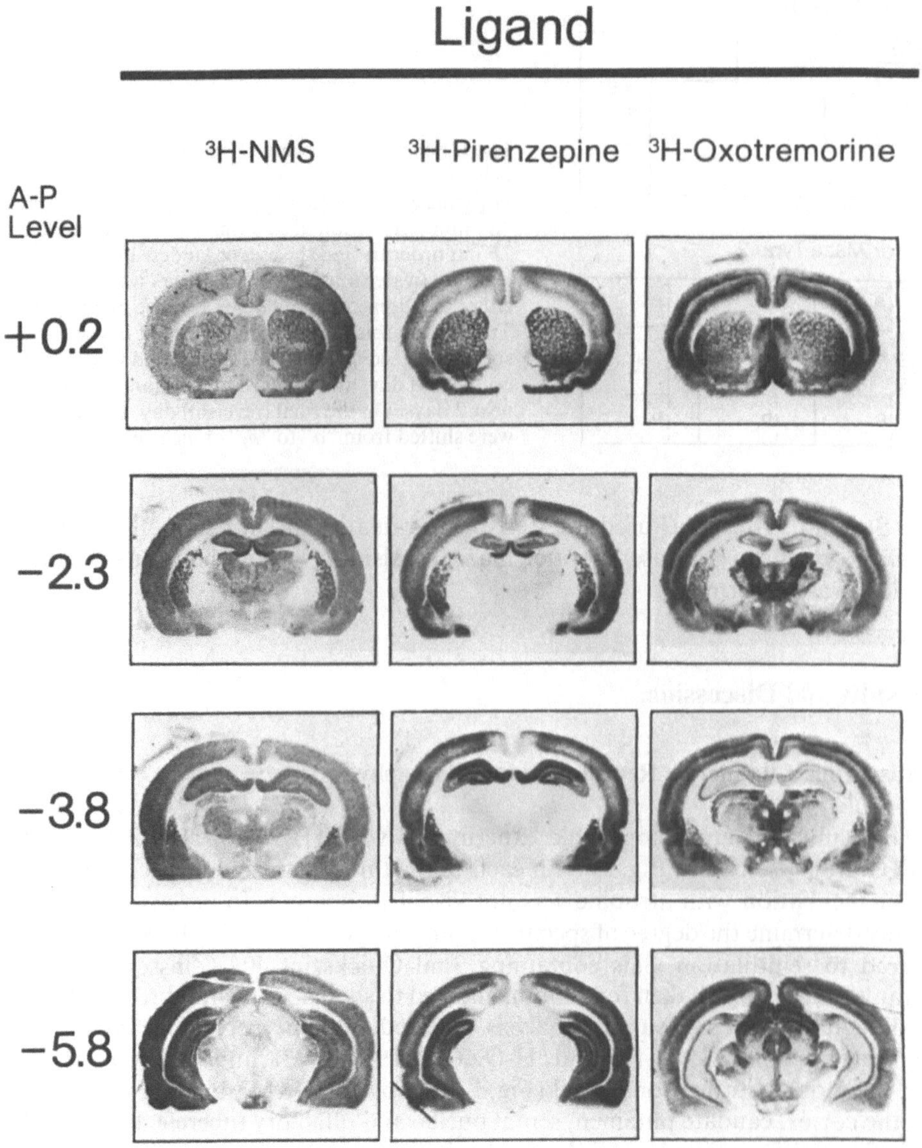

Fig. 2. Coronal rat brain sections showing the binding of three muscarinic cholinergic agents. *A-P level* refers to the rostral-caudal position of the slice relative to bregma (Paxinos and Watson 1982)

cortex, but bound only weakly in the cingulate cortex. The pattern of cerebral cortical lamination with ^{3}H-OXO continued at this level, but the pattern was discontinuous with that observed in the cingulate cortex. All three ligands again bound to the caudate putamen, but, whereas both ^{3}H-*N*MS and ^{3}H-OXO bound to the diencephalic thalamic and hypothalamic nuclei, ^{3}H-PZ did not.

More caudally, at bregma A-P level −3.8 mm, cortical binding patterns for the three ligands were the same as described above, but interesting differences in hippocampal binding began to emerge. ^{3}H-*N*MS was found throughout the entire hippocampal formation, but ^{3}H-PZ binding was strongly concentrated in CA1 and the dentate gyrus. Conversely, ^{3}H-OXO binding was relatively weak in this structure; labelling was evident in the subiculum, areas CA1 and CA2, only weakly apparent in CA3, and virtually absent in the dentate gyrus. ^{3}H-*N*MS binding was present in the amygdala, and amygdalar binding was evident with both ^{3}H-PZ and ^{3}H-OXO, especially in the basolateral amygdaloid nucleus. A concentration of ^{3}H-OXO binding was noted more laterally, in the deep layers of the perirhinal cortex. At the most caudal level studied (Fig. 2, bottom row), the binding differences among the three muscarinic cholinergic ligands described above continue to be apparent. The fine lamination of ^{3}H-OXO binding that was found more rostrally in the cingulate cortex was also found in the retrosplenial cortex. In addition, ^{3}H-OXO bound intensely to the superior and inferior gray layers of the superior colliculus and bound to a lesser extent to the periaqueductal gray. Although data are not shown, ^{3}H-OXO binding was present in the inferior colliculus and brainstem cranial nerve nuclei (e.g., the trigeminal and vagal nuclei), as well as in the medial layer of the olfactory bulbs (where ^{3}H-PZ displayed an equally striking opposite affinity for the lateral aspect).

The results of autoradiographic determination of M1 receptor distribution using ^{3}H-PZ agree well with those described in previous reports. In particular, the M1 distribution in the hippocampus and the superficial layers of the cerebral cortex has already been described (Yamamura et al. 1983; Wamsley et al. 1984), but the present findings provide additional detail, especially with regard to the discontinuity between parietal and cingulate cortical binding. The pattern of M2 binding seen with ^{3}H-OXO also agrees with previous reports using carbachol displacement of labelled antagonist binding (Wamsley et al. 1980; Potter et al. 1983) and ^{3}H-OXO itself (Potter et al. 1983). However, several novel aspects of M2 distribution patterns have emerged in the present study: the lamination of cerebral cortical binding, the differentiation from the fine lamination seen in the cingulate and retrosplenial cortex, the concentration of receptors near the rhinal fissure, and the detailed pattern of thalamic and hypothalamic distribution. Even so, the present data also support the conclusion made by Potter and co-workers that M2 receptors appear to be better markers than M1 receptors for cholinergic cell nuclei in the rat central nervous system. It is therefore possible that a large proportion of M2 receptors exist on cholinergic cells themselves and play a role in the regulation of cholinergic cell activity.

Anterograde Tracing Using PHA-L

When stained for AChE, the rat nBM appears as a diffuse conglomeration of unusually large cells (Fig. 3). Iontophoretic injections of PHA-L into this area resulted in two sorts of labelled projections. One type terminated in the thalamus and the substantia nigra and was clearly the result of PHA-L transport by neurons of the extrapyramidal motor system. The other type terminated in the

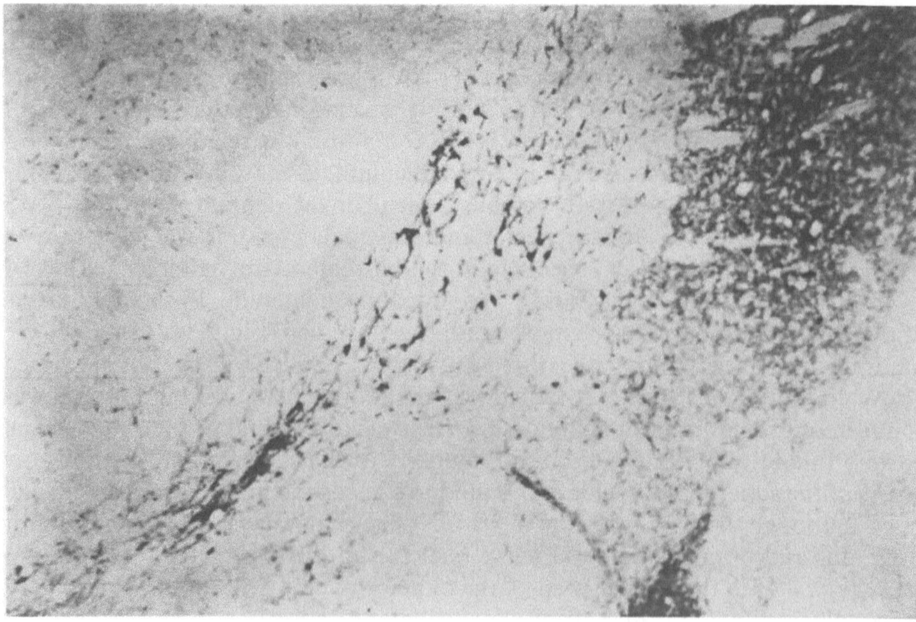

Fig. 3. The nucleus basalis magnocellularis of the rat, as revealed by AChE stain. Subjects were pretreated with diisopropyl fluorophosphate before sacrifice in order to suppress the cholinesterase enzyme in regions outside the cholinergic cell bodies

cortex and amygdala (particularly in the basolateral amygdaloid nucleus). PHA-L injections in areas surrounding the nBM never gave rise to such cortical projections. PHA-L–labelled projections to the neocortex were of fine detail and complexly organized (Fig. 4). The cortical areas most densely innervated from the nBM were the frontal, entorhinal, and perirhinal cortices. Within the frontal cortex, fibers were predominantly oriented parallel to the pial surface in layers I and VI, whereas a more radial fiber orientation was seen in layers III and IV. Terminal swellings from these fibers were often seen in association with cresyl-violet–counterstained neocortical cell bodies, and such terminals were most frequent in cortical layers I, II, and V. Terminals in the perirhinal cortex were observed in primarily superficial layers, while the entorhinal cortex was densely innervated throughout its extent.

The following lines of evidence support the hypothesis that within the rat basal forebrain, it is only the cholinergic magnocellular neurons of the nBM that project to the neocortex. First, lesions of this ventral globus pallidus region result in appreciable decreases in neocortical ChAT activity (45%–55%, Johnston et al. 1981; 65%, McKinney et al. 1983). Second, these magnocellular cells are retrogradely labelled by tracers such as horseradish peroxidase injected in the cortex and undergo retrograde degeneration when the neocortex is ablated (Lehmann et al. 1980). Third, studies combining retrograde tracers from the neocortex with AChE or ChAT histochemistry indicate the cholinergic nature of these cells (Bigl

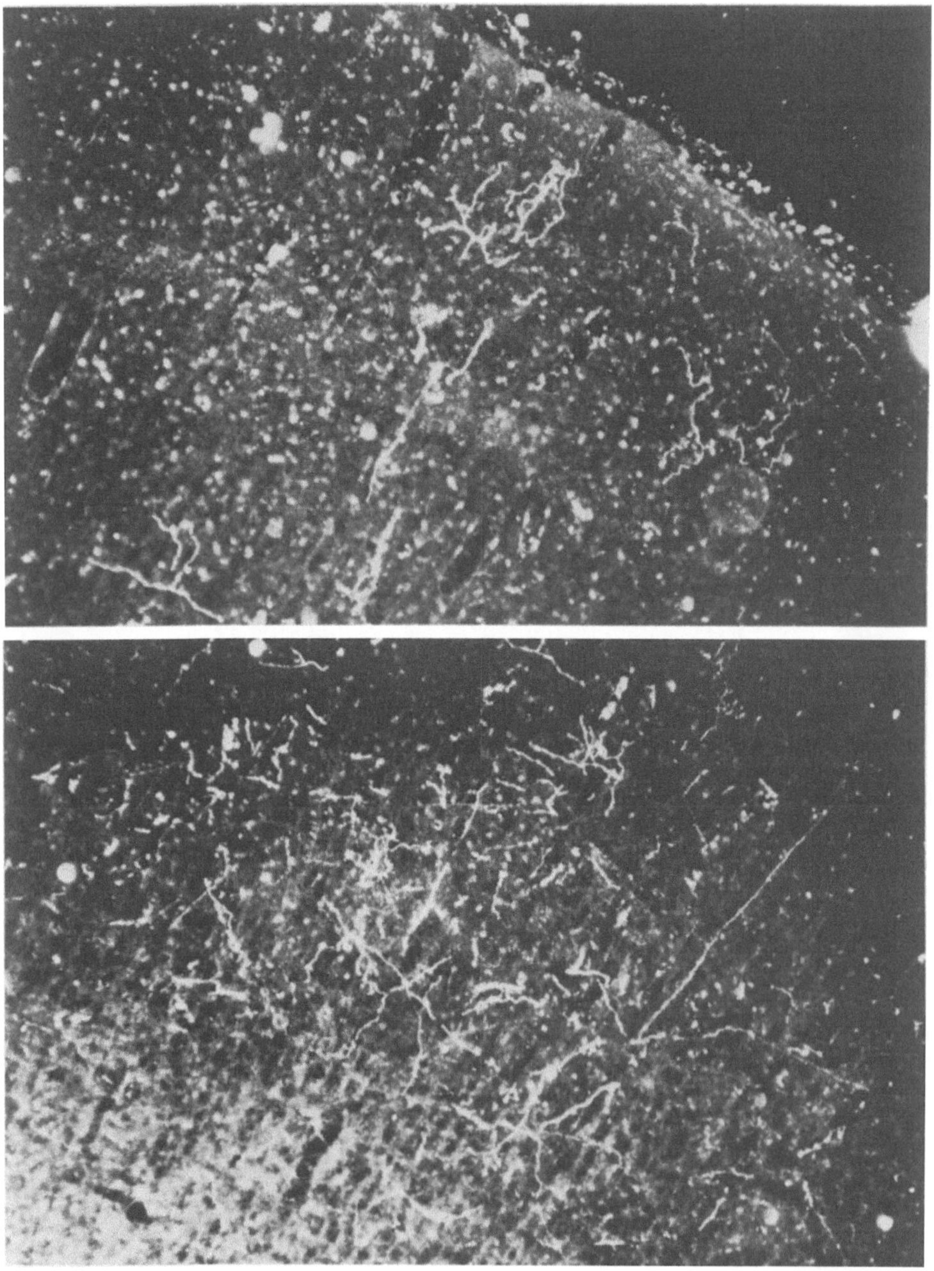

Fig. 4. Projections of the nBM to the neocortex, as revealed by dark-field microscopy of PHA-L–labelled fibers. The *top section* depicts frontoparietal cortical projections in the most superficial layers (I–IV), whereas the *bottom micrograph* shows the deepest layers (IV–VI)

et al. 1982; Woolf et al. 1983; Wahle et al. 1984). The same methodology, when applied to retrograde transport from the amygdala, indicates that cholinergic cells in the area of the nBM also project to the basolateral amygdala.

The present data based on the PHA-L technique reveal a previously unknown level of organization of the nBM-cortical projections. Information thus derived should be of great help in defining more precisely the anatomical regions where neurochemical and electrophysiological changes resulting from nBM lesions should arise. Additionally, the PHA-L technique provides material with sufficient detail for the determination of the microneurocircuitry of the nBM-cortex connection and the nature of the cortical cells that preferentially receive these projections.

Morphological and Behavioral Consequences of Chemical Lesions of Cholinergic Nuclei

The morphological consequences 2 weeks after AF64A injection (1 nmol in 0.5 μl saline) in the nBM and medial septum are shown in Fig. 5 (top and bottom respectively). Cresyl violet histologic examination revealed clear cellular destruction, but there was no evidence of any sort of tissue specificity of the lesion.

Response to a Novel Environment. The frequencies of observation of the various behaviors of bilaterally lesioned and vehicle control animals is shown in Table 1. Animals with AF64A lesions of the medial septum did not differ significantly from animals with vehicle injections into this area, nor were those with vehicle injections in the nBM different from the other two groups. However, nBM-lesioned rats engaged in significantly more locomotion ($t(10)=3.2$, $P<0.01$) and licking/sniffing ($t(10)=3.0$, $P<0.02$) than control rats, and they groomed ($t(10)=3.2$, $P<0.01$) and slept ($t(10)=4.9$, $P<0.001$) less. Since behavioral frequency rather than intensity was measured, these data indicate that nBM-lesioned rats did not

Table 1. Behavioral response of rats with vehicle or AF64A brain infusions to a novel environment

Behavior	Infusion site			
	Medial septum		nBM	
	vehicle	AF64A	vehicle	AF64A
Locomotion	16	19	11	54
Rearing	0	1	1	3
Grooming	45	32	49	22
Licking/sniffing	17	20	21	49
Gnawing	0	1	1	0
Hunched posture	0	0	0	9
Sitting	63	81	49	57
Sleeping	58	47	68	5

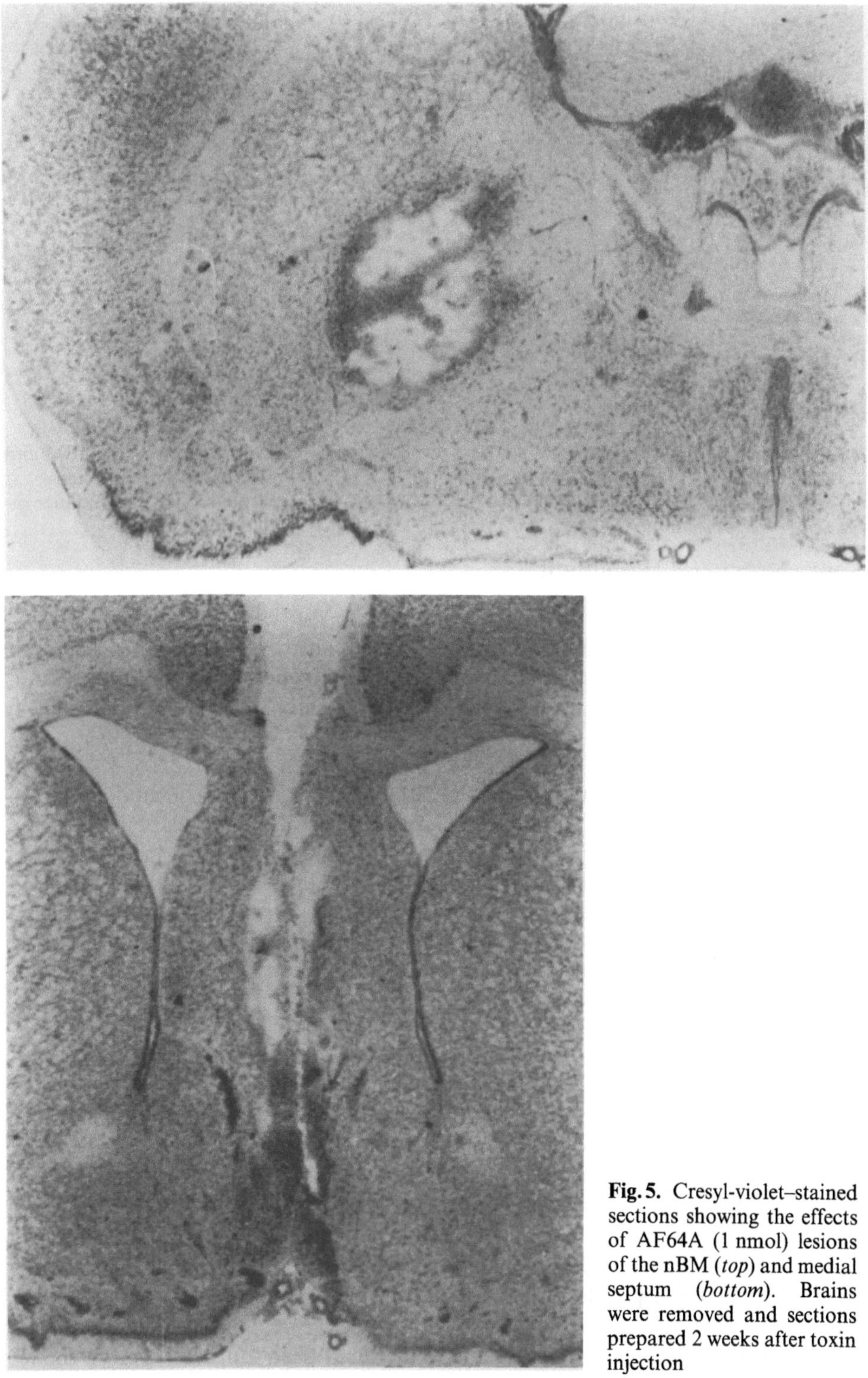

Fig. 5. Cresyl-violet–stained sections showing the effects of AF64A (1 nmol) lesions of the nBM (*top*) and medial septum (*bottom*). Brains were removed and sections prepared 2 weeks after toxin injection

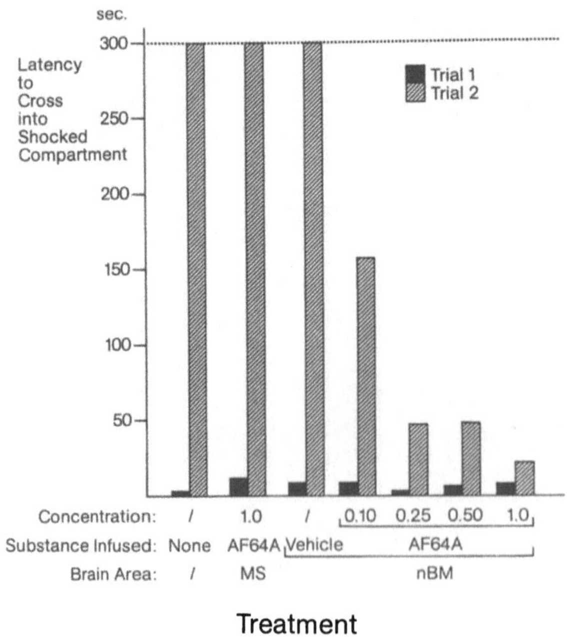

Fig. 6. Effects of AF64A-induced lesions of the nBM and medial septum on a step-through passive avoidance of foot shock task

become habituated to the environment as did controls (Gispen and Isaacson 1981); exploratory behaviors remained dominant throughout the 50-min session in the lesioned rats. In addition, there was no evidence of motor impairment in the lesioned rats.

Passive Avoidance. Bilateral injections of 1.0 nmol AF64A into the medial septum did not disrupt the passive avoidance behavior, whereas injections of 0.1 (nonsignificant), 0.25 ($t(18)=2.7$, $P<0.02$), 0.5 ($t(15)=2.8$, $P<0.02$), and 1.0 nmol ($t(18)=4.3$, $P<0.001$) into the nBM dose-dependently reduced the time required for lesioned rats to enter a compartment that they had previously been shocked in (see Fig. 6). Since the entrance latencies of the nBM-lesioned rats on the first trial were not different from those of control rats, there was again no evidence of motor dysfunction.

Active Avoidance. No deficit was observed in medial septal-lesioned rats of acquisition speed of active avoidance behavior (see Table 2). However, rats with nBM lesions were significantly slower than vehicle-injected control rats to learn the avoidance task (third session performance difference: $t(17)=3.0$, $P<0.01$). Even after 7 days of training, usually resulting in 90%–100% active avoidance responses in normal rats, nBM-lesioned rats had still not acquired the behavior. A separate group of rats were trained to stability on active avoidance and then received either vehicle or AF64A injections in the medial septum or nBM. After treatment, medial septal-lesioned rats performed as well as controls (Table 3). Rats with nBM lesions performed fewer avoidance responses, but greatly increased their intertrial crossing activity, which had been quite low before the le-

Table 2. Effects of vehicle or AF64A brain infusions on acquisition of active avoidance behavior in rats, as measured by percentage active avoidance responses

Session	Infusion site			
	Medial septum		nBM	
	vehicle	AF64A	vehicle	AF64A
1	27	33	41	43
2	50	60	59	38
3	60	71	82	41
.	.	.	.	.
.	.	.	.	.
.	.	.	.	.
7	n.t.	n.t.	n.t.	47

n.t., not tested

Table 3. Effects of vehicle or AF64A brain infusions on retention of previously acquired active avoidance behavior in rats, as measured by percentage active avoidance responses

Session	Infusion site			
	Medial septum		nBM	
	vehicle	AF64A	vehicle	AF64A
Preinfusion	97	97	81	85
Postinfusion[a]	90	95	83	67[b]

[a] First session, 2 weeks after operation
[b] Accompanied by a large increase in intertrial activity (from 1.4 to 23 mean counts)

sion. It is therefore likely that a portion of the 67% avoidance responses in the nBM-lesioned rats were due to chance, therefore increasing the likelihood that the nBM lesion was responsible for a retention deficit in this task.

Water Maze. Rats with nBM lesions were significantly worse than vehicle-injected control rats (session 4: $U(10)=16$, $P<0.01$; session 5: $U(10)=18$, $P<0.01$; session 6: $U(10)=19$, $P<0.01$; session 11: $U(10)=6$, $P<0.001$) in learning to navigate water maze type 1 (see Table 4), continuing to make many more turning errors than control rats even after 11 days of training. Rats with medial septal lesions acquired the initial configuration of water maze type 2 more slowly than control rats (session 2: $t(18)=2.2$, $P<0.05$, session 3: $t(18)=3.2$, $P<0.01$) and made significantly more turning errors than control animals when the configuration was reversed ($t(18)=3.7$, $P<0.01$; see Table 5). Typically, the number of errors made by control rats on the reversal session of this procedure is proportional

Table 4. Effects of vehicle and AF64A infusions into the nBM of rats on turning errors during initial acquisition in a water maze

Session[a]	Infusion condition	
	vehicle	AF64A
1	18	20
2	18	18
3	14	16
4	6	17
5	3	13
6	1	8
.	.	.
.	.	.
.	.	.
11	0	13

[a] One trial per session

Table 5. Effects of vehicle and AF64A medial septal infusions in rats on number of turning errors in initial and reversal learning conditions in a water maze

Session[a]	Infusion condition	
	vehicle	AF64A
Initial # 1	3.7	6.8
Initial # 2	1.8	4.4
Initial # 3	0.8	3.5
Reversal	5.4	12

[a] Five trials per session

to their accuracy on the initial maze configuration. Thus, the increased number of errors that the medial septal-lesioned rats made relative to controls was not due to the poorer level of performance in the initial configuration. Rather, the data indicate that the medial septal lesion resulted in a genuine reversal learning deficit of the sort that has been often previously reported for lesions of the hippocampus (Winocur 1980; Cormier 1981) to which the medial septum projects.

The behavioral data presented here indicate that lesions of the basal forebrain area, including the nBM, result in profound performance reductions in tasks requiring learning, memory, and habituation. In general, these findings are consistent with previous reports of nBM lesions induced in different ways. Accordingly, both bilateral excitotoxin (Flicker et al. 1983; Friedman et al. 1983) and unilateral electrolytic (Lo Conte et al. 1982) lesions of the nBM in rats result in passive avoidance retention deficits, whereas the latter manipulation also leads to poorer acquisition of the shuttlebox active avoidance task.

In the present experiments, AF64A was used to produce the lesions. Contrary to previous reports using intraventricular administration (Mantione et al. 1981; Fisher et al. 1982; Walsh et al. 1984) and striatal injection (Sandberg et al. 1984 a, 1984 b), no evidence was found for the claim of selective cholinotoxicity of this compound in doses as low as 0.1–1.0 nmol. Jarrard et al. (1984) and Levy et al. (1984) have also reported a lack of specificity of this compound when given either intraventricularly or locally. In the present report, we therefore claim only that the behavioral results described above pertain to lesions including, but not specifically limited to, the magnocellular cholinergic neurons of the nBM and the medial septum.

Conclusion

The results of autoradiographic studies with ^{3}H-PZ and ^{3}H-OXO provide strong evidence for an anatomical separation in the distribution of muscarinic cholinergic M1 and M2 receptors in the rat brain. Regions in which this differentiation was observed to be particularly marked are the olfactory bulbs, cerebral and cingulate cortices, hippocampal formation, thalamus, superior colliculus, and brainstem. The cerebral cortical distribution of M2 receptors was found to have interesting similarities to the cortical projection pattern of the nBM, as revealed by anterograde transport of lectin. The behavioral effects of lesions of the nBM were compared with those of another forebrain cholinergic nucleus, the medial septum. Lesions of both structures produced behavioral disruptions: medial septal lesions resulted primarily in reversal learning deficits, while nBM lesions produced more general and profound disturbances of performance requiring habituation, learning, and memory.

Autoradiography with specific pharmacologic agents and novel tracing methods such as the PHA-L technique increasingly allow histochemical neuroanatomy and functional neuropharmacology to be combined. As our ability to localize and manipulate receptor function grows, so will be opportunity to intervene specifically, efficaciously, and therapeutically in the depredations wrought by aging and disease in humans. The invention of empirically valid physiologic and behavioral model systems in animals of such human pathologies is a vital step in the process of developing novel therapeutic approaches.

References

Ader R, Weinen JAWM, Moleman P (1972) Retention of a passive avoidance response as a function of the intensity and duration of electric shock. Psychon Sci 26:125–128

Bartus RT, Johnson HR (1976) Short-term memory in the rhesus monkey: Disruption from the anti-cholinergic scopolamine. Pharmacol Biochem Behav 5:39–46

Bauer RH (1982) Age-dependent effects of scopolamine on avoidance, locomotor activity, and rearing. Behav Brain Res 5:261–279

Bevan P (1984) (^{3}H)oxotremorine-M binding to membranes prepared from rat brain and heart: evidence for subtypes of muscarinic receptors. Eur J Pharmacol 101:101–110

Bigl V, Woolf NJ, Butcher LL (1982) Cholinergic projections from the basal forebrain to frontal, parietal, temporal, occipital, and cingulate cortices: a combined fluorescent tracer and acetylcholinesterase analysis. Brain Res Bull 8:727–749

Birdsall NJM, Hulme EC (1983) Muscarinic receptor subclasses. Trends Pharmacol Sci 459–463

Birdsall NJM, Hulme EC, Burgen ASV (1980) The character of the muscarinic receptors in different regions of the rat brain. Proc R Soc Lond [Biol] 207:1–12

Blozovski D (1979) PA-Learning in young rats with dorsal hippocampal- and hippocampo-entorhinal atropine. Pharmacol Biochem Behav 10:369–372

Carlton PL (1983) Cholinergic mechanisms in the control of behavior by the brain. Psychol Rev 70:19–39

Cormier SM (1981) A match-mismatch theory of limbic system function. Physiol Psychol 9:3–36

Crow TJ, Grove-White IG (1973) An analysis of the learning deficit following hyoscine administration to man. Br J Pharmacol 49:322–327

Douglas RJ (1967) The hippocampus and behavior. Psychol Bull 67:416–442

Drachman DA (1978) Central cholinergic system and memory. In: Lipton MA, DiMascio A, Killam KF (eds) Psychopharmacology: a generation of progress. Raven, New York, pp 651–662

Fisher A, Mantione CR, Abraham DJ, Hanin I (1982) Long-term central cholinergic hypofunction induced in mice by ethylcholine aziridinium ion (AF64A) in vivo. J Pharmacol Exp Ther 222:140–145

Flicker C, Dean RL, Watkins DL, Fisher SK, Bartus RT (1983) Behavioral and neurochemical effects following neurotoxic lesions of a major cholinergic input to the cerebral cortex in the rat. Pharmacol Biochem Behav 18:973–981

Friedman E, Lerer B, Kuster J (1983) Loss of cholinergic neurons in the rat neocortex produces deficits in passive avoidance learning. Pharmacol Biochem Behav 19:309–312

Gilbert R, Rattan S, Goyal RK (1984) Pharmacologic identification, activation and antagonism of two muscarine receptor subtypes in the lower esophageal sphincter. J Pharmacol Exp Ther 230:284–291

Gispen WH, Isaacson RL (1981) ACTH-induced excessive grooming in the rat. Pharmacol Ther 12:209

Goyal RK, Rattan S (1978) Neurohumoral, hormonal and drug receptors for the lower esophageal sphincter. Gastroenterology 74:598–619

Hammer R, Giachetti A (1982) Muscarinic receptor subtypes: M1 and M2 biochemical and functional characterization. Life Sci 31:2991–2998

Hammer R, Berrie CP, Birdsall NJM, Burgen ASV, Hulme EC (1980) Pirenzepine distinguishes between different subclasses of muscarinic receptors. Nature 283:90–92

Harden TK, Meeker RB, Martin MW (1983) Interaction of a radiolabelled agonist with cardiac muscarinic cholinergic receptors. J Pharmacol Exp Ther 227:570–577

Hearst E (1959) Effects of scopolamine on discriminated responding in the rat. J Pharmacol Exp Ther 126:349–358

Heise GA, Conner R, Martin RA (1976) Effects of scopolamine on variable intertrial interval spatial alternation and memory in the rat. Psychopharmacology (Berlin) 49:131–137

Hrbek J, Komenda S, Siroka A, Macakova J (1971) On the interaction of scopolamine and physostigmine in man. Act Nerv Super 13:200–201

Hulme EC, Berrie CP, Birdsall NJM, Jameson M, Stockton JM (1983) Regulation of muscarinic agonist binding by cations and guanine nucleotides. Eur J Pharmacol 94:59–72

Jarrard LE (1975) Role of interference in retention by rats with hippocampal lesions. J Comp Physiol Psychol 89:400–408

Jarrard LE (1976) Anatomical and behavioral analysis of hippocampal cell fields in rats. J Comp Physiol Psychol 90:1035–1050

Jarrard LE, Kant GJ, Meyerhoff JL, Levy A (1984) Behavioral and neurochemical effects of intraventricular AF64A administration in rats. Pharmacol Biochem Behav 21:273–280

Johnson CT, Olton DS, Gage FH III, Jenko PG (1977) Damage to hippocampus and hippocampal connections: Effects on DRL and spontaneous alternation. J Comp Physiol Psychol 91:508–522

Leaton RN, Rech RH (1972) Locomotor activity increases produced by intrahippocampal and intraseptal atropine in rats. Physiol Behav 8:539–541

Lehmann J, Nagy JI, Atmadja S, Fibiger HC (1980) The nucleus basalis magnocellularis: the origin of a cholinergic projection to the neocortex of the rat. Neuroscience 5:1161–1174

Leith NJ, Barrett RJ (1975) Effects of hippocampal microinjections of *d*-amphetamine and scopolamine on active avoidance behavior in rats. J Comp Physiol Psychol 88:285–299

Levy A, Kant GJ, Meyerhoff JL, Jarrard LE (1984) Non-cholinergic neurotoxic effects of AF64A in the substantia nigra. Brain Res 305:169–172

Lo Conte G, Bartolini L, Casamenti F, Marconcini-Pepeu I, Pepeu G (1982) Lesions of cholinergic forebrain nuclei: changes in avoidance behavior and scopolamine actions. Pharmacol Biochem Behav 17:933–937

Luthin GR, Wolfe BB (1984) Comparison of (^{3}H)pirenzepine and (^{3}H)quinuclidinylbenzilate binding to muscarinic cholinergic receptors in rat brain. J Pharmacol Exp Ther 228:648–655

Mantione CR, Fisher A, Hanin I (1981) The AF64A-treated mouse: Possible model for central cholinergic hypofunction. Science 213:579–580

Martin MW, Smith MM, Harden TK (1984) Modulation of muscarinic cholinergic receptor affinity for antagonists in the rat heart. J Pharmacol Exp Ther 230:424–430

McKinney M, Coyle JT, Hedreen JC (1983) Topographic analysis of the innervation of the rat neocortex and hippocampus by the basal forebrain cholinergic system. J Comp Neurol 217:103–121

Mewaldt SP, Ghoneim MM (1979) The effects and interactions of scopolamine, physostigmine and methamphetamine on human memory. Pharmacol. Biochem Behav 10:205–210

Milar KS (1981) Cholinergic drug effects on visual discriminations: a signal detection analysis. Psychopharmacology (Berlin) 74:383–388

Milner TA, Loy R, Amaral DG (1983) An anatomical study of the development of the septo-hippocampal projection in the rat. Dev Brain Res 8:343–371

Moore JW, Goodell NA, Solomon PR (1976) Central cholinergic blockade by scopolamine and habituation, classical conditioning, and latent inhibition of the rabbit nictitating membrane response. Physiol Psychol 4:395–399

Myhrer T (1975) Locomotor, avoidance, and maze behavior in rats with selective disruption of hippocampal output. J Comp Physiol Psychol 89:759–777

Ostfeld AM, Aruguete A (1962) Central nervous system effects of hyoscine in man. J Pharmacol Exp Ther 137:133–139

Paxinos G, Watson C (1982) The rat brain in stereotaxic coordinates. Academic, New York

Potter LT, Flynn DD, Hanchett HE, Kalinoski DL, Luber-Narod J, Mash DC (1983) Independent M1 and M2 receptors: ligands, autoradiography and functions. Trends Pharmacol Sci [Special Issue] 22–31

Ross JF, Grossman SP (1974) Intrahippocampal application of cholinergic agents and blockers: effects on rats in differential reinforcement of low rates and Sidman avoidance paradigms. J Comp Physiol Psychol 86:590–600

Ross JF, McDermott LJ, Grossman SP (1975) Disinhibitory effects of intrahippocampal or intrahypothalamic injections of anticholinergic compounds in the rat. Pharmacol Biochem Behav 3:631–639

Sandberg K, Hanin I, Fisher A, Coyle JT (1984a) Selective cholinergic neurotoxin: AF64A's effects in rat striatum. Brain Res 293:49–55

Sandberg K, Sanberg PR, Coyle JT (1984b) Effects of intrastriatal injections of the cholinergic neurotoxin AF64A on spontaneous nocturnal locomotor behavior in the rat. Brain Res 299:339–343

Sinnamon HM, Freniere S, Kootz J (1978) Rat hippocampus and memory for places of changing significance. J Comp Physiol Psychol 92:142–155

Solomon PR, Gottfried KE (1981) The septohippocampal cholinergic system and classical conditioning of the rabbit's nictitating membrane response. J Comp Physiol Psychol 95:322–330

Spencer DG Jr, Lal H (1983) Effects of anticholinergic drugs on learning and memory. Drug Dev Res 3:489–502

Spencer DG Jr, Pontecorvo MJ, Heise GA (in press) Central cholinergic involvement in learning and memory: effects of scopolamine on continuous non-matching and discrimination performance in the rat. Behav Neurosci

Ter Horst GJ, Groenewegen HJ, Karst H, Luiten PGM (1984) Phaseolus vulgaris leuco-agglutinin immunohistochemistry: A comparison between autoradiographic and lectin tracing of neuronal efferents. Brain Res 307:379–383

Traber J, Klein HR, Gispen WH (1982) Actions of antidepressant and neuroleptic drugs on ACTH- and novelty-induced behavior in the rat. Eur J Pharmacol 80:407–414

Waelbroek M, Robberecht P, Chatelain P, Christophe J (1982) Rat cardiac muscarinic receptors. I. Effects of guanine nucleotides on high- and low-affinity binding sites. Mol Pharmacol 21:581–588

Wahle P, Sanides-Buchholtz C, Eckenstein F, Albus K (1984) Concurrent visualization of choline acetyltransferase-like immunoreactivity and retrograde transport of neocortically injected markers in basal forebrain neurons of cat and rat. Neurosci Lett 44:223–228

Walker DW, Messer LG, Freund G, Means LW (1972) Effect of hippocampal lesions and intertrial interval on single alternation peformance in the rat. J Comp Physiol Psychol 80:469–477

Walsh TJ, Tilson HA, DeHaven DL, Mailman RB, Fisher A, Hanin I (1984) AF64A, a cholinergic neurotoxin, selectively depletes acetylcholine in hippocampus and cortex, and produces long-term passive avoidance and radial arm maze deficits in the rat. Brain Res 321:91–102

Wamsley JK, Zarbin MA, Birdsall NJM, Kuhar MJ (1980) Muscarinic cholinergic receptors: autoradiographic localization of high and low affinity agonist binding sites. Brain Res 200:1–12

Wamsley JK, Gehlert DR, Roeske WR, Yamamura HI (1984) Muscarinic antagonist binding site heterogeneity as evidenced by autoradiography after direct labelling with (^{3}H)-QNB and (^{3}H)-pirenzepine. Life Sci 34:1395–1402

Warburton DM, Heise GA (1972) Effects of scopolamine on spatial double alternation in rats. J Comp Physiol Psychol 81:523–532

Watson M, Roeske WR, Yamamura HI (1982) (^{3}H)pirenzepine selectively identifies a high affinity population of muscarinic cholinergic receptors in the rat cerebral cortex. Life Sci 31:2019–2023

Watson M, Yamamura HI, Roeske WR (1983) A unique regulatory profile and regional distribution of (^{3}H)pirenzepine binding in the rat provides evidence for distinct M1 and M2 muscarinic receptor subtypes. Life Sci 32:3001–3011

Wesnes K, Warburton DM (1984) Effects of scopolamine and nicotine on human rapid information processing performance. Psychopharmacology (Berlin) 82:147–150

Winocur G (1980) The hippocampus and cue utilization. Physiol Psychol 8:280–288

Woolf NJ, Eckenstein F, Butcher LL (1983) Cholinergic projections from the basal forebrain to the frontal cortex: a combined fluorescent tracer and immunohistochemical analysis in the rat. Neurosci Lett 40:93–98

Yamamura HI, Wamsley JK, Deshmukh P, Roeske WR (1983) Differential light microscopic autoradiographic localization of muscarinic cholinergic receptors in the brainstem and spinal cord of the rat using (^{3}H)pirenzepine. Eur J Pharmacol 91:147–149

Immunologic Factors Related to Cognitive/Behavioral Dysfunctions in Aging*

H. LAL [1], M.J. FORSTER[1], and K. NANDY[2]

Introduction

The loss of synapses (Bondareff 1976, 1980), the disappearance of neurotransmitter binding sites (Finch 1982; Lal and Carroll 1979; Severson and Finch 1980), and the mortality of neurons themselves (Colon 1973; Vogel 1969; Johnson and Erner 1972) are conspicuous changes observed in the normally aging mammalian CNS, and they have long been recognized as possible immediate causes for senescence-related declines in the capacity for adaptive behavior of both humans and animals (Landfield 1983; Rapport and Karpiak 1978). Continued research will no doubt further clarify the nature of degenerative changes in the normally aging brain, their contributions to normal senescence-related behavioral changes, and their relevance to senescence-related neuropsychopathology in humans.

The etiologic mechanisms involved in CNS degenerative changes remain highly speculative, although identification of those mechanisms will be necessary for a complete understanding of senescence-related cognitive disorders and may well be critical to their effective prevention or therapy. In general, any senescence-linked pathologic process contributing to functional degeneration is of significance. In this review, we wish to propose that autoimmune reactions within the CNS may be responsible for such alterations, as has been pointed out earlier (Chaffee et al. 1978; Nandy 1977, 1978, 1981 c). If immune reactions affect those CNS constituents critical to complex behavioral processes, a relationship between immunologic factors and behavioral degeneration should be apparent. The purpose of this monograph is to review available evidence implicating immunologic factors in the etiology of senescence-related cognitive deterioration and to describe our recent attempts to identify correlational or empirical links between immunologic factors and senescence-related behavioral changes using inbred mouse models.

Immunologic Mechanisms as an Etiologic Factor in the Neuropsychopathology of Aging

A recently formulated hypothesis is that immunologic factors may be involved in the pathogenesis of senile dementia (Nandy 1981 c). It has been suggested that

* This research was supported by research funds of the Veterans Administration, US Public Health Service Grant NS-129624, and National Institute of Aging Grant 1 RO 3 AGO3623

1 Department of Pharmacology, Texas College of Osteopathic Medicine, Fort Worth, TX 76107, USA

2 Veterans Administration Hospital, Bedford, MA 01730 and Department of Anatomy, Boston University School of Medicine, Boston MA 02118, USA

Senile Dementia of the Alzheimer Type
Ed. by J. Traber and W.H. Gispen

amyloid fibrils associated with senile plaques of dementia patients are immunoglobulin derivatives (Glenner 1978), based upon immunoelectron-microscopic (Ishii and Haga 1976) and other circumstantial evidence (Glenner 1978). High serum Ig levels are associated with the incidence of senile dementia and are often correlated with the degree of cognitive impairment in demented individuals (Eisdorfer et al. 1978), as are densities of senile plaques (Blessed et al. 1968). These findings have led to some speculation that an infectious viral or autoimmune mechanism is involved in the deposition of amyloid in senile brains (Ishii and Haga 1976; Ishii et al. 1983).

There is sufficient experimental precedent to warrant the proposal that senescence-related declines in the functioning of the immune system result in the formation of autoantibodies capable of interacting with CNS constituents. With aging, there is an increase in humoral autoantibodies (Delespesse et al. 1980; Hijmans et al. 1984) and a heterochronic deterioration of certain immune functions (Makinodan 1976; Weksler 1983). Moreover, there is an age-related increase in the tendency of human serum to bind against neural tissues (Ingram et al. 1974; Nandy 1978, 1981 c). The neuron-binding properties of sera taken from aged persons are thought to reflect the presence of specific and/or cross-reactive antineural antibodies which have been referred to collectively as brain-reactive antibodies (BRA). Ingram et al. (1974) compared frequencies of individuals showing significant in vitro binding of their sera to human brain tissue within age groups of psychiatrically and neurologically normal hospital patients. They reported BRA (i.e., significant binding) in 74% of individuals aged 55–80 years, as compared with 12% of individuals aged 20–39 years.

There would also appear to be a correlation between the incidence of dementia and abnormally high serum BRA levels among aged individuals. Nandy (1978) reported an overall increase in serum BRA with age, but also noted that patients with the clinical diagnosis of Alzheimer's disease or senile dementia had higher serum BRA levels than aged-matched, healthy individuals (Table 1).

BRA also occur with increasing frequency in sera of aging mice (Nandy 1972 a; Threatt et al. 1971; Blumenthal et al. 1984), rats (Feden et al. 1979; Miller and Blumenthal 1978), and nonhuman primates (Nandy 1981 a) (Table 2). Furthermore, a declining capacity for adaptive behavior as a function of aging in

Table 1. BRA of senile dementia patients[a] and age-matched controls[b]

Age group (years)	Controls		Senile dementia	
	(*n*)	Serum-reactive cells (%)	(*n*)	Serum-reactive cells (%)
40–50	7	12±7.0	4	33±4.5
51–60	10	24±6.2	5	44±6.7
61–70	10	33±7.2	10	52±7.2
71–80	9	44±8.4	6	60±6.8
81–90	6	52±8.0	4	70±7.9

[a] Including Alzheimer-type dementia
[b] Based upon Nandy (1978)

Table 2. BRA in sera of nonhuman primates (Nandy, 1981a)

Donor age (year)	Brain cells reacting to sera (mean ± S.E.) (%)	*P*
4	37.3 ± 1	–
10	55.5 ± 9	0.05
20	80.4 ± 12	0.01

these mammalian species has been documented (Bartus et al. 1980; Campbell et al. 1980; Dean et al. 1981).

The presence of humoral BRA in both humans and animals in conjunction with senescence-related behavioral dysfunctions provides some circumstantial support for an autoimmune hypothesis of senescence-related CNS degeneration. However, the plausibility of such a hypothesis also depends on the validity of two important assumptions. First, some senescence-related mechanism must permit deposition of BRA in sufficient concentrations into CNS tissue, and second, BRA must have the potential for producing functional neurologic impairment in those CNS components involved with cognitive functions.

Potential of Humoral BRA for Impairing CNS Function

Numerous findings attest to the ability of antineural antibodies to produce neuropathologic changes and behavioral effects (including memory impairment) when introduced into the CNS of animals (Kobiler et al. 1976; MacPherson and Chinerman 1971; Rapport and Karpiak 1978; Simon and Simon 1975), and studies of humoral BRA suggest that these antibodies may have the potential for similar effects. Humoral BRA from aging C57BL/6 mice are cytotoxic (with complement) in vitro (Nandy et al. 1983). Furthermore, evidence of morphological damage to the CNS tissue of C57 mice is found following intracerebral injection of serum from aged mice into young mice and following damage (cold probe) to the blood-brain barrier (BBB) of aged mice. It was found that, following either of these procedures, 25% of cells showing antigen-antibody reactions by immunofluorescence also had severe morphological damage (Nandy 1972b). In addition to the potential of BRA for direct cytolytic actions, it has been suggested (Nandy 1978) that binding of BRA to CNS tissue would attract miroglia, resulting in eventual damage to cells.

Accessibility of Humoral BRA to CNS Tissue

A number of recent studies have provided evidence of BRA within CNS tissues of aged rats (Feden et al. 1979) and aged C57BL/6 mice (Blumenthal et al. 1984; Finger et al. 1984). These findings suggest that BRA may have access to CNS tissue as a result of some age-related weakening of blood-CNS permeability barriers. Another theory is that BRA are perhaps produced within the brain itself

(Blumenthal 1976). A number of mechanisms might permit penetration of serum BRA into CNS tissue. Senescence-related pathologic conditions such as atherosclerosis or chronic hypertension have the ability to increase the permeability of neural tissue to circulating autoantibodies, as do numerous transient pathologic conditions (Rappoport 1977). In fact, structures which contribute to the BBB have been shown to undergo senescence-related alterations (Burns et al. 1981; Scott and Sladek 1981), and increased vascular permeability has been reported in some senile dementia patients (Wisniewski and Koslowski 1982). However, a number of attempts to demonstrate a weakening of the BBB in normally aging mice and rats have thus far failed to provide positive findings (Buell and Rudick 1983; Feden et al. 1979). On the other hand, recent evidence has indicated that levels of circulating immune complex can affect permeability of the blood-CSF barrier, but not of the BBB proper (Hoffman et al. 1983). Circulating immune complexes have been shown to increase with aging in normal humans (Delespesse et al. 1980) and may constitute one mechanism contributing to senescence-related weakening of the blood-CSF barrier.

Links Between BRA and Senescence-Related Behavioral Dysfunction in Aging C57BL/6 Mice

The study of causative mechanisms in senile dementia has been difficult because of the apparent lack of short-lived, animal model systems exhibiting senescence-related neurologic or behavioral degeneration similar in magnitude or nature to that of senile dementia (Finch 1982; Ritger 1983; Sprott 1980). Nevertheless, CNS alterations (Lal and Carroll 1979; Lal et al. 1973) and declines in adaptive behavioral capacities (Campbell et al. 1980; Dean et al. 1981) occur with age in short-lived rodent species, and studies involving these species could uncover causative mechanisms applicable to both mild and severe forms of senescence-related cognitive dysfunction.

To evaluate the rodent as an autoimmune model system, we have conducted a number of studies exploring the links between senescence-related behavioral deterioration and the presence of BRA in sera of inbred mouse strains. The C57BL/6 mouse strain was chosen because it had been shown to exhibit declines in numerous behavioral functions (including learning and memory) (Dean et al. 1981; Freund and Walker 1971) as well as increases in BRA with aging (Nandy 1972a).

Correlation of Impaired Avoidance Learning and Serum BRA in Aging C57BL/6 Mice

The findings of a recent study suggest a systematic, inverse relation between age-related changes in BRA levels and performance of a learning task in C57BL/6 mice (Nandy et al. 1983). In this study, separate groups of C57 mice aged 2–5, 10–12, 18–20, or 24–25 months were tested for their ability to acquire a one-way

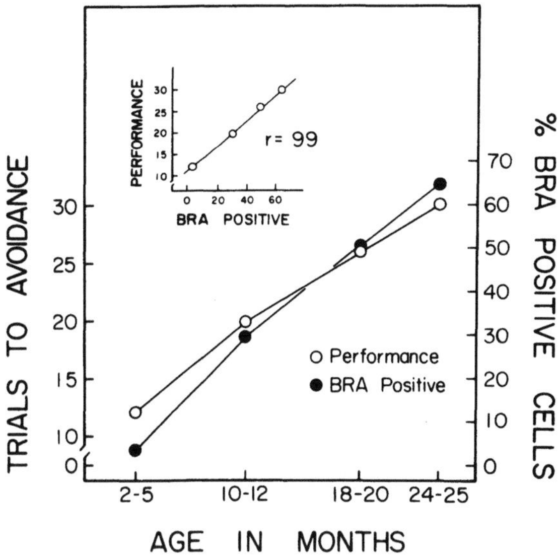

Fig. 1. Mean number of trials to fulfill avoidance response criterion and percentage of BRA-positive cells as a function of age group for C57BL/6 mice. The *inset* shows mean number of trials to fulfillment of criterion as a simple function of BRA-positive cells. (Extrapolated from Nandy et al. 1983)

active avoidance response. After testing, their sera were assayed for BRA. The behavioral testing procedure consisted of active avoidance training to elicit an avoidance response by the animal in 8 of 10 trials. In a given trial, each mouse was able to avoid foot shock by reaching a safe platform at one end of the apparatus within a 10-s period of tone presentation preceding the onset of foot shock. An avoidance response was recorded if the mouse reached the platform with a latency of less than 10 s from tone onset and if shock did not occur. If the mouse failed to reach the platform within the 10-s period, shock and tone continued until the safe platform had been reached (an escape trial). Serum BRA determinations were made by an indirect immunofluorescence procedure (Nandy et al. 1983), with BRA levels estimated by counting serum-reactive cells in sections of mouse cerebral cortex.

The relation between age, BRA, and avoidance performance (extrapolated from Nandy et al. 1983) is depicted in Fig. 1. As shown, the number of trials required to fulfill the avoidance criterion increased as a function of age group, as did BRA level, suggesting an inverse relation between avoidance performance and age-related changes in BRA. When chronological age was not considered as a variable (see inset Fig. 1), there was a surprisingly strong linear relationship ($r = 0.99$) between BRA levels and the number of trials required to fulfill the avoidance response criterion.

Behavioral Effects of Experimental Immune Manipulations

The high correlation of BRA and learning dysfunction in C57 mice prompted a study designed to test the effects of immune factors from aged C57BL/6 mice introduced into the sera of young mice on BRA levels and learning ability. In this study, bone marrow cell and spleen cell suspensions were transferred from aged

Table 3. Effects of bone marrow and spleen cell transfers on recipient mice (Nandy et al. 1984)

Age group		Mean ± S.E.	
Donor	Recipient	BRA serum levels (%)	Trials to learn avoidance response (*n*)
none	young	0	17±1
young	young	0	15±1
old	young	64±2	28±3
none	old	67±2	27±3
young	old	59±3	27±2
old	old	87±3	28±4

mice (20–21 months) to young mice (3–4 months) which had been irradiated to inactivate their immune system prior to transfer. The transfers were mady by injecting 1:1 bone marrow and spleen cell suspensions into the tail vein of the recipient mice, as described previously (Nandy and Bennett 1983). Three months following the transfer, these recipient mice were tested for their ability to acquire the active avoidance response and were assayed for BRA, as were aged recipients of young cells, untreated control groups, and control groups receiving age-matched transfers. We expected that the ability of young mice to acquire the avoidance response would vary with changes in BRA levels brought about by the immune manipulation, based on the high correlation between these variables in the previous study.

In accordance with this prediction, young recipients of cell suspensions from old mice showed substantially higher serum BRA and slower avoidance response acquisition when compared with young or age-matched transfer groups or untreated control groups (Table 3). Moreover, young recipients of old transfers were nearly identical in performance and BRA levels to the old recipient groups, all of which showed higher BRA and slower acquisition than the young control groups.

Because the immune manipulation resulting in BRA formation in young mice also resulted in behavioral deterioration, the findings provide empirical support for the possible role of immune factors in behavioral deterioration related to senescence in mice. Although it is not certain that BRA was directly involved in

Table 4. Neuropsychiatric manifestations in systemic lupus erythematosus (SLE) (Carr et al. 1978)

	Patients affected with symptoms (%)
Disorders of mental function	12–60
Seizures	7–57
Cranial nerve disorders	5–42
Pareses	5–25
Peripheral neuropathy	3–18
Movement disorders	2– 5

the avoidance deficits, the effect obtained was clearly some consequence of the aged-young immune manipulation. There was no detectable effect of the procedures per se (i.e., irradiation, transfer of cells), as evidenced by the absence of behavioral effects following the age-matched transfer.

Relations Between Behavioral Dysfunction and BRA in New Zealand Black (NZB) Mice

We initiated our studies of NZB mice for two reasons. First, we wished to test further the relationship between BRA and behavioral dysfunction in aging by comparing differences in behavior throughout the life spans of different mouse strains which exhibit heterochronic changes in BRA levels. Second, it was thought that NZB mice could perhaps be a convenient model system for future studies of immune mechanisms in aging by virtue of the relatively early appearance of BRA in sera of these mice (Nandy et al. 1983).

BRA are found in association with a variety of psychoneuropathologic conditions (Baldinger and Blumenthal 1982), including systemic lupus erythematosus (SLE) (Bluestein and Woods 1982). It has been estimated that 60% of SLE patients suffer some mental dysfunction (Table 4), and the presence of BRA has been proposed as an etiologic factor in the CNS manifestations of this disease (Bluestein and Woods 1982). The onset of autoantibody formation in existing mouse models of SLE is known to occur in periadolescence (Quimby and Schwartz 1982), and BRA have been demonstrated with high frequency during adulthood in the model strains investigated (Hoffman et al. 1978; Nandy et al. 1983). The New Zealand Black (NZB) mouse, a strain which is genetically prone to autoimmune disorder (Howie and Helyer 1968), has a shorter life span than the C57Bl/6 mouse and also exhibits precocious development of humoral BRA levels when compared with the C57BL/6 strain (Fig. 2).

In a recent study (Harris et al. 1984), we compared the developmental time course of active avoidance response acquisition in NZB and C57BL/6 mice in

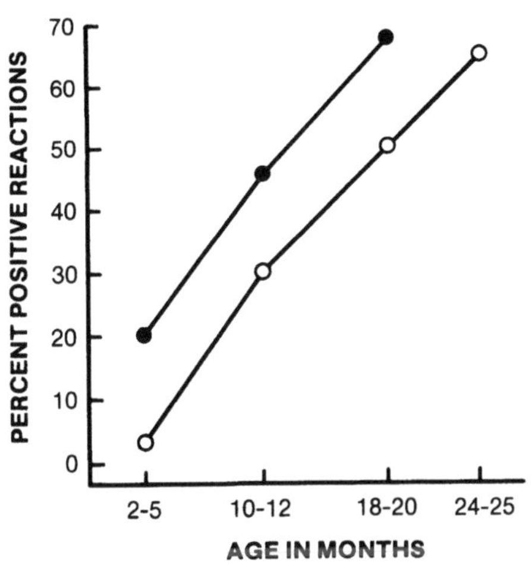

Fig. 2. Mean percentage of BRA-positive cells as a function of age group for C57BL/6 (o) and NZB (●) mice

order to determine whether the time course for each strain can be correlated with the presence of serum BRA. Based on the previous demonstration that autoimmune disorder becomes manifest between 1 and 3 months of age in the NZB strain (Quimby and Schwartz 1982) and our own findings of elevated BRA by the age of 2.5 months (Fig. 2), it was predicted that a declining ability to acquire the avoidance response would become evident within this time period. It was expected that acquisition difficulty would be detectable by 6 months of age for C57BL/6 mice, in accordance with previous findings.

Separate groups of NZB mice, aged 1.5, 2–4, 6–8, and 10–14 months, and C57BL/6 mice, aged 2–4, 6–8, or 10–14 months, were tested for active avoidance acquisition according to the procedure used in the previous study.

Each age group was also administered a retention test 48 h after the original training in order to test for age-related changes in memory abilities among the strains. The retention test consisted of five avoidance trials, and the measure of retention was the latency to reach the platform on the first trial of the retention test.

Acquisition and retention of active avoidance learning are summarized in Fig. 3 as a function of strain and age (log units). The NZB strain showed an abrupt increase in the number of trials required for avoidance acquisition which occurred between 1.5 and 2–4 months of age. A smaller, more graded increment in the number of trials to acquisition was evident for C57BL/6 mice, as indicated by comparison of C57BL/6 mice aged 2–4 months with those aged 10–14 months. The appearance and development of these avoidance acquisition deficits appear to correspond roughly to the developmental time course of BRA accumulation for each strain (Fig. 2).

It is also evident that there was an age-related decline in avoidance performance during retention tests for C57BL/6 mice, beginning sometime after 3

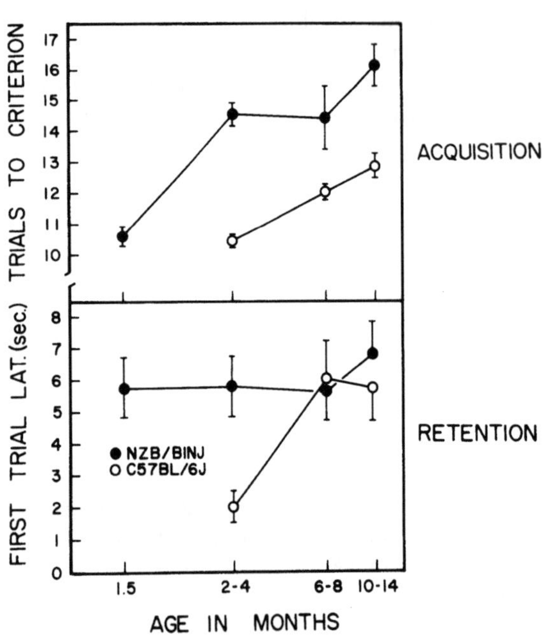

Fig. 3. Acquisition (mean number of trials to fulfillment of avoidance response criterion, *top panel*) and retention (first-trial latency in seconds, *bottom panel*) performances of NZB and C57BL/6 mice as a function of age

months of age. Retention performance of NZB mice was equivalent to that exhibited by the oldest (12- to 14-month-old) C57BL/6 mice, even at the youngest age tested (1.5 months). This finding perhaps reflects the fact that NZB mice show retention performance comparable to aged mice even when tested at early chronological ages. However, it was not possible to make such a judgement based on our comparisons of the genetically unrelated strains in the absence of any significant age-related change in retention performance of the NZB strain. Therefore, it was tentatively concluded that only the retention performance of C57BL/6 mice was clearly related to age and changes in BRA levels (Fig. 2). However, it should be pointed out that an improvement in retention between 1 and 3 months of age can be expected as a normal consequence of maturational processes continuing into periadolescence (Campbell and Spear 1972; Nagy et al. 1977). Because significant changes in serum BRA levels of NZB mice also occur within the same time span, firm conclusions regarding the relation of changes in BRA levels to retention capacities in the NZB strain would require additional age groups and behavioral analysis.

Status of NZB and C57BL/6 Mice as Model Systems of Aging

Overall, our observations support the hypothesis that immunologic factors constitute a pathologic mechanism contributing to the decline of adaptive behavioral capabilities with normal aging. Our findings may indicate that BRA is related to cognitive deterioration with aging, although, based only on our preliminary studies of avoidance learning, this interpretation would be premature. A variety of CNS-dependent processes (e.g., sensory, motor, cognitive) are thought to contribute to avoidance performance, and our data may reflect age-related deterioration of functions not directly involved in cognitive abilities per se. However, the differences in the performances of NZB and C57BL/6 mice at various ages do not appear to be trivial consequences of strain, age differences in sensorimotor abilities, or shock aversiveness, as judged by initial and asymptotic performance of the mice in our avoidance studies (Nandy et al. 1983) and in a number of control experiments (Spencer and Lal 1983).

Deterioration of the ability to acquire an active avoidance response appears to be a normal consequence of aging in C57BL/6 mice (Freund and Walker 1971) which, based on our own findings, is closely associated with increases in serum BRA levels. The NZB mouse strain displays a parallel between behavioral dysfunction and BRA levels at an earlier developmental stage.

The mechanisms contributing to the formation of BRA in young NZB and aging C57 mice are related to the extent that these strains show similar responses to a number of treatments affecting their life spans and immune functions. For example, C57 and NZB mouse strains respond to certain dietary restriction regimens with concurrent increases in life span and delays of normal age-related changes in autoantibody production (Fernandes et al. 1971, 1976; Gerbase-DeLima et al. 1975; Nandy 1981 b, 1982). Drug treatments affecting immune system activity can also produce these effects (Schwartz et al. 1984; Walker et al. 1982).

Currently available information indicates that the NZB mouse strain warrants consideration as a potential model system for behavioral dysfunctions in aging.

As such, this strain could be useful in the identification of immunologically based neurodegenerative changes, etiologic mechanisms, and therapeutic measures. The validity of the NZB strain as a model would be further enhanced if NZB mice were found to exhibit morphological or neurochemical abnormalities similar to those arising in normal aging or senile dementia. One such parallel exists, based on the recent finding (Zilles, this volume) of localized cholinergic cell deficiencies in the brains of NZB mice.

Acknowledgements. The contributions of M. Bennett, D. Bennett, K. Retz, and D. Spencer, Jr. are gratefully acknowledged.

References

Baldinger A, Blumenthal HT (1982) Neuroimmunology of the aging brain. In: Platt D (ed) Geriatrics. Springer, Berlin Heidelberg New York, pp 283–299

Bartus RT, Dean RL, Beer B (1980) Memory deficits in aged cebus monkeys and facilitation with central cholinomimetics. Neurobiol Aging 1:145–152

Blessed G, Tomlinson BE, Roth M (1968) The association between quantitative measures of dementia and of senile change in the central gray matter of elderly subjects. Br J Psychiatry 144:797–811

Bluestein HG, Woods VL (1982) Antineuronal antibodies in systemic lupus erythematosus. Arthritis Rheum 25:773–778

Blumenthal HT (1976) Immunological aspects of the aging brain. In: Terry RD, Gershon S (eds) Neurobiology of aging, vol 3. Raven, New York, pp 313–334

Blumenthal HT, Young D, Wozniak D, Finger S (1984) Effects of age, brain damage and stress on antibody binding to the brain. J Gerontol 39:552–560

Bondareff W (1976) Loss of synapses in the dentate gyrus of the senescent rat. Am J Anat 145:129–136

Bondareff W (1980) Compensatory loss of axosomatic synapses in the dentate gyrus of the senescent rat. Mech Ageing Dev 12:221–229

Buell SJ, Rudick RA (1983) Integrity of blood-brain barrier to peroxidase in senescent mice. Neurobiol Aging 4:283–287

Burns EM, Kruckeberg TW, Gaetano PK (1981) Changes with age in cerebral capillary morphology. Neurobiol Aging 2:285–291

Campbell BA, Spear NE (1972) Ontogeny of memory. Psychol Rev 79:215–236

Campbell BA, Krauter EE, Wallace JE (1980) Animal models of aging: Sensory-motor and cognitive function in the aged rat. In: Stein (ed) The psychobiology of aging: problems and perspectives. Elsevier, Amsterdam, pp 201–226

Carr RI, Shucard DW, Hoffman SA, Hoffman AW, Bardana EJ, Harbeck RJ (1978) Neuropsychiatric involvement in systemic lupus erythematosus. In: Bergsma D, Goldstein AL (eds) Neurochemical and immunologic components in schizophrenia. Liss, New York, pp 209–235

Chaffee J, Nassef M, Bobin S (1978) Cytotoxic autoantibody to the brain. In: Nandy K (ed) Senile dementia: A biomedical approach. Elsevier, Amsterdam, pp 61–72

Colon EJ (1973) The cerebral cortex in presenile dementia: a qualitative analysis. Acta Neuropathol 23:281–290

Dean RL, Scozzafava J, Goas JA, Regan B, Beer B, Bartus RT (1981) Age-related differences in behavior across the life span of the C57BL/6J mouse. Exp Aging Res 7:427–451

Delespesse G, Guasset PH, Sarfati M, Dubi-Rucquoy M, Debisschop MJ, Van Haelst L (1980) Circulating immune complexes in old people and diabetics: Correlation with autoantibodies. Clin Exp Immunol 40:96–102

Eisdorfer C, Cohen D, Buckley CE III (1978) Serum immunoglobulins and cognition in the impaired elderly. In: Katzman R, Terry R, Bick K (eds) Alzheimer's disease–Senile dementia and related disorders. Raven, New York, pp 401–407 (Aging, vol. 7)

Feden G, Baldinger A, Miller-Soule D, Blumenthal HT (1979) An in vivo and in vitro study of an aging-related neuron cytoplasmic binding antibody in male Fischer rats. J Gerontol 34:651–660
Fernandes G, Yunis EJ, Smith J, Good RA (1971) Dietary influence on breeding behavior, hemolytic anemia, and longevity in NZB mice. Proc Soc Exp Biol Med 139:1189–1196
Fernandes GE, Yunis J, Good RA (1976) Influence of protein restriction in immune functions in NZB mice. J Immunol 116:782–790
Finch CE (1982) Rodent models for aging processes in the human brain. In: Corkin S, Davis KL, Growdon JH, Usdin E, Wurtman RJ (eds) Alzheimer's disease: A report of progress in research. Raven, New York, pp 249–257 (Aging, vol 19)
Finger S, Wozniak D, Blumenthal H (1984) Longevity, disease, and autoimmune reactions following focal cortical injuries. In: Scheff SW (ed) Aging and recovery of function in the central nervous system. Plenum, New York, pp 1–21
Freund G, Walker DW (1971) The effect of aging on acquisition and retention of shuttle box avoidance in mice. Life Sci 10:1343–1349
Gerbase-DeLima N, Liu RK, Cheney KE, Mickey R, Walford R (1975) Immune function and survival in a long-lived mouse strain subjected to undernutrition. Gerontologia 21:184–202
Glenner GG (1978) Current knowledge of amyloid deposits as applied to senile plaques and congophilic angiopathy. In: Katzman R, Terry RD, Bick KL (eds) Alzheimer's disease: Senile dementia and related disorders. Raven, New York, pp 493–501 (Aging, vol 7)
Harris CM, Forster MJ, Retz KC, Frantz N, Lal H (1984) Deficient retention of appetitive and aversive learning in New Zealand Black mice. Soc Neurosci Abs 10:451
Hijmans W, Radl J, Bottazzo GF, Doniach D (1984) Autoantibodies in highly aged humans. Mech Ageing Dev 26:83–89
Hoffman SA, Hoffman AA, Shucard DW, Harbeck RJ (1978) Antibodies to dissociated cerebellar cells in New Zealand mice as demonstrated by immunofluorescence. Brain Res 142:477–486
Hoffman SA, Arbogast DN, Day TT, Shucard DW, Harbeck RJ (1983) Permeability of the blood cerebrospinal fluid barrier during acute immune complex disease. J Immunol 130:1695–1698
Howie JB, Helyer BJ (1968) The immunology and pathology of NZB mice. Adv Immunol 9:215–223
Ingram CR, Phegan KJ, Blumenthal HT (1974) Significance of an aging-linked neuron binding gamma globulin fraction of human sera. J Gerontol 29:20–27
Ishii T, Haga S (1976) Immuno-electron microscopic localization of immunoglobulin in amyloid fibrils of senile plaques. Acta Neuropathol 36:243–250
Ishii T, Haga S, Tajima M (1983) Viral antigens in senile plaques: an immunofluorescence study. In: Hirano A, Miyoshi K (eds) Neuropsychiatric disorders in the elderly. Igaku-Shoin, Tokyo, pp 32–38
Johnson HA, Erner S (1972) Neuron survival in the aging mouse. Exp Gerontol 7:111–117
Kobiler D, Fuchs S, Samuel D (1976) The effect of antisynaptosomal plasma membrane antibodies on memory. Brain Res 115:129–138
Lal H, Carroll PT (1979) Alterations in brain neurotransmitter systems related to senescence. In: Nandy K (ed) Geriatric Psychopharmacology. Elsevier, New York, pp 3–15
Lal H, Pogacar S, Daly P, Puri S (1973) Behavioral and neuropathological manifestations of nutritionally-induced central nervous system "aging" in the rat. Prog Brain Res 40:129–140
Landfield PW (1983) Mechanisms of altered neural function during aging. In: Gispen WH, Traber J (eds) Aging of the brain. Elsevier, New York, pp 51–60 (Developments in neurology, vol 7)
MacPherson CFC, Chinerman J (1971) Effect of intraventricular injections of brain isoantibodies on learning. Exp Neurol 31:45–52
Makinodan T (1976) Immunobiology of aging. J Am Geriatr Soc 24:249–252
Miller DT, Blumenthal HT (1978) Neuron-thymic lymphocyte binding by serum IgG of 90and 500 day old female Wistar albino rats. J Gerontol 33:329–336
Nagy ZM, Thaller K, Massaferri TA (1977) Acquisition and retention of a passive avoidance task as a function of age in mice. Dev Psychobiol 10:563–573
Nandy K (1972a) Brain-reactive antibodies in mouse serum as a function of age. J Gerontol 27:173–177

Nandy K (1972 b) Neuronal degeneration in aging and after experimental injury. Exp Gerontol 7:303–311

Nandy K (1975) Significance of brain-reactive antibodies in serum of aged mice. J Gerontol 30:412–416

Nandy K (1977) Immune reactions in aging brain and senile dementia. In: Nandy K, Sherwin I (eds) The aging brain and senile dementia. Plenum, New York, pp 181–196 (Advances in behavioral biology, vol 23)

Nandy K (1978) Brain-reactive antibodies in aging and senile dementia. In: Katzman R, Terry R, Bick K (eds) Alzheimer's disease–Senile dementia and related disorders. Raven, New York, pp 503–512

Nandy K (1981 a) Brain-reactive antibodies in aging non-human primates. Mech Ageing Dev 16:141–146

Nandy K (1981 b) Effects of caloric restriction on brain-reactive antibodies in sera of old mice. Age 4:117–121

Nandy K (1981 c) Senile dementia: a possible immune hypothesis. In: Mortimer JA, Shuman M (eds) Epidemiology of senile dementia. Oxford University Press, New York, pp 87–100

Nandy K (1982) Effects of controlled dietary restriction on brain-reactive antibodies in sera of aging mice. Mech Ageing Dev 18:97–102

Nandy K, Bennett M (1983) Immune manipulations and brain-reactive antibody formation in aging mice. Mech Ageing Dev 22:287–293

Nandy K, Lal H, Bennett M, Bennett D (1983) Correlation between a learning disorder and elevated brain-reactive antibodies in aged C57BL/6 and young NZB mice. Life Sci 33:1499–1503

Nandy K, Lal H, Bennett M, Bennett D (1984) Bone marrow transplant from aged to young mice produces brain reactive antibodies and concurrent acceleration of learning/memory deficits. Soc Neurosci Abs 10:721

Quimby FW, Schwartz RS (1982) Systemic lupus erythematosus in mice and dogs. In: Lachman PJ, Peters DK (eds) Clinical aspects of immunology, vol. 2. Blackwell, Oxford, pp 1217–1230

Rappoport SL (1977) Reversible modification of blood-brain barrier permeability to proteins. In: Nandy K, Sherwin J (eds) The aging brain and senile dementia. Plenum, New York, pp 197–209 (Advances in behavioral biology, vol 3)

Rapport MM, Karpiak SE (1978) Immunological perturbation of neurological functions. In: Nandy K (ed) Senile dementia: A biomedical approach. Elsevier, New York, pp 73–88

Ritger H (1983) Pitfalls in behavioral ageing research in animals. In: Gispen WH, Traber J (eds) Aging of the brain. Elsevier, New York, pp 197–208 (Developments in neurology, vol 7)

Schwartz AG, Nyce JW, Tannen RH (1984) Inhibition of tumorigenesis and autoimmune development in mice by dehydroepiandrosterone. In: Cristofalo VJ, Baker III GT, Andelman RC, Roberts J (eds) Altered endocrine status during aging. Liss, New York

Scott DE, Sladek JR Jr (1981) Age-related changes in the endocrine hypothalamus: I. Tanycytes and the blood-brain cerebrospinal fluid barrier. Neurobiol Aging 2:89–94

Severson JA, Finch CE (1980) Reduced dopaminergic binding during aging in the rodent striatum. Brain Res 192:147–162

Simon J, Simon O (1975) Effect of passive transfer of antibrain antibodies to a normal recipient. Exp Neurol 47:523

Spencer DG Jr, Lal H (1983) Specific behavioral impairments in associational tasks in mice with an autoimmune disorder. Soc Neurosci Abs 9:1146

Sprott RL (1980) An appraisal of the utility of genetic techniques for the study of neurobiology and aging in mice. In: Stein DG (ed) The psychobiology of aging: Problems and perspectives. Elsevier, New York, pp 21–33

Threatt J, Nandy K, Fritz F (1971) Brain-reactive antibodies in serum of old mice demonstrated by immunofluorescence. J Gerontol 26:316–323

Vogel FS (1969) The brain and time. In: Busse EW, Pfeiffer E (eds) Behavior and adaptation in later life. Little Brown, Boston, pp 251–262

Walker SE, Solsky M, Schnitzer B (1982) Prolonged lifespans in female NZB/NZW mice treated with the experimental immunoloreguatory drug Frentizole. Arthritis Rheum 25:1291–1297

Weksler ME (1983) Senescence of the immune system. Med Clin North Am 67:263–272

Wisniewski HH, Koslowski (1982) Evidence for blood-brain barrier changes in senile dementia of the Alzheimer type (SDAT). In: Sinex FM, Merrill CR (eds) Alzheimer's disease, Down's syndome, and aging. New York Academy of Sciences, New York, pp 119–129

Morphological Studies on Brain Structures of the NZB Mouse: An Animal Model for the Aging Human Brain?

K. ZILLES [1]

Introduction

The need for animal models that exhibit brain aging phenomena similar to those of humans is among the most urgent methodological problems confronting research on aging. Extensive work has been done by numerous authors on brains of very old animals. These studies have not only provided valuable new insights into processes of aging, but also raised some questions: Is the process of aging in experimental animals (e.g., rats) really comparable to human aging at all, and more specifically, is the normal aging of animal brains comparable to the normal aging of the human brain? Is it really useful to compare the brains of animals (e.g., rodents) and those of humans with disorders like Alzheimer's disease or other dementias?

The list of questions could be extended, and some have been discussed elsewhere. Furthermore, it is impossible at this point to propose the ideal animal model for *all* aspects of brain aging because the subject to be imitated by an animal model, the aging human brain, is far from being completely defined. However, an animal model should reflect at least a few of the phenomena also found in human brain aging.

Alzheimer's disease has of late become one of the most intensively studied phenomenon in human brain aging. Functional, morphological and biochemical bases of some aspects of this disease have been described. The validity of an animal model must therefore be tested with respect to each of these criteria.

Memory and learning deficits are typical symptoms of Alzheimer's disease. Diffuse atrophy of the brain, senile plaques, neurofibrillary tangles, and neuronal cell death are well-known morphological signs of the disease. Deficiencies in cortical choline acetyltransferase (ChAT) activity as well as changes in other neurotransmitter systems and in neuropeptides like somatostatin constitute some of the biochemical signs. Morphologically, the basal nucleus of Meynert, which is the main source of cholinergic innervation in the human cortex, shows a severe neuronal loss. An animal model for Alzheimer's disease should present at least some of these symptoms.

NZB Mouse as a Model

The New Zealand Black mouse (NZB) might be an appropriate model for Alzheimer's disease. The following paper concentrates first on possible morpho-

1 Anatomisches Institut, Joseph-Stelzmann-Str. 9, 5000 Köln 41, FRG

Senile Dementia of the Alzheimer Type
Ed. by J. Traber and W.H. Gispen

logical correlates of memory and learning deficits and secondly on some simple quantitative results of studies investigating the cholinergic basal forebrain area and the caudate-putamen complex. These preliminary morphological studies, though far from being complete, may prove useful if analyzed with respect to the psychological results of other authors.

Learning deficits in young NZB mice are at least as marked as in very old specimens of other strains (Nandy et al. 1983). Spencer et al. (to be published) compared the sensorimotor competence and performance of NZB mice with that of Carworth Farm Webster strain (CFW) mice. This comparison was based on tasks requiring learning and memory. Pronounced deficits in performance noted for passive and active shock avoidance responses are too great to be accounted for by the slight sensorimotor disadvantage of the NZB mice.

The fact that the senile plaques of Alzheimer's disease contain immunoglobins (Ishii and Haga 1976) and cholinergic markers (Struble et al. 1982) leads to the supposition that the autoimmunologic involvement underlying plaque formation in Alzheimer's disease is related to a cholinergic decline. The NZB mouse might be a useful model in this context because a close correlation has been found between immunologic disorders and deficits in learning and memory (Nandy et al. 1983). Morphological and, in particular, quantitative data on the brain of the NZB mouse have been unknown until now. The study discussed here attempts to provide such data.

Material and Methods

Two groups consisting of 21 male NZB mice aged 4–6 months and 21 CFW mice of the same sex and age were used. One group of animals was perfused with Bodian's fixative. The brains were removed, paraffin-embedded, and histologically processed according to standard procedures. Serial sections with thicknesses of 4 µm and 20 µm were Nissl-stained with cresyl-fast-violet. The outlines of the Ammon's horn region, the dentate gyrus, the anterodorsal thalamic nucleus, and the medial and lateral parts of the mammillary body were drawn on paper using a camera lucida system. The areas of the outlined structures of at least 12 equidistant sections per region were measured with a digitizer and corrected for histologic shrinkage. This procedure permits estimation of the volume of any of these regions with a maximal error of less than 5% (Zilles et al. 1982).

Furthermore, the numer of nucleolated pyramidal cells in the CA1 region of Ammon's horn were counted, and their density was calculated for a 100-µm-long region of the pyramidal layer. In this and in the following cases, a randomized sampling procedure was used. The number of nucleolated neurons per mm^3 were determined for the anterodorsal thalamic nucleus and the mammillary body. This factor is called the „neuron packing density“ in the diagrams to follow. The number of neurons in the latter two brain regions can be calculated by multiplying the volume by the packing density.

Ammon's horn, the dentate gyrus of the hippocampus, and the medial and lateral parts of the mammillary body were analyzed because these regions are the main stations of the Papez circuit. The latter is a neuronal system which plays an important role as a recall circuit in learning and memory functions (Meissner 1966, 1977). Moreover, the mammillary body has been found to be affected in cases of Korsakoff's psychosis, which is characterized, among other symptoms, by memory dysfunctions. Degenerative neuronal changes together with severe losses of neurons in the mammillary body have been described (for a review, see Barbizet 1963).

Quantitative Aspects of Brain Regions in the Papez Circuit

Figure 1 shows the volumes of the whole brains, which were 441 ± 14 mm^3 for the CFW mice and 435 ± 23 mm^3 for the NZB mice. The 6-mm^3 difference between the brain volume of the NZB mice and that of the CFW mice is statistically insignificant. Similarly, the differences in the volumes of Ammon's horn, the dentate gyrus, the medial and lateral parts of the mammillary body and the anterodorsal thalamic nucleus of the two mice strains were also without statistical significance (Fig. 1, 2). In short, it is possible to say that the brain regions of the Pa-

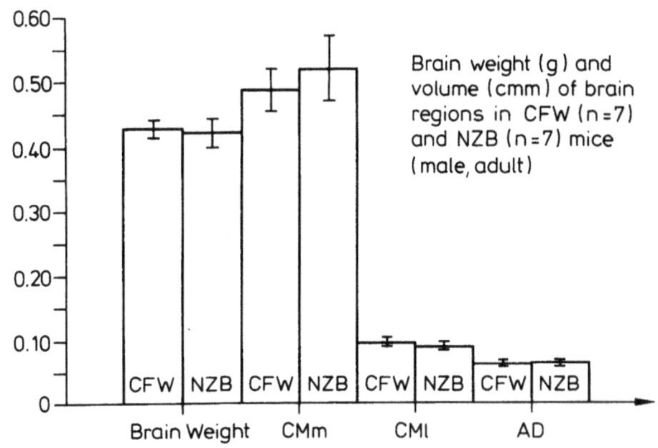

Fig. 1. Brain weights (in g) and volumes (in mm^3) of NZB and CFW mice in the medial (*CMm*) and lateral (*CMl*) parts of the mammillary body and in the anterodorsal thalamic nucleus (*AD*)

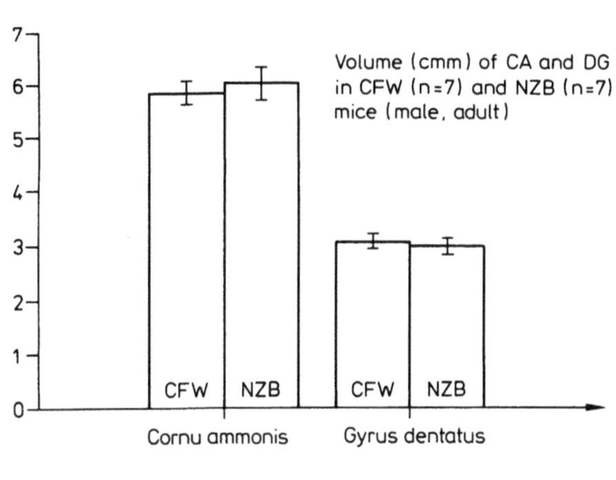

Fig. 2. Volumes (in mm^3) of the Ammon's horn (*CA*) and the dentate gyrus (*DG*) in NZB and CFW mice

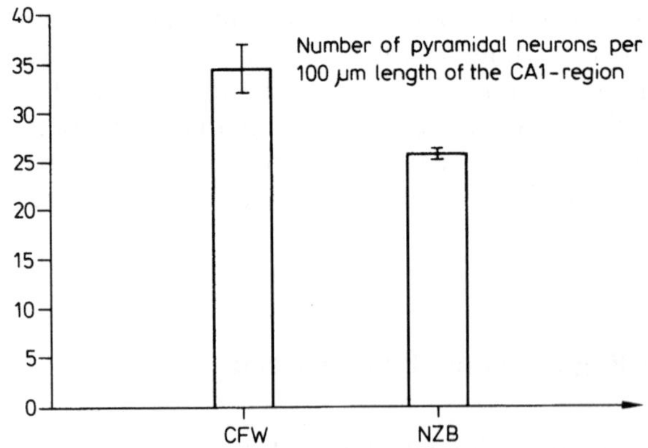

Fig. 3. Number of pyramidal neurons per 100-μm length in the CA1 region of the Ammon's horn in NZB and CFW mice

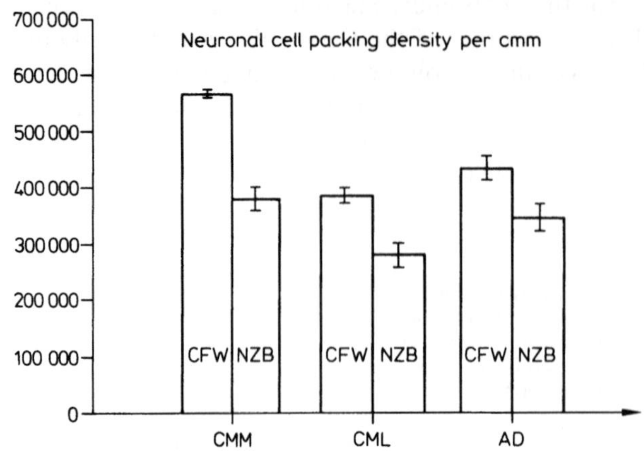

Fig. 4. Neuronal cell packing density (neurons per mm^3) in the medial (*CMM*) and lateral (*CML*) parts of the mammillary body and in the anterodorsal (*AD*) thalamic nucleus of NZB and CFW mice

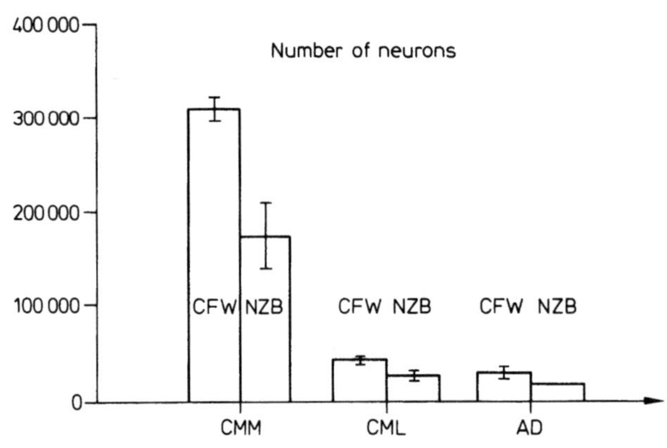

Fig. 5. Total number of neurons in the medial (*CMM*) and lateral (*CML*) parts of the mammillary body and in the anterodorsal (*AD*) thalamic nucleus of NZB and CFW mice

pez circuit and of the brain as a whole are volumetrically comparable for both strains.

Quite a different relation was found after measuring the neuronal cell packing density. Figure 3 shows that there are 25% fewer pyramidal cells per 100-μm length in the CA1 region of NZB mice than in the controls. This is a statistically significant difference (Mann-Whitney U-test). Furthermore, the NZB mice were also found to have significantly lower neuronal cell packing densities in other brain regions than the control CFW mice (Fig. 4): 33% lower in the medial part of the mammillary body, 27% lower in the lateral part, and 20% lower in the anterodorsal thalamic nucleus.

After the absolute neuronal counts had been calculated (Fig. 5), the neuronal deficit of the NZB mice amounted to 44% in the medial part of the mammillary body, 39% in the lateral part of the mammillary body, and 40% in the anterodorsal thalamic nucleus. Thus, the NZB mice manifest a severe neuronal cell deficit in brain regions involved in learning and memory, which could represent a possible morphological correlate of the previously described learning dysfunctions.

Cholinergic Neurons in the Forebrain

Methodological Considerations

The second half of this paper concentrates on cholinergic neurons in the forebrain of the NZB mouse because salient feature of Alzheimer's disease is the destruction of neuronal cells in the cholinergic basal forebrain regions. This cell loss is accompanied by a decrease in cholinergic innervation in the cortex (Whitehouse et al. 1982; Arendt et al. 1983) and a correlated increase in the number of cortical plaques (Arendt et al. 1984).

A neuron's cholinergic nature can be shown by using the immunohistochemical choline acetyltransferase (ChAT) method. In many cases, the simple histochemical demonstration of acetylcholinesterase (AChE) activity is insufficient to determine whether a neuron is cholinergic or not. This is because some brain regions exhibit AChE activity without containing cholinergic neurons. The more convenient cholinesterase method can be applied in the caudateputamen complex and in the basal nucleus of Meynert because, at least for these two regions, both methods demonstrate the same neuronal populations. This has been verified by comparative investigations of ChAT- and cholinesterase-positive neurons (Satoh et al. 1983).

To demonstrate a cell's cholinergic nature using the AChE method, it is first necessary to treat the living specimens with diisopropylfluorophosphate (DFP) several hours before the analysis is to be carried out. Because DFP is an irreversible inhibitor of AChE, only those cells which have a high capacity for synthesizing AChE can be stained in animals which have been previously injected with DFP. As Satho et al. (1983) have shown, both the caudate-putamen complex and the magnocellular basal nucleus, which is the rodent equivalent of the human basal nucleus of Meynert, contain cholinergic neurons which can be demonstrated by the immunohistochemical method or by DFP histochemistry for AChE. The latter method permits fast and easy identification of the cholinergic neurons in these regions.

Since the magnocellular neurons of the forebrain are scattered over a large area, it was not feasible to delineate the whole region in a way comparable to de-

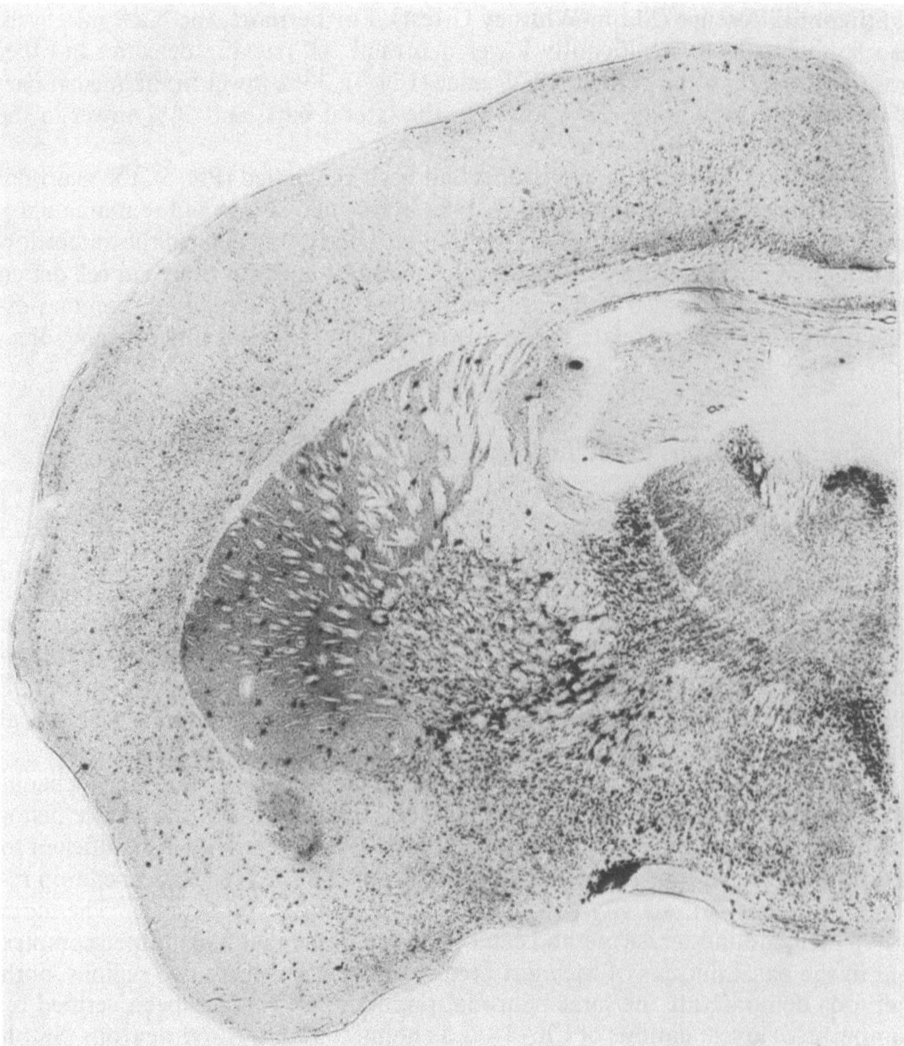

Fig. 6. Micrograph of a hemisphere of a DFP-treated NZB mouse after AChE staining. The heavily stained magnocellular neurons of the basal nucleus equivalent are visible at the medial and ventral contours of the *globus pallidus*

lineations of compact nuclei. Consequently, it was possible to calculate the cell packing density of cholinergic neurons only by random sampling. In addition to these measurements, the packing density, volume, and cholinergic neuron count were determined for the caudate-putamen complex of the same material. Figure 6 shows an AChE preparation in the forebrain of an NZB mouse which had been treated with DFP. Even at this low magnification, the large, intensely stained cholinergic cells of the basal nucleus equivalent are easily recognizable. This magnocellular region in the NZB and CFW mice is shown at a higher magnification in Fig. 7.

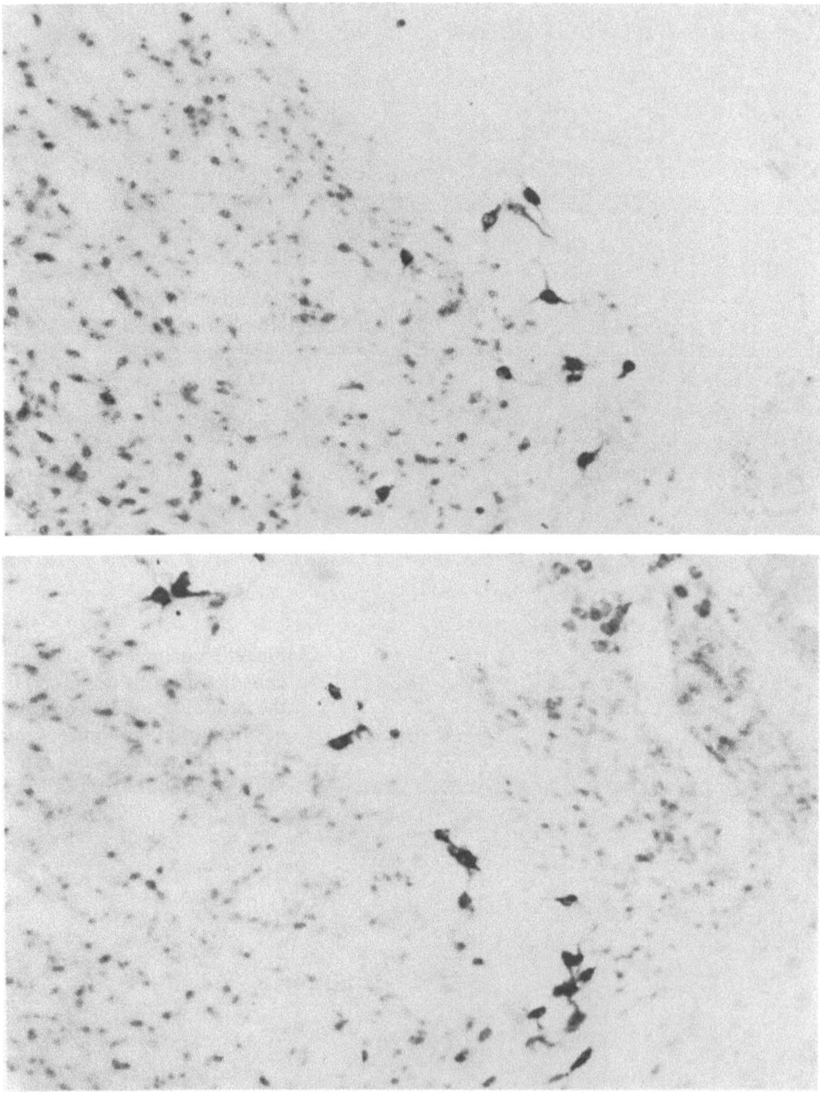

a

b

Fig. 7 a, b. Micrograph of large, AChE-stained neurons of the basal nucleus equivalent after DFP treatment of **a** NZB and **b** CFW mice

Caudate-Putamen Complex

The results of the quantitative analysis of the caudate-putamen complex are presented in Fig. 8–10. The volume of the caudate-putamen complex in NZB mice is 11% lower than in CFW mice. This difference is small but significant (Fig. 8). There is, however, no significant difference between the two strains in the cell packing density of AChE-positive neurons (Fig.). Thus, the total number of cholinergic neurons in the caudate-putamen complex of the NZB mice is 11% lower

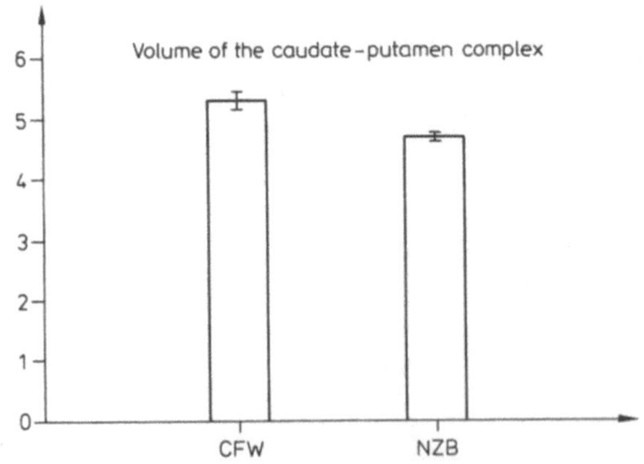

Fig. 8. Volume (in mm^3) of the caudate-putamen complex of NZB and CFW mice

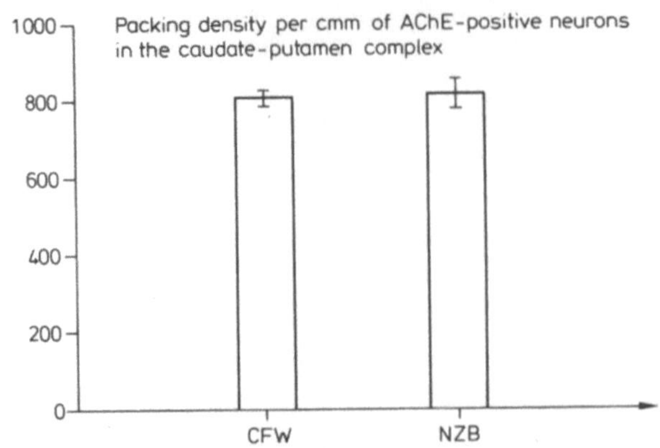

Fig. 9. Neuronal cell packing density (neurons per mm^3) in the caudate-putamen complex of NZB and CFW mice. Only AChE-positive neurons after DFP treatment are counted

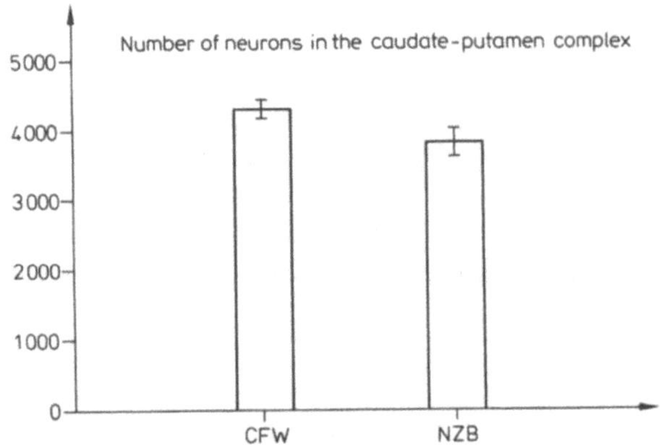

Fig. 10. Total number of AChE-positive neurons in the caudate-putamen complex NZB and CFW mice

than that of the CFW control mice (Fig. 10). Because it is connected with almost the entire cortex, the caudate-putamen region is involved in many complex functions aside from extrapyramidal motor activities (Divac 1972). As a result, no precise description of the influence of the cholinergic neuron deficit in this region can be given at this time.

Magnocellular Basal Forebrain Region

An even more interesting finding resulted from the investigation of the packing density of cholinergic projection neurons in the basal forebrain region (Fig. 11). Here, a statistically significant drop of 21% in cholinergic neuron packing density was found for the basal nucleus equivalent. This neuronal loss is also observed in Alzheimer's disease, which results in the atrophy and destruction of 20%–80% of the cholinergic neurons of the basal nucleus. This loss of cholinergic basal forebrain neurons could be the basis of a very useful parallel between the NZB mice and Alzheimer's disease in humans, if the cortical effects of the neuron deficiency can be demonstrated.

We found no signs of neurofibrillary tangles or plaques, which seem to be restricted to human brains. To test this possibility, we measured the neocortical volume of NZB and CFW mice. We found a significant drop of 14% in the volume of the NZB cortices (Fig. 12). This indicates a diffuse shrinkage of the cortices of the NZB mice. Hypothetically, this decrease in cortical volume might be attributed to the premature loss of 21% of cholinergic forebrain neurons.

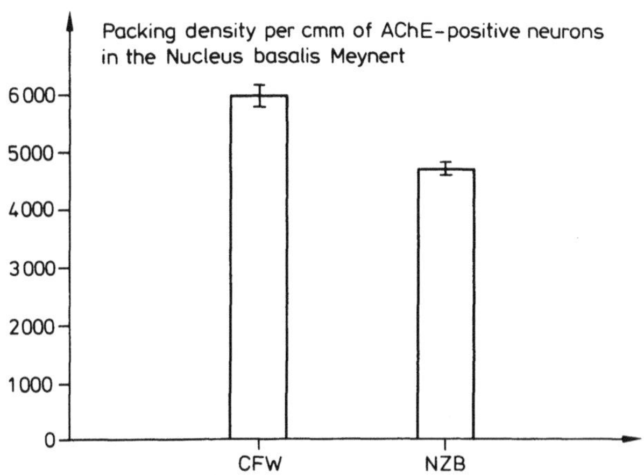

Fig. 11. Neuronal cell packing density (neurons per mm^3) in the basal nucleus equivalent after DFP treatment and AChE staining in NZB and CFW mice

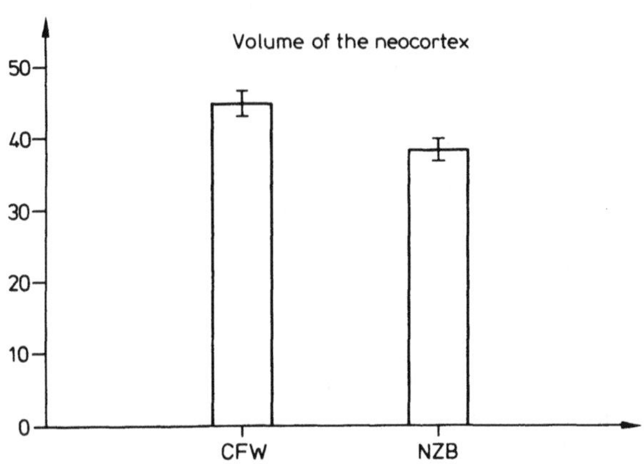

Fig. 12. Volume (in mm^3) of the neocortex of NZB and CFW mice

Conclusion

The NZB mouse shows elevated brain-reactive antibody levels during young adult life, a condition which is normally found only in very old specimens of other strains. Experimental studies have verified that the NZB mouse shows severely reduced learning and memory capabilities. Both whole-brain and regional volumes are in most cases comparable in the NZB and CFW strains. The only exceptions are the neocortex and the caudate-putamen complex. The volumes of these two regions are smaller in the NZB mouse.

The NZB mouse shows a 20%–44% lower nerve cell count than the CFW mouse in brain regions of the Papez circuit. There are significantly fewer cholinergic neurons in the basal nucleus equivalent of the forebrain of the NZB mouse than in that of the CFW mouse.

As for the question of whether the NZB mouse is an appropriate animal model of the aging human brain, the NZB mouse exhibits some phenomena found in aging human brains, especially those afflicted with Alzheimer's disease. However, several typical Alzheimer features such as neurofibrillary tangles and senile plaques are not found in this model. Consequently, although the NZB mouse does not reflect all phenomena observed in the aging human brain, it is a promising model for investigating certain age-related changes.

Acknowledgements. This study was supported by the *Verein der Freunde und Förderer der Universität zu Köln.* I thank Dr. J. Traber, Cologne, for providing me with NZB and CFW animals, and Dr. Bauschulte, Cologne, for technical assistance.

References

Arendt T, Bigl V, Arendt A, Tennstedt A (1983) Loss of neurons in the *nucleus basalis* of Meynert in Alzheimer's disease, paralysis agitans and Korsakoff's disease. Acta Neuropathol 61:101–108

Arendt T, Bigl V, Tennstedt A, Arendt A (1984) Correlation between cortical plaque count and neuronal loss in the nucleus basalis in Alzheimer's disease. Neurosci Lett 48:81–85

Barbizet J (1963) Defect of memorizing of hippocampalmammilary origin: a review. J Neurol Neurosurg Psychiatry 26:127–135

Divac I (1972) Neostriatum and functions of prefrontal cortex. Acta Neurobiol Exp 32:461–477

Ishii T, Haga S (1976) Immuno-electron microscopic localization of immunoglobulins in amyloid fibrils of senile plaques. Acta Neuropathol 36:243–249

Meissner WW (1966) Hippocampal functions in learning. J Psychiatr Res 4:235–304

Meissner WW (1967) Hippocampus and learning. Int J Neuropsychiatry 3:298–310

Nandy K, Lal H, Bennet M, Bennet D (1983) Elevated brainreactive antibodies and a learning deficit co-occur in young NZB mice. Life Sci 33:1499–1503

Satoh K, Armstrong DM, Fibiger HC (1983) A comparison of the distribution of central cholinergic neurons as demonstrated by acetylcholinesterase pharmacohistochemistry and choline acetyltransferase immunohistochemistry. Brain Res Bull 11:693–720

Spencer DG, Humphries K, Mathis D, Lal H (to be published) Behavioral impairments related to cognitive dysfunction in the NZB mouse: potential for an autoimmunological animal model for pre-senile dementia. Behav Neurosci

Struble RG, Cook LC, Whitehouse PJ, Price DL (1982) Cholinergic innervation in neuritic plaques. Science 216:413–415
Whitehouse PJ, Pric DL, Struble RG, Clark AW, Coyle JT, DeLong MR (1982) Alzheimer's disease and senile dementia: loss of neurons in the basal forebrain. Science 215:1237–1239
Zilles K, Schleicher A, Pehlemann FW (1982) How many sections must be measured in order to reconstruct the volume of a structure using serial sections? Microsc Acta 86:339–346

Subject Index

MIX
Papier aus verantwortungsvollen Quellen
Paper from responsible sources
FSC® C105338

If you have any concerns about our products,
you can contact us on
ProductSafety@springernature.com

In case Publisher is established outside the EU,
the EU authorized representative is:
Springer Nature Customer Service Center GmbH
Europaplatz 3, 69115 Heidelberg, Germany

Printed by Libri Plureos GmbH
in Hamburg, Germany